D0905205

Issues in Cost Accounting for Health Care Organizations

Second Edition

Steven A. Finkler, PhD, CPA
Program in Health Policy and Management
Robert F. Wagner Graduate School of Public Service
New York University
New York, New York

David M. Ward, PhD
Department of Health Administration and Policy
College of Health Professions
Medical University of South Carolina
Charleston, South Carolina

AN ASPEN PUBLICATION®
Aspen Publishers, Inc.
Gaithersburg, Maryland
1999

This publication is designed to provide accurate and authoritative information in regard to the Subject Matter covered. It is sold with the understanding that the publisher is not engaged in rendering legal, accounting, or other professional service. If legal advice or other expert assistance is required, the service of a competent professional person should be sought. (From a Declaration of Principles jointly adopted by a Committee of the American Bar Association and a Committee of Publishers and Associations.)

Library of Congress Cataloging-in-Publication Data

Issues in cost accounting for health care organizations / edited by Steven A. Finkler, David M. Ward.—2nd ed.
p. cm.
Includes bibliographical references and index.
ISBN: 0-8342-1010-X
I. Health facilities—Costs—Accounting. 2. Hospitals—Cost of operation—Accounting. 3. Cost accounting. I. Finkler, Steven A.
HF5686.H7F564 1999
658.8'8—dc21
98-54116
CIP

Copyright © 1999 by Aspen Publishers, Inc.
All rights reserved.

Aspen Publishers, Inc., grants permission for photocopying for limited personal or internal use. This consent does not extend to other kinds of copying, such as copying for general distribution, for advertising or promotional purposes, for creating new collective works, or for resale. For information, address Aspen Publishers, Inc., Permissions Department, 200 Orchard Ridge Drive, Suite 200, Gaithersburg, Maryland 20878.

Orders: (800) 638-8437
Customer Service: (800) 234-1660

About Aspen Publishers • For more than 35 years, Aspen has been a leading professional publisher in a variety of disciplines. Aspen's vast information resources are available in both print and electronic formats. We are committed to providing the highest quality information available in the most appropriate format for our customers. Visit Aspen's Internet site for more information resources, directories, articles, and a searchable version of Aspen's full catalog, including the most recent publications: **http://www.aspenpublishers.com**
Aspen Publishers, Inc. • The hallmark of quality in publishing
Member of the worldwide Wolters Kluwer group.

Editorial Services: Ruth Bloom
Library of Congress Catalog Card Number: 98-54116
ISBN: 0-8342-1010-X

Printed in the United States of America

1   2   3   4   5

WX
157
I86
1999

40.51

To Gary and Gabrielle

404 0 8 9 2 0

Table of Contents

Preface

Cost Accounting has become an essential part of health care management. The growth of managed care in the 1990s heightened the awareness of the critical role of cost measurement and cost management. You cannot manage care effectively unless you know the costs of different alternative approaches to providing care. Those costs can only be known if the organization has the knowledge and capability to measure costs. All health care managers, not just accountants, are becoming more and more aware of the importance of understanding as much as they possibly can about costs.

Issues in Cost Accounting for Health Care Organizations, Second Edition, consists of a collection of articles that focus on critical issues in health care cost accounting. Each article provides insight about a specific potential problem area in the management of health care organizations. This is the most complete compilation of articles on the topic of health care cost accounting. Many of the articles are recent, incorporating the latest costing techniques such as the application of Activity Based Costing to health care. Some of the articles are classics—seminal articles that lay the foundation for health care costing, and that have weathered the passage of time.

The reader may wish to combine the discussions provided in this book with *Essentials of Cost Accounting for Health Care Organizations, Second Edition.*[*] The *Essentials* text provides a

complete, up-to-date discussion of cost accounting for the health care industry. It de-emphasizes cost accounting for manufacturing: the process of converting raw materials into finished goods. Such inventory tracking is a major theme of most cost accounting books. Instead, *Essentials* emphasizes cost accounting methods more relevant to organizations in the health care field. It covers the basic tools of cost accounting common to all industries, using health care examples. It also focuses on costing issues and concepts peculiar to the health care field. The *Essentials* book is supported by a Web-site which offers a variety of helpful features, including tutorials on using spreadsheets to solve costing problems, updates on the book, a method for contacting the authors, links to other cost accounting sites, and other features.

This book is broken down into four parts that parallel the sections in the *Essentials* text. The articles in each section may be read on a stand-alone basis, or be used to provide supporting applications for the concepts discussed in the parallel part of the *Essentials* book. **Part I** focuses on issues related to the foundations of cost accounting. **Part II** addresses the use of cost accounting for planning and control. **Part III** provides additional cost accounting tools to aid in decision-making, and **Part IV** considers the latest trends and techniques in cost accounting.

The primary change in this second edition has been recognition of the increasing role of health care providers other than hospitals. Hospitals continue to dominate the health care literature.

[*] Steven A. Finkler and David M. Ward, *Essentials of Cost Accounting for Health Care Organizations, Second Edition*, Aspen Publishers, Inc., Gaithersburg, MD, 1999.

However, with the growth of managed care and other changes in the health care system, the role of nonhospital health care organizations has been increasing substantially. This edition has added a number of articles that apply health care cost accounting issues to organizations other than hospitals. We believe that all of the articles contained in this book provide valuable concepts and techniques for use in all types of health care organizations.

Steven A. Finkler
David M. Ward

Part I

Cost Accounting Foundations

Part I of both this book and of the companion text, *Essentials of Cost Accounting for Health Care Organizations, Second Edition*,[1] deal with the foundations of cost accounting. The chapters in this section provide an introduction to costing and cost definitions. Various approaches to product costing and cost allocation are discussed. Techniques for making nonroutine decisions are also discussed in this section, along with tools for breakeven analysis.

Chapter 1 is introductory in nature. The first article in that chapter addresses the issue of the value of a cost accounting system. Why have one? What can it do for the health care manager and health care organization? Cost accounting information is useful for managers in a number of areas. Just a few specific examples are for the management of department-level costs, for pricing decisions in negotiations with health maintenance organizations (HMOs) and preferred provider organizations (PPOs), for purposes of strategic planning, and for profitability analysis. These examples are discussed in Reading 1–1, "The Value of a Cost Accounting System," by Mark Toso.

Knowing why we need a cost system is just the first step. The second is to begin to gain an understanding of the process of cost accounting. Bryan Dieter provides an overview and introduc-

tion to this topic in Reading 1–2, "Understanding the Hospital Cost Accounting Process." This article provides the reader not only with a framework for understanding the cost accounting process, but also a sense of what information a good cost accounting system needs to provide.

Often accounting is viewed as a numbers oriented field. In reality, people are a critical element in all aspects of financial management. Cost accounting requires explicit recognition of people and their goals and interests, as well as those of the organization. Managers must consider not just the calculation of costs, but also the incentives and motivations of the people working for the organization. In cost accounting, we record the results of actions taken by people. Understanding their motivations and likely responses to incentives is essential to the design of an effective cost accounting system. This issue is addressed in "The Human Element in Cost Accounting," Reading 1–3.

Chapter 2 looks at cost measurement. The concepts of full costs, average costs, cost objectives, direct and indirect costs, fixed, variable, marginal, total, and joint costs are applied to the issue of departmental costing versus product-line costing. The first article in Chapter 2 is Bryan Dieter's, "The Identification of Surgical Services Costs," which provides a detailed look at departmental costing.

In contrast to the departmental focus on costing, Reading 2–2, "Cost Finding for High-Technology, High-Cost Services: Current Practice

---

[1]Steven A. Finkler and David M. Ward, *Essentials of Cost Accounting for Health Care Organizations, Second Edition*, Aspen Publishers, Inc., Gaithersburg, MD, 1999.

1

and a Possible Alternative," raises the issue of focusing on the cost of the product, rather than the cost of the department. Another costing approach that is receiving growing attention relates to the issue of value-added costs. Rather than considering the costs of a department or the costs of a product, Reading 2–3, "Horizontal Accounting Considered for the Hospital Setting," considers the issue of providing quality services without spending money on anything that does not add value for the customer.

Few things in cost accounting are totally black or white. The area of departmental versus product costing is no exception. Departmental costing may well be insufficient under managed care. But product costing that truly focuses on differential costs for different types of patients may result in tremendous data collection costs. In many cases, health care organizations try to seek a happy balance between the two. Two examples of attempts to develop a hybrid approach are offered in "Costing Out Nursing Services," and "Cost Accounting for Emergency Services." These articles are Readings 2–4 and 2–5. They each attempt to improve product costing, within the sphere of a department in a health care organization.

Chapter 3 introduces the conflict between the job-order and process costing approaches to product costing. It also provides an examination of standard costing, a cost tool that is likely to be of growing importance throughout the remainder of this century. The technique of micro-costing is also discussed.

An example of job-order costing is provided in Reading 3–1 by Lorelei Cheli, "Job Order Costing in Physician Practice." Job-order costing examines the specific resources consumed by a patient or type of patient in great detail. In contrast, process costing relies on broad averages to assign costs to patients.

The extremes of job costing and process costing rarely find complete applicability. For example, the product costing discussion in Leonard Scinto's article, "Product Cost Analysis in the Clinical Laboratory," Reading 3–2, merges the two approaches. In that article, the

laboratory cost for treating a diabetes patient consists of the costs for each type of test consumed. Taking a job-costing approach, the quantity of each test for that type of patient are aggregated in the article. This distinguishes the patient from other types of patients with different mix and volume of laboratory tests. On the other hand, as the article describes, the cost for each test is calculated on a process costing approach. The labor and materials for all glucose tests are averaged to find the cost per glucose test.

In a seminal work, William Cleverley opened the door for standard costing in health care with his "Product-Costing for Health Care Firms," Reading 3–3. Cleverley has proposed that health care organizations cost their products using a standard costing approach that is centered around service units, standard cost profiles, and standard treatment protocols. For any specific type of patient, there would be a standard treatment protocol specifying the various intermediate hospital services that should be employed in providing that patient's care. These intermediate products are called service units. For each service unit, a standard cost profile details the expected costs of providing that care.

Standard costs provide estimates of what costs should be for different types of patients. Although they can be reasonably accurate, if an application requires extremely specific and accurate product cost information, one potentially useful approach is microcosting. That is the process of closely examining the actual resources consumed by a particular patient or service. A detailed view of microcosting is presented in Reading 3–4.

Chapter 4 addresses the complex issue of cost allocation. In the companion book, *Essentials of Cost Accounting for Health Care Organizations, Second Edition,* the reasons for allocating costs are explained, and guidelines for cost allocation are provided. Cost allocation techniques are discussed, including cost pools and cost bases. The chapter also reviews the Medicare Cost Report and the relative merits of ratio of cost to charges (RCC) costing versus relative value unit (RVU) costing. The chapter ends with a discussion of the difficulties concerning allocation of joint costs. The readings in this book for this chapter focus on some of the critical concerns in the area of cost allocation.

The steps in traditional cost-finding are examined in Reading 4–1, "The Distinction between Cost and Charges." That article examines the reasons that costs and charges cannot be considered to be synonymous. Much discussion in health care uses charge information as a proxy for cost. Often, this usage is not even made explicit because of a mistaken impression that costs and charges are nearly the same thing. That myth is dispelled by this reading.

Cost allocations often substitute expediency for accuracy. One reaction to this has been the widespread introduction of Activity Based Costing (ABC). That approach is addressed in Chapter 17. A more modest approach to improving the accuracy of information resulting from cost allocation is adoption of the reciprocal allocation technique. This technique and its advantages for management decision making are explained in Reading 4–2 by Lawrence Metzger.

Many would argue that the Metzger approach to improving cost allocation does not go nearly far enough. Although it would improve the accuracy of cost allocation by moving away from the step-down allocation technique toward a better approach, it still leaves many of the problems that were discussed in Reading 4–1. These are likely to be inherent in any "ratio of cost to charges (RCC)" system. Some have called for the use instead of a "relative value unit (RVU)" system for costing. An RVU approach performs a special study to determine the resources consumed by each activity (such as a service unit in the Cleverley model discussed in Reading 3–3). The various activities (or service units) are then compared to each other and relative costs determined. Based on the relative costs, a relationship is established that becomes the basis for allocation of future costs.

The RVU approach is explained in Kirk Mahlen's article, Reading 4–3, "RVU's: Relative Value Units or Really Very Useful?" Leslie

Davis Weintraub and Richard Dube go beyond this, discussing the results of a fairly sophisticated RVU system in Reading 4–4, "Alternative Costing Methods in Health Care."

Cost allocation is not only an issue for in-patient care in hospitals. Reading 4–5, "Accounting for the Move to Ambulatory Patient Groups," addresses the challenges of establishing a good costing method for use in reimbursement of outpatient visits. The chapter finishes with Reading 4–6, "Cost Allocation in the Emergency Department," which considers problems of associating costs with specific patients in the emergency department setting.

Next, Chapter 5 addresses the issue of developing cost information for nonroutine decisions. The identification of alternatives and the issue of relevant costs are considered. "HMO Negotiations and Hospital Costs," Reading 5–1, provides an example of cost data concerns related to a potential expansion in the quantity of services offered by a hospital.

A controversy today exists over the proper management of health care organizations in a capitated environment. Is it better to be busy or slow when you receive capitated payments? Reading 5–2, "Capitated Hospital Contracts: The Empty Beds versus Filled Beds Controversy" arrives at an unexpected conclusion.

There are many possible uses for nonroutine decision analyis. "Privatization in Health Care Institutions," by Yehia Dabaa and colleagues, presents an application of relevant costing to the topic of privatization in Reading 5–3.

One technique for nonroutine decision analysis that is widely used is cost-effectiveness analysis. Two examples of this approach are given in Readings 5–4 and 5–5, "Considering Cost Effectiveness in the Hospital Setting," and "Cost-Effectiveness Analysis in Health Care."

Chapter 6, the last chapter in this part of the book, focuses on cost-volume-profit analysis. The fundamentals of breakeven analysis, central to cost-volume-profit analysis can be found in any financial management text. Formulas for breakeven and definitions of contribution margin are readily available elsewhere. The readings in this chapter go beyond these basics.

The first two readings focus on issues related to breakeven analysis and managed care. Reading 6–1, "Breakeven Analysis for Capitated Arrangements," focuses on the need to adjust the denominator of the breakeven formula to determine the breakeven number of covered lives. Calculating the number of patients or visits is counter-productive when capitated. By changing the equation to focus on the required number of members, breakeven analysis continues to provide useful results. Reading 6–2, "Managed Care and Breakeven Analysis: A Clarification," tries to overcome the misconception that revenue becomes fixed in a capitated environment. As discussed in that article, total revenue increases with the number of members, just as total revenue increases with the number of discharges in a prospective payment DRG environment. In both cases one wants to minimize the cost of providing services to any given patient. But in both cases the organization can focus on efforts to increase volume.

"Using Breakeven Analysis with Step-Fixed Costs," Reading 6–3, explores the issue of step-fixed costs. Although costs are often treated as if they are fixed or variable, that is a simplification. While some costs (e.g., rent or depreciation) will be fixed, and some costs (e.g., clinical supplies) will be variable, in health care one of the most significant cost elements cannot be so simply defined. That is labor. Most staff costs are in fact neither strictly fixed nor variable. They do not increase patient by patient, but they are not fixed over the relevant range of activity. This reading explores the problem of breakeven analysis when some costs are step-fixed.

The importance of contribution margin is well known. The price of a unit of service less its variable cost is the contribution margin. Each extra unit of service provided will benefit the organization by that contribution margin. The contribution can be used to cover fixed costs or to provide a profit. This is an important measure for any health care organization. In situations in which a health care organization is near capacity of any resource (beds, clinic visit capacity, etc.), contribution margin is no longer an adequate basis for decision making. Instead, one should use the contribution margin per unit of the most constrained resource. This concept is explored in "Alternative Contribution Margin Measures," Reading 6–4.

1

Introduction to Cost Accounting

Reading 1–1

Reader's Forum: The Value of a Cost Accounting System

Mark E. Toso

The question has been raised as to the value of a cost accounting system to a hospital. It has been asserted that management of a hospital is unlike the management of any other business and that hospital management cannot make decisions regarding a particular disease entity due to the interrelationship of hospital activities that support all disease entities. The cost/benefit of cost accounting information has been challenged due to the uniqueness of the hospital operation and the perceived inability of managers to demonstrate how the costs of implementing and maintaining a cost accounting system are offset by new revenues or cost reductions.

In order to address the broad issue of the value of a cost accounting system when managing a hospital, it is important to review the perceived uses of cost accounting information in a thoughtful and pragmatic manner. We can then make an assessment as to whether we, as health care managers, can use this information to achieve the goal of managing the hospital in a more effective

and efficient manner—in decision making, planning and control, and profitability.

Until the advent of the prospective payment system (PPS) in 1983, hospitals were paid for their services based on their cost; therefore, a hospital manager did not have to behave in the same way as a manager of a traditional business. Since 1983 the health care industry has evolved from being a regulated industry to one that is very competitive. The dominant theme has changed from one of growth for all hospitals to one of decline for inpatient hospital services. This has led to an emphasis on increased market share and to the reduction of operating costs.

The emphasis on controlling and understanding costs led to the development of cost accounting systems by numerous vendors and hospitals. These cost accounting systems accommodate detailed clinical and financial information collected at a procedural level. The clinical and financial database can provide information that can be used for a variety of purposes:

- cost management at a departmental level
- pricing decisions with HMOs and PPOs
- strategic planning
- physician management
- profitability analysis

Source: Reprinted from Mark Toso, "Reader's Forum: The Value of a Cost Accounting System," *Hospital Cost Management and Accounting,* Vol. 1, No. 4, July 1989, pp. 5–7. Copyright 1989, Aspen Publishers, Inc.

COST MANAGEMENT AT A DEPARTMENTAL LEVEL

The development of a cost accounting system requires the development of standards at a procedural level. The development of these standards, in turn, contributes to the development of flexible budgeting and productivity monitoring. These budgeting and monitoring tools help to manage operations in the context of declining inpatient services and payers who are adopting capitation systems similar to Medicare. The ability to adjust staffing and spending patterns based on volume and case-mix will become even more important as state regulators (Medicaid and Blue Cross) and HMOs/PPOs adopt case-mix payment systems similar to Medicare. Therefore, the departmental standards that are created by the development of the cost accounting system serve as valuable managerial tools.

PRICING DECISIONS WITH HMOs AND PPOs

Although most HMOs and PPOs have negotiated with hospitals on the basis of per diems or a percentage of charges, many are now beginning to adopt the case basis of payment. In addition, many payers are looking for specialized pricing for specific types of services (for example, children's hospitals and open heart surgery programs). In negotiations with HMOs and PPOs, as well as with other payers, it will be important to have the cost per case broken down between fixed and variable components for product-specific pricing analyses. In a cost accounting system the procedural cost information is broken down into a number of components of cost such as fixed and variable, salary and nonsalary, and overhead.

STRATEGIC PLANNING IN TODAY'S COMPETITIVE ENVIRONMENT

Hospital managers need to know how much it costs to deliver a specific service and/or product line. A hospital would not want to embark on an expansion of a service or product line that was losing a substantial amount of money. In fact, for the first time hospitals are beginning to close both services and entire facilities where volume is not sufficient to cover the costs of delivering the service.

Strategic financial planning is the theme of today's hospital planners. Financially driven strategic planning is based on the assumption that the planning efforts should improve the health care system's financial position. Strategic financial planning recognizes that health care systems are generally nonprofit and are often affiliated with a religious organization where financial performance is not the primary indicator of success; however, a health care system cannot achieve the organization's statement of purpose or mission unless financial viability is achieved.

PHYSICIAN MANAGEMENT

A cost accounting system will be of little value if physician input is not obtained. Assuming that physicians have been part of the process that developed the utilization standards for the case-mix measure employed by the cost accounting system, management has a powerful tool to control physician behavior. A cost accounting system will provide information to review physician efficiency through a comparison of individual physician treatment protocols for varying types of patients with protocols of other physicians at the same hospital or through other acceptable standards. Additionally, if the system can provide profitability analysis about a physician's clinical practice patterns, management can alter physician behavior based upon what the system has determined it can afford to pay. Managing average length of stay does not mean that the physician will release a patient before it is clinically appropriate; it does, however, make the physician aware of the financial realities management must deal with in order to maintain hospital viability.

PROFITABILITY ANALYSIS

A goal of the cost accounting system is to establish the costs of providing service by

- case type or DRG
- department
- specialty or product line
- physician
- patient

In addition, the cost accounting system would provide management with payer and net revenue information by the same categories mentioned above. This will allow hospital management to identify profit margins by payer, by physician, by service, or by product line and make the appropriate decisions about resource allocation based upon the goal of maintaining the financial viability of the hospital. This does not mean that because a specific procedure or case type is losing money that the procedure will no longer be provided or the case type no longer can be treated.

This information has to be used in the context of how the hospital operates all of its services. Cost accounting information does not replace management; rather, it provides a tool that allows management to understand how its hospital provides health care services. In a competitive environment it is critical for hospital managers to understand the hospital production function and to work with physicians to improve the quality of provided services while at the same time providing those services in a more effective and efficient manner. Cost accounting information provides hospital managers with the necessary knowledge to do this. In conclusion, there are several points that are important to mention:

- In today's competitive environment, hospitals that can control their costs will be the survivors. Market share is very important, but the realities of today's environment indicate that many hospitals will be downsizing, with financial performance as the most important variable. The only exception might be the large teaching hospitals, which have a different purpose and also have development capabilities that can raise substantial amounts of money.

- The cost of implementing a cost accounting system is declining every year. Hardware and software are available on mini-computers, microcomputers, or on in-house mainframe computers. Hospital management has now had the opportunity to work with this type of information over the last several years and it is beginning to utilize the information more effectively to make decisions and control hospital operations.

- Information is a very important strategic tool, and cost accounting information provides management with information that will allow it to understand the actual costs of delivering services. If management does not understand the hospital production function, how can it make decisions that will reduce the cost of providing a service without having a negative impact on the quality of that service?

Reading 1–2

Understanding the Hospital Cost Accounting Process

Bryan B. Dieter

As more pressure is exerted on hospitals to negotiate prices, reduce costs, and market services competitively, the accurate identification of costs per service becomes imperative. Since hospital management is beginning to recognize this need, this article will not address the "current environment" and why hospitals need a cost accounting system, but will focus on where and how to begin the whole cost accounting process.

In theory, cost accounting is fairly basic: identify resources consumed in the production/provision of goods or services and the corresponding costs of those resources. Applying the theory to a real hospital setting can be complex and time consuming. However, if this is done properly, the resulting information will be extremely informative and applicable, giving administrators, financial managers, and department heads an edge in everyday decision making.

The implementation of a cost accounting system requires preparation that vendors do not generally cover when presenting system features. This article will cover some of the groundwork to be completed prior to and during the course of a system installation, and features to look for in the selection of a system, to ensure that the information generated has a high degree of accuracy and proves valuable as a management tool.

Source: Reprinted from Bryan B. Dieter, "Understanding the Hospital Cost Accounting Process," *Hospital Cost Accounting Advisor,* Vol. 2, No. 2, July 1986, pp. 1–6. Copyright 1986, Aspen Publishers, Inc.

THE CHARGE DESCRIPTION MASTER

The driving force of any cost accounting system is the hospital's charging mechanism, usually referred to as the charge description master (CDM). The CDM should be the initial focal point in the initiation of cost accounting. This is especially true since "fee for service" and cost-based reimbursement methodologies have encouraged manipulation of the CDM to maximize revenue. With the inception of the prospective payment system (PPS), there will be a shift from many departmental revenue centers to *one* revenue center—the hospital itself. As a result of this shift, the charge description master should soon be considered the *cost* description master. Therefore, the CDM should be reviewed to determine charges that must be added, deleted, or revised in order to accurately reflect the manner in which the services are provided.

Specifically, the charges should reflect resource consumption in the provision of service, and therefore the cost. A common comment from hospitals on recommended charging changes is, "We can't charge different amounts for those services since we won't be reimbursed for them." That may be true. However, you still need to identify which services vary from the standard and cost you more than they should. You may decide to establish new/revised charges and assign no dollar value to them, yet be generating the information necessary to monitor utilization and costs accurately.

Another consideration is whether or not, in marketing your hospital's services, you will be offering "packaged prices." If so, charges need to be established to monitor costs and revenue separately for those packages.

Some common revisions to CDMs include

- Routine services. Revise the room-charging mechanism to include patient acuity levels (staff utilization) identified in the nursing acuity system, e.g., establishing a charge for Med/Surg Unit 4E, Semiprivate, Level 2. The semiprivate and other occupancy designations should be retained to facilitate the allocation of overhead expenses.
- Surgical services. Common revisions to Surgical Services CDMs:

    Removal of charge explosion system, a system that generates charges automatically based upon customary resource utilization for the procedure performed. These systems usually charge all patients equally for the same procedure without regard for *actual* resources or services provided to the patient. This type of system does not allow for utilization/costs identification and monitoring by surgeon, surgical team, or anesthesiologist.

    Acuity-based room charges. Room charges should be based on the number of staff members involved in the procedure and the length of time for each case. Usually three or four levels of base charges (for example, 15-min., 30-min., or one hour minimum) and incremental charges (each additional one, five, or 15 minutes) are appropriate.

    Capital equipment. Separate equipment charges should be established based on those pieces of equipment that are used only for specific cases. Costs should be determined by the frequency of use of the equipment and its rate of depreciation. Maintenance contract costs should be associated with equipment when possible.

    Suture charges. The hospital should charge for sutures individually, yet in classifications based on type and cost (e.g., ophthalmic, strand, micro, wire).

    Tray charges. Tray charges should be established for each type of tray since instrument and supply costs vary greatly.

    Additional labor. Establish a charge for additional staff (usually RN or tech) who may float through the room during the procedure to provide assistance only as needed—usually an incremental time charge of 10 or 15 minutes.

    After-hours or emergency charges. These charges would reflect pay differentials for overtime, on-call, and call back. This charge may also help to identify surgeons who routinely schedule at more costly times.

- Emergency room. ER visits should be acuity based and reflect time actually spent "hands-on" with the patient or on functions directly related to that patient (e.g., triage, arranging for transport/admission, paperwork, communication with outside agencies). Studies have shown little, if any, relationship between the amount of time a patient spends in the ER and the actual amount of staff time related to him or her.
- Laboratory. Establish stat charges to reflect cost increase over batched tests.
- Pharmacy. Establish administration mode charges (e.g., injectable, iv). These charges should reflect pharmacist time in preparation of the pharmaceutical. Charge separately for the actual drugs dispensed.
- Physical therapy. Charges should reflect both time and modality. The current charging system may not recognize the skill level and cost of staff involved or of supplies utilized in providing the various treatments.
- All departments. In all departments, review for duplicate and unused charges and delete them. Also, "miscellaneous" charges reflecting proportionately large amounts of reve-

nue should be carefully researched to identify which services provided are being coded as "miscellaneous," and should be revised as necessary.

This is only a partial list of commonly suggested revisions to the CDM. The emphasis is on the importance of reviewing the CDM to ensure that charges *do* reflect resource consumption and, ultimately, costs. In addition, charges should be specific enough to result in equitable charges to patients based upon actual goods and services received and to diminish the occurrence of some patients subsidizing others.

DEPARTMENTAL GENERAL LEDGERS

The next step in the process is a review of the general ledger of each department by the materials manager, the accounting department, and each department head. This activity is essential to identify costs that may be accumulating in inappropriate natural classifications (sub-accounts) or cost centers. The hospitalwide natural classification of expense categories should also be assessed to determine whether additional classifications should be added. For example, if the hospital groups labor costs into one or two categories designated "labor" or "salaries," it is recommended that they break them out into categories such as "management/supervision," "technical/specialist," "RN," "clerical," etc. Another example is separating "radiology films" from "general supplies" in the radiology department and separating other specific, high cost supplies in other departments.

After the general ledger has been reviewed and revised as needed, the accounting department and each department head should review each natural classification *departmentally* to classify expenses as fixed, variable, or semivariable for each department. If the expense is semivariable, an amount or a percentage should be identified as either fixed or variable. This determination may initially be difficult, but on the "first cut," a best educated guess is usually fairly accurate. As

more information is available, or as studies of each expense are completed, the amounts or percentages can be refined, thus making the information more accurate.

RESOURCE UTILIZATION STUDIES

To be conducted concurrently with the three steps outlined above are the departmental and service-specific resource utilization/consumption studies. These studies identify the "standard" list of materials utilized in the provision of each service. The service referred to is any charge listed in the CDM. Many hospitals are currently grappling with the question, "Which services should be studied and to what level of detail should studies be conducted?" Generally, the 80/20 rule (80 percent of revenues or costs come from 20 percent of services—closer to 90/20 in actuality) is recommended in the selection of services to be studied specifically. An identification of direct labor (by classification), supplies, and equipment (minor and capital) utilized in the provision of each service selected for study would establish the *minimum* basis for meaningful cost accounting information. However, it is recommended that these studies be regarded as the groundwork and that cost accounting be a "living" system. Additional studies *do* improve the accuracy of the cost accounting information and can, in some cases, significantly alter the identified costs. Other cost classifications recommended for study include service contracts, professional fees, additional supply studies, purchased services, and rental/lease costs. Also, indirect cost studies should be completed where a relationship can be identified between an indirect expense and specific services/procedures.

The main intent in cost accounting is to quantitatively identify how each service benefits from each natural classification of expense. This is the most important point in understanding the cost accounting process. If this concept is understood, hospital cost accounting itself will be more easily comprehended, and the selection of a system becomes greatly simplified.

For the cost accounting system, a relationship needs to be identified between the services provided within each department and the expenses, both direct and indirect, incurred. For some of those expenses, the relationship is fairly clear—for example, RN and technical labor, physician fees (if service-specific), medical supplies, prostheses, radiology films, instruments (minor equipment), depreciation on movable equipment, and some maintenance contracts. For the other direct expenses where the relationship may not be as evident, discussions should be initiated or studies performed to determine the most accurate statistic for recognizing how each service benefits (whether equally or variably) from each expense (resource).

SELECTING A COST ACCOUNTING SOFTWARE SYSTEM

The next major step is the selection of a software system that will take the information you have developed and determine and maintain your cost-per-service information base. The development of a system internally is no longer a cost-justified alternative to purchasing a system, although it may have been the only viable alternative as recently as a year ago. Today, it could take more than two years and millions of dollars to develop a sophisticated system in-house, whereas there are excellent systems available for around $75,000. With numerous vendors, accounting firms, and consulting companies selling their systems and/or consulting services under the "cost accounting" umbrella, it is becoming increasingly difficult to understand the real features and applications of each and how each differs operationally from the others.

There are some features that should be considered important in the selection of a system. Few, if any, systems will meet all of these criteria, but the goal in selecting a system should be to choose one that has the capability to meet your changing and increasingly sophisticated informational requirements in the future. Some recommended features of a cost accounting system include

- capability to handle and process detailed resource utilization studies for every natural classification of expense for all departments, direct and/or indirect (overhead)
- reconciliation of identified expenses to actual financial statements
- internal indirect cost allocations to both the departmental and service levels. This is very important, since the indirect expenses allocated to the departments often exceed their direct expenses. The allocation of these expenses to the departments and to the services is a critical point in monitoring full costing and is often not given the detailed review it deserves.
- ability to maintain a very large number of statistical bases for allocating costs
- updating of information quickly. The cost accounting system should interface with the other financial systems software operating on the same hardware, thus eliminating a second manual entry of current financial information.
- interface with the case-mix system. The cost accounting system should be able to pass cost information to the case-mix system (which ideally would accept five cost fields per service: direct, indirect, fixed, variable, and total) and accept information from the case-mix system to review profitability of service and cost variances from standard (by product line, case, physician, payer, etc.).
- budget system interface—preferably flexible product line budgeting
- support of multihospital users on the same system (if applicable)
- forecasting capabilities and "what-if" situation forecasting
- ability to support both standard and allocated costing methodologies for *all* services
- exception reporting—reports identifying new services on the CDM or costs that have not been accounted for
- variance reporting—reports comparing standard and actual costs and corresponding variances

- base data file—a file that contains resource utilization study information from national averages or standards, to be used to allocate costs to those services not directly studied
- grouping or "roll-up" feature—allows for easy comparison of departments and administrative responsibility areas as well as inter-hospital comparisons, etc.
- extensive security features—identifying and limiting users as desired
- data entry ease. A data entry person should be able to enter the information directly from input forms.
- general ledger reclassifications—should allow reclassifications inter- and intradepartmentally.
- support of fixed, variable, and semivariable classification of expenses by department
- rapid recalculation response time. You should be able to recalculate entire hospital information or each department individually.
- maintenance of the hospitalwide cost accounting information base within the singular system. The cost accounting system should support the whole hospital's cost information base. Avoid systems that have only the capability to maintain departments as separate entities.

The system you select should be designed and have the capability to support you as your informational needs become more refined. The system should not soon become obsolete or require a great deal of staff time to maintain. The system should have the capability of being fully operational within one month of installation, using whatever information you currently have available, and support future refinements. It should share information internally with your other financial systems and support both standard and allocated costing methodologies. Contrary to seemingly popular belief, a mini- or mainframe-based system does not have a longer implementation time frame than a PC-based system, and in

some instances it is considerably less. There are currently one or two vendors who have systems that meet most of the selection criteria outlined. Most of them do not, and you should approach the selection process critically. Avoid "simple" systems designed mainly to generate consulting revenue.

USING CONSULTANTS

You may wish to use consultants to assist in the implementation of your system. If the system is designed well and has easily comprehensible input forms, consultants may not be necessary. However, a few who have had extensive experience in hospital cost accounting can facilitate a successful system installation, and you may benefit from their experience in conducting studies and assisting in the development of standards. Consultants would also expedite the installation, a very important consideration in generating timely information, and may also identify immediate cost-saving opportunities.

SUMMARY

Some hospitals today are actually faring well financially under PPS and are questioning the urgency of implementing a cost accounting system. The system would prove beneficial to those hospitals as well, since the information would allow them to review their margin per product line, DRG, or service. This would assist in making decisions about which services or products to promote through physician recruitment and marketing, and which services or products require further cost containment efforts, and in formulating "make or buy" decisions while recognizing and understanding the financial implications of each alternative.

As both a consultant to hospitals and a vendor, I find that hospitals are often misled by vendors as to the preparation and work required to properly implement a cost accounting system that will generate *meaningful* information. However, the implementation and monitoring of a properly developed cost accounting system will provide information valuable in containing costs, reviewing the profitability of services, and contracts. Accurate cost accounting information can also promote informed hospital leadership and assist in responding to today's health-care payment initiatives. A flexible, so-phisticated system with standards developed "from the bottom up" will have the capability to continue to monitor cost behavior and profitability of service in any payment system, prospective or otherwise, that impacts on health care providers in the future.

Reading 1–3

The Human Element in Cost Accounting

Steven A. Finkler

Cost accounting is a field in which we often become buried in the numbers. Determining what something costs can be a totally absorbing task. One risk in cost accounting is that we tend to lose touch with the various human beings who are involved in the different parts of the process. If we don't closely consider the individual people involved in the cost accounting process, we may calculate accurate costs, but we may be causing things to cost more than they ought to.

GOAL CONGRUENCE

It is the basic nature of individuals that their own personal goals will generally be divergent from the goals of the organization they work for. This does not mean that human nature is bad; just that there is such a thing as human nature and we are foolish if we refuse to recognize it as such.

For example, other things being equal, most employees of a hospital would prefer a salary that is substantially larger than what they are currently receiving. Most would be quite content if the hospital were to double their salary overnight. There's nothing particularly bad about such people or wrong in their wanting more

Source: Reprinted from Steven A. Finkler, "The Human Element in Cost Accounting," *Hospital Cost Management and Accounting,* Vol. 2, No. 10, January 1991, pp. 1–4. Copyright 1991, Aspen Publishers, Inc.

money. In fact, ambition is probably a desirable trait among employees.

On the other hand, most hospitals are reluctant to provide employees with substantial raises, because they lack the revenues to pay for those raises. While the employees are not wrong to desire the raises, the hospital is not wrong to deny such raises. Inherently however, a tension or conflict exists.

Most hospital managers would like more office space. They would like nicer office space with new furniture and remodeled facilities. They would certainly like more staff to carry out their existing functions. Introductory economics books clearly indicate that society simply has limited resources. All organizations must make choices concerning how to spend their limited resources.

In fact, if we were to find a hospital in which the vast majority of managers were content with the size of their salary, office, and staff, then we probably will have identified a hospital that is failing in its mission. Perhaps there is a small percentage of all hospitals that is so well endowed as to be able to provide all health services their communities could dream of, and also provide their employees with all of their desires.

Perhaps. But for the at least ninety-nine percent of all hospitals with limited resources, providing unlimited amenities to employees certainly means some patient service limitations must be taking place. The hospital, in allocating its scarce resources, by giving in to the wants of its employees must place limits on the amount of health care services it provides. In most hospitals there are some concessions to employees, and there are some patient service limitations.

Thus we must face the fact that in the majority of hospitals, even where morale is generally excellent and is not considered to be a problem, an underlying tension will naturally exist. Even though the employees may want to achieve the mission of the hospital in providing care, their personal desires will be for things the hospital will not choose to provide.

Perhaps surprisingly, to a great extent it is the accountants of the hospital who have to deal with this divergence and develop means of creating congruency. The hospital must bring together the interests of the individual and the hospital so that they can work together. And cost accounting systems are one area in which we can work on creating that common bond of interest.

In the budgeting and costing process we are attempting to control the amount the organization spends. We don't want to measure costs just because it is nice to know what things cost. The reason we spend time and money on the measurement process is so that we have information for decision making and for control. But it is not the cost information that actually controls costs; it is the human beings involved in the process.

It is in the direct interests of the hospital for costs to be controlled. In order to be sure that the human beings will in fact want to control costs, we need to make sure that it is somehow in their direct best interests for costs to be controlled. The key is to establish some way that the normally divergent desires of the hospital and its employees become convergent or congruent. We want both the hospital and the employee to want the same thing.

Since congruent goals are not always the norm, and since divergent goals frequently exist, we need to formally address how convergence is to be obtained. Organizations generally achieve such convergence or congruence by setting up a system of incentives that make it serve the best interests of the employees to serve the best interests of the organization.

MOTIVATION AND INCENTIVE

Developing a set of incentives to motivate people is not something that most cost accountants are likely to think of as part of their job. However, since cost accountants are at least to some extent "cost managers," we must consider what things can be done to provide incentives to motivate managers to control costs.

In industry, one common motivating tool is the use of bonus systems. Since managers have many desires that relate to spending money (e.g., larger offices, fancier furniture, larger staffs), we need to develop formalized incentives to spend less money. For example, we can tell a manager that last year his department spent $200,000, and that next year his budget is $208,000 (a four percent increase). However, for any amount that his department spends below $208,000, he can keep 10 percent. So, if the department spends only $180,000, he gets a personal bonus of $2,800. The total cost to the organization is $182,800, including the bonus, as opposed to the $208,000 budgeted. The employee benefits and the organization benefits.

However, incentives are tricky to work with, as the federal government seems to find out every time it tries to control overall spending. When an incentive is given to accomplish one end, sometimes the responses to that incentive are unexpected. In the case of the federal government, we have found that DRGs, intended to reduce health care spending, increase spending on nursing homes and home care agencies. In the case of a 10 percent bonus on spending reductions from budget, a manager may have an incentive to treat fewer patients to keep costs down. If that also reduces revenue, the outcome may be very undesirable.

Hospitals are also concerned about the quality of care. If incentives cause managers to reduce staff to save money, that savings is not very worthwhile if it unexpectedly reduces quality of care.

These are not insurmountable problems. They merely point out some of the complexities in developing an incentive system. The quality issue requires that the hospital have a strong internal quality assurance program. Part of the bonus process would have to be restrictions on bonuses when quality of care has declined.

The volume-of-patients problem can be solved by making the incentive depend on a flexible budget, which adjusts automatically for changes in volume. For example, if a department has a budget of $104,000 of fixed costs, and $104,000 of variable costs, for a total budget of $208,000 (as above), then we could adjust the budget prior to calculating the bonus. If volume of patients drops by 10 percent, we would expect costs to fall by $10,400 (i.e., 10 percent of the variable costs). Therefore, costs should have been $208,000 less $10,400, or a total of $197,600. If actual costs were $180,000, the bonus would be based on the $17,600 difference between the flexible budget of $197,600 and the actual cost, rather than being based on the full difference between the original budget and the actual result.

A flexible budget adjustment should be particularly appealing to managers if workload is rising. It is hard to convince a manager that a bonus based on reduced costs will help him, if each year our patient volume increases, and costs rise with patient load. In the above example, suppose that the number of patients rises by 20 percent above expectations when the $208,000 budget was prepared. The flexible budget would allow the variable portion to increase by 20 percent, or a total of $20,800 ($104,000 × 20%). If actual spending is $220,000, which is $12,000 over budget, the manager will still get a bonus, since the flexible budget will be the original $208,000, plus $20,800 allowed for the volume increase, or a total budget of $228,800. The actual spending of $220,000 will result in a bonus of $880, even though spending went over the original budget.

This does not mean that bonuses are the solution to all motivational problems. Bonus systems have a variety of other problems as well. Some bonus systems reward all employees if spending is down. But, if everyone gets a bonus, then no one feels that individual actions have much impact. As long as they believe everyone else is keeping spending down, some individuals may feel that they don't have to work particularly hard to reap the benefits of the bonus. In that case, probably very few will work hard to control costs.

On the other hand, if bonuses are given only to some employees, it may create a competitive environment in a situation in which teamwork is needed to provide quality care.

There are alternatives to bonuses. For example, one underused managerial tool is a letter from supervisor to subordinate. All individuals responsible for controlling costs should be explicitly evaluated with respect to how well they do in fact control costs. That evaluation should be communicated in writing. This approach, which is both the carrot and the stick, costs little to implement, but can have a dramatic impact.

Telling managers that they did a good job and that their boss knows that they did a good job can be an effective way to get the manager to try to do a good job the next year. In the real world, praise is both cheap and, in many cases, effective. On the other hand, criticism, especially in writing, can have a stinging effect that managers will work hard to avoid in the future.

UNREALISTIC EXPECTATIONS

While motivational devices can work wonders at getting an organization's employees to work hard for the organization and its goals, they can also backfire and have negative results. This occurs primarily when expectations are placed at unreasonably high levels.

There is no question that many workers do attempt to *satisfice*—to do just enough to get by. One thing we use incentives to accomplish is to motivate those individuals to work harder. A target that requires hard work and stretching, but is achievable, can be a useful motivating tool. If the target is reached, there might be a bonus, or there should be at least some formal recognition of the achievement, such as a letter. At a minimum, the worker will have the self-satisfaction of having worked hard and reached the target.

But all of those positive outcomes can occur only if the target can in fact be reached. Some organizations have adopted the philosophy that if a high target makes people work hard, a higher target will make them work harder. This may not be the case. If targets are placed out of reach, this will probably not result in people reaching to their utmost limits to come as close to the target as possible.

It may seem as if we are short-changing ourselves whenever a subordinate achieves a target. We may think to ourselves, "We set the target too low. Perhaps if the target was higher, this person would have achieved the higher target. Since the target we set was achieved, we really don't know just how far this person can go. We haven't yet realized all of the potential." The problem with that logic is that there are risks associated with failure.

If managers fail to meet a target because they are not very competent or because they do not work very hard, the signal of failure that we send is warranted. In fact, repeated failure may be grounds for replacement of that individual in that job. But if a manager is both competent and hard working, failure is not a message that we want to send. Even though our intent may be simply to encourage the individual to achieve even more, the signal of failure will be discouraging.

When people work extremely hard, and fail, they often question why they bothered to work so hard. If hard work results in failure to achieve the target, they think, "Why not ease off? If you're going to fail anyway, must it be so painful?" Thus we must be extremely judicious to ensure that all goals assigned to managers are reasonable, or results may be less favorable than they otherwise would be.

CONCLUSION

Accountants can prepare budgets and cost reports to their heart's content. However, it is usually other managers and workers who must be counted upon to make those plans become a reality. Why would they want to do that?

It may seem like a flippant question, but in fact it is both serious and critical. When we ask a manager to accomplish something, we must be concerned with whether there is any reason in the world that he would want to do it.

Perhaps he will do it out of loyalty to the organization. Perhaps he will do it out of fear of losing his job. Perhaps he will do it in the hope of earning a promotion. Perhaps he will do it because he's just such a good guy.

Getting an understanding of what people will want to do and what they won't want to do is important. And once we know what they won't want to do, we should carefully attempt to develop some clear motivational device that will give them an incentive to do what they otherwise might not want to. After all, how many of us would work if we didn't get paid at all? Paychecks are simply a bribe to get people to come to work. Once they are at work, we need to provide additional incentives to make sure that the hospital benefits from their efforts to the greatest extent possible.

2

Cost Definitions

Reading 2–1

The Identification of Surgical Services Costs

Bryan B. Dieter

The Surgery Department is generally one of the hospital's highest revenue-producing areas and also one of the most difficult in which to determine service-level costs. The services provided vary greatly depending upon each patient's condition, the surgeon's preferences, the hospital and surgery director's policies, and the anesthesiologist's practices. All of these factors can also impact upon the cost of providing services to each patient.

The most important mechanism for accurately identifying costs is a well-defined and representative Charge Description Master (CDM). The CDM should accurately reflect the resources utilized and the cost of services provided. It should be specific enough to promote equitable patient charges, yet not too cumbersome to use.

We will therefore begin with a review of an effective CDM. We aren't advocating this as the only acceptable methodology, but the charge structure discussed in this article has been implemented very successfully in a number of hospitals. More importantly, the charge structure and

Source: Reprinted from Bryan B. Dieter, "The Identification of Surgical Services Costs," *Hospital Cost Accounting Advisor,* Vol. 2, No. 8, January 1987, pp. 1–5. Copyright 1987, Aspen Publishers, Inc.

cost accounting methodology discussed can be applied in determining service-level costs in any well-defined CDM.

THE CHARGE DESCRIPTION MASTER

In the past, charge structures for surgical services have been poor and frequently did not accurately represent resource utilization. Often, charges were grouped into gross categories, were generated through a charge-explosion system, or had no incremental time or acuity designations. A well-designed surgical services charge system should include

- acuity-related base and incremental time charges
- tray charges
- capital equipment charges
- suture and patient chargeable supply charges
- inpatient and outpatient designations

We will discuss the direct costing of these classifications of charges followed by various suggestions for allocating remaining direct and indirect expenses.

ESTABLISHING ACUITY-BASED CHARGES

In surgery, the acuity-related charges are not necessarily designed to reflect a patient's actual physical condition, but rather the acuity of the case from the standpoint of the surgery department itself—namely, how many and what type of staff are involved in the case and for how long. An example of acuity-related charges follows:

- Level 1—Base 15 Min. (1 RN for up to 15 min.)
- Level 1—Ea Add Min. (1 RN for each minute over 15)
- Level 2—Base 30 Min. (1 RN & 1 technician for up to 30 min.)
- Level 2—Ea Add 5 Min. (1 RN & 1 technician for each 5 min. over 30)
- Level 3—Base 1 Hour (2 RNs for up to 1 hour)
- Level 3—Ea Add 5 Min. (2 RNs for each 5 min. over 1 hour)
- Level 4—Base 1 Hour (2 RNs & 1 technician for up to 1 hour)
- Level 4—Ea Add 5 Min. (2 RNs & 1 technician for each 5 min. over 1 hour)
- Emergency Surgery—Base 2 Hours (2 RNs for up to 2 hours)
- Emergency Surgery—Ea Add 15 Min. (2 RNs for each 15 min. over 2 hours)
- Circulating RN—Each 5 Min. (1 RN for 5 min.)

In determining the base charges that would be most appropriate for your department, review your general staffing practices. The base charges that you establish should be related to your usual staff assignments. You may have as few as two or three levels, or up to 10 or 12 depending upon your staffing patterns/requirements. The time designations (15 min., 30 min., 1 hour) associated with the base charges should reflect the mode, or the most frequent amount of time, for a case with that number of staff. A log or a record review will help determine what the base levels should be.

The incremental time charges are intended to account for those cases that exceed the mode. The emergency charge is designed to capture the expense for "on-call" and the pay differential for call-back. The base time for the emergency surgery is usually set at a time that the staff may be guaranteed by contract if they are called in. If there is no guaranteed paid time for call-back, then a shorter base time may be appropriate for your hospital. You may encounter a situation in which your staff is called in for a procedure that takes only 20 minutes. However, the actual expense to the hospital is still for two RNs for two hours at time and a half. The charge structure should be able to reflect this actual cost. The 5-minute circulating charges are established for those instances when an additional nurse is required for only a limited portion of the procedure, perhaps to get the case started, or at a particularly difficult point in the procedure. This charge should be assessed only for the time actually spent by that nurse preparing for or assisting in the case.

These charges would account for the majority of the variable departmental labor per procedure. Additionally, a factor should be added to each base charge for turnaround functions related to opening up a room, cleaning up after a procedure, moving equipment, etc. These times could be determined from running a room log or from your productivity system if your hospital has one.

To determine the actual standard cost for each of your types of labor for each of your acuity levels, you could use the following formula (illustrated using Level 1 Base Charge):

Base Time 15 Min. + Turnaround Time 10 Min.	Number of Staff	Labor Cost/Hour	Standard Labor Cost
25 Min.	× 1	× $12.00	= $5.00

For the purposes of cost accounting, it will be necessary to retrospectively estimate service volumes for the newly created charges. The easiest way to do this is to use work sampling. Select cases randomly from your surgery logbook. You should select cases only from the period of time you have established as your base period for the cost accounting information. With the cases you select at random, you should assign each of them an acuity-based charge under the new CDM and the additional incremental time charges that would be associated with each case (the difference between the time allowed for in the base charge and the actual case time). You would then determine what percent of the total case volume each of the acuity charges represents. Then, using your total volume of cases over this same period of time, you would estimate what your case volume would have been for each acuity level during this base period of time. You will also have developed the volumes for the incremental time charges in this process.

You have now determined your service volumes for each of the labor-related charges and the times for each type of labor to provide each of those services. The next step is to allocate your actual expenses for each type of labor based upon the standard labor cost you identified for each charge. This is accomplished by multiplying the standard cost for each charge (as determined in the example above) by its corresponding volume. To determine your actual cost of providing these services during your base period of time, you would use this total standard cost information as a basis for allocating the actual expense from the general ledger.

It is important that whenever possible in the cost accounting process you keep the cost categories (i.e., RNs, technicians, film, sutures, clerks, aides, housekeeping) separate with their own standard costs. There is significant value in not grouping expenses for allocation purposes. The major advantage is in providing department managers with utilization variance reporting by specific expense type. When you allocate an actual expense based upon the standard cost determined for that specific type of expense, you greatly increase the value of the cost accounting information. One of the primary purposes of implementing a cost accounting system should

be to promote cost control at the department management level. The more finite the cost categories are, the greater the opportunity the department manager has to identify *specific* expenses that require additional cost containment efforts.

CAPITAL EQUIPMENT CHARGES

Capital equipment charges should be established for those major (as determined by cost) pieces of equipment that are used only for specific procedures. Examples include monitors, special lighting, scopes, saws, drills, and special tables. You should begin your determination of which pieces of equipment require charges by obtaining a copy of the department's capital assets report and identifying the use of each piece of equipment. This will also provide an opportunity to verify the listing and to correct or modify it as needed.

If your department hasn't used capital equipment charges in the past, you will need to have the surgery staff project as accurately as possible the service volumes for each of the charges you have established. The cost per use for these pieces of equipment is determined by dividing the depreciation of the equipment by the number of projected uses for the same period of time. Pieces of equipment that could be used interchangeably should be grouped together and one cost per use determined for the group. (See Table 2–1–1.)

Maintenance contract costs should be identified with the capital equipment the contracts are intended to cover. The costs for these contracts should be determined using the same methodology as for the capital equipment. They would then become a part of the cost for the capital equipment charge.

TRAY CHARGES

Determining the costs of trays is the most time-consuming and difficult task in identifying your surgery costs per charge. The concept is actually fairly simple: determine the replacement

Table 2–1–1 Determining Monitor w/Recorder Capital Equipment Cost/Use

Number	Description	Annual Depreciation Cost	Annual Usage	Cost/ Use
15862	Cardiac Monitor	$1,100		
15863	Cardiac Monitor	1,100		
15866	Cardiac Monitor	1,100		
17415	Cardiac Monitor	1,260		
15881	Recorder	900		
15882	Recorder	900		
15883	Recorder	900		
		$7,260	2,500	$2.90

cost of the tray, multiply by the total number of that type of tray, divide by its expected life, and then divide by the anticipated number of times that tray would be used. The difficulty is in determining the replacement cost of the tray. Having spent many, many, many hours flipping through instrument catalogues, I've sworn never to undertake this venture again. A Kelly clamp is not *just* a Kelly clamp. It is certainly best left to the surgery staff, at least to identify catalogue numbers, so you just have to look up the prices.

Some may question the need to develop capital equipment and tray charges and argue for keeping the cost buried as an "other" expense. Yet, it makes a substantial difference in the identified cost for the acuity levels as well as in your review of costs by surgeon for providing each of your various surgical cases. All surgeons certainly do not use the same resources when performing similar cases. For apparently similar cases one surgeon may take longer and use a varying number and type of staff in addition to different equipment and supplies (chargeable and nonchargeable) and may request special and more expensive trays. If this information is buried in your "procedure based" charge system, you will not have the capability to accurately determine costs or provide *meaningful* product-line and physician-cost analysis.

SUPPLY COSTS

Patient-chargeable supplies are costed out at their actual purchase price. Any labor required

will be accounted for in the acuity charges. In certain cost accounting systems, such as Hospital Cost Consultant's (HCC), you have the capability to reference these costs directly from your materials management system. This provides you with a much less maintenance-intensive system.

Nonchargeable supplies should also have standards developed for their normal use. Items such as caps, gowns, shoe covers, masks, gloves, etc., can all be identified in relation to the acuity-based charges. Other nonchargeable supplies, not directly accounted for as a "standard" cost, are allocated to the acuity-related charges based upon the standard supply usage that was identified. In studies I have completed, a direct correlation has consistently been identified between a procedure's acuity level and length and its utilization of nonchargeable supplies.

OTHER DIRECT COSTS

You may wish to continue on and develop standards for other types of direct expenses. If so, it is worth the effort in most cases, since there truly can be benefits realized from continuing on to greater levels of detail, especially in the area of cost containment. However, it does require additional time, which many hospital staffs do not seem to have enough of lately. That brings us to "What happens with the other departmental costs?"

These costs, from the general ledger, need to be allocated to the procedures based upon a cost/benefit relationship. For example, if management labor is perceived as an expense from which all patients benefit equally, then this cost can be reasonably allocated only to each base charge. For monitoring purposes, you may also wish to keep these expenses separate from one another. This would give you the capability to monitor these "fixed" expenses on a per-procedure basis for the purpose of trend analysis and to identify possible methods of reducing your fixed expenses on a per-use basis.

INDIRECT EXPENSES

Indirect expenses are often grossly overlooked in determining procedure-level costs, primarily because most of the cost accounting systems available are inadequate in their ability to handle indirect costs. Indirect expenses will, in most cases, increase the total departmental expenses 40 to 110 percent over their direct general ledger costs. Grouping these expenses together and allocating them based upon one or two statistics only dilutes the accuracy of the information developed for your direct departmental expenses.

Some systems, such as the HCC System, allow for the development of standards for indirect as well as direct expenses. The HCC System also allows indirect expenses to be stepped down by natural classification of expense and does not require that each indirect department's expenses be stepped down in the same step.

In the surgery department this is helpful, since it allows the hospital to establish standard costs for housekeeping labor to turn around rooms after the surgical procedures, and even to develop standards for the specific housekeeping supplies that are used. It also allows you to allocate the other indirect costs of surgery based upon thousands of potential allocation statistics to improve the accuracy of the information. Some other examples include

- Personnel   The total labor time per charge
- MIS   Equally to each charge
- Building Maint. Minutes per case
- Administration   Equally to each patient in base charge

- Admitting   Inpatient cases only
- OP Registration Ambulatory cases only
- Materials Mgmt/ Number or cost of
  Purchasing   supplies

THE IMPORTANCE OF ACCURATE DATA

This article was intended to provide the reader with some thoughts on alternative methods of developing accurate procedure-level cost information. This database of information will come to play an increasingly important role in the day-to-day operations of the hospital. If properly implemented, accurate cost accounting data can directly help you with management decisions intended to improve the financial performance of your hospital. It can also be very misleading if the information is inaccurate.

Many hospital management teams are implementing cost accounting in their hospitals to support product line and DRG analysis. That is indeed a very important use for the information, but too often too little attention is paid to how the building blocks of this aggregate information are developed. The adage "garbage in, garbage out" certainly applies to hospital cost accounting systems and methodologies. I am attempting in this series to provide *Hospital Cost Accounting Advisor* readers with some methods for developing more meaningful management tools. I also hope to encourage hospitals to step beyond the "good enough" attitude and establish more aggressive systems and databases.

Reading 2–2

Cost Finding for High-Technology, High-Cost Services: Current Practice and a Possible Alternative

Steven A. Finkler

Economic theory indicates that the cost of producing a unit of a product or service will change as the volume produced changes. In large part this results from the sharing of the resources required in a set amount for production at any volume. In hospitals these "fixed costs" remain the same regardless of the number of patients treated, whereas according to economic theory the more patients, the less fixed cost any patient must bear.

In a free market environment a producer would be forced to cease production of any product produced at an uneconomically low volume. Such production would not spread fixed costs sufficiently and would therefore result in a high average cost. Producers operating at a sufficiently large volume would have lower unit costs, and therefore be able to undersell the low-volume, high-cost producers. Rather than cease business completely, a producer, knowing the average costs were high, could just stop producing a product.

In hospitals, cost reimbursement has somewhat restricted this free market mechanism. A hospital producing a low volume of product re-

Source: Reprinted from Steven A. Finkler, "Cost Finding for High-Technology, High-Cost Services: Current Practice and a Possible Alternative," *Health Care Management Review,* Summer 1980, pp. 17–29. Copyright 1980, Aspen Publishers, Inc.

ceives a higher price (reimbursement) and is thus enabled to keep producing the product inefficiently. The market mechanism does not force the hospital to produce at efficient volumes or cease production.

Hospital administrators and regulators alike are well aware of this, and have tried diligently to keep utilization of facilities high. Nevertheless, there have been persistent reports of underutilized facilities and excessive duplication of highly sophisticated, high-cost technology at too many hospitals.

PARADOX EXPLAINED

How does this apparent paradox arise? Apparently physicians have been quite willing to attempt to maximize utilization of facilities that they have. However, they have been reluctant to pass by some new technologies simply because there is a relatively low demand for them. Certainly there are medical justifications for these actions. Physicians would like the hospitals they are affiliated with to offer the highest possible quality of care, and bringing in new technology raises the quality of care.

In addition, the cost analysis of new technology has centered on direct cost and a "can we afford it" approach. Rather than look at the total additional cost a hospital will incur in each department if a new program is added, the analysis typically looks at the new capital outlays. Capital costs, however, are but a small fraction of the overall costs of a hospital. Furthermore, the question of "can we afford it" depends a lot on who pays. Currently, 94 percent of hospital costs are paid by third party payers on cost-reimbursement systems.[1] The costs *can* be passed on to these third party payers, so the answer to the affordability question is often yes, irrespective of the potential demand for the service at that hospital.

As a result, hospitals offer high-technology, high-cost services at widely varying levels of utilization. Thus a major cause of different hospitals having different costs for the same service is simply the degree to which fixed costs are spread across patients.

Regulatory agencies have tried to combat the problem of inefficient production with a variety of flexible charging schedules based on different patient types. The aim of this approach is to cause hospitals to lose money on services offered inefficiently. Those hospitals would either have to become efficient or else cease production of the product to avoid such losses. The most recent program of that type is a project being tried in New Jersey that uses prospective reimbursement based on diagnosis-related groups.

A major problem these approaches have had is that they focus on prospective reimbursement of costs without in-depth investigation of appropriate cost data. Frequently, an average of charges made by hospitals for treatment of a patient type is used as the basis for the reimbursement rate for that patient type. Since charges are based on costs, this averaging should result in some average or reasonable cost for offering the service. However, cross-subsidizations within the hospital cost-finding system may prevent this method from reflecting the true economic costs of the patient type.

Cross-subsidies within the accounting system result from simplifications made to reduce the bookkeeping costs of data collection. The cost information produced is adequate for the uses for which the cost-finding system was designed. However, there are problems when the data are used to determine a uniform cost per patient for a specific service at different hospitals with different levels of utilization. To improve hospital efficiency, regulators need estimates that give the cost per patient for a service at alternative volumes of production, based on economic resources utilized specifically for that service.

TWO APPROACHES TO HOSPITAL COST FINDING

Hospitals use cost information to establish rates, apply for cost-based reimbursement, and comply with governmental and hospital association reporting requirements. This has resulted in the compilation of different types of information than that used by most industries. However, current accounting literature has emphasized that there is not one "true" cost that can be measured;[2] different measures of cost are appropriate for different needs. Nevertheless, hospital information requirements have stressed cost-finding methods for both the control of departmental costs and external reporting needs, with only limited cost-finding efforts concerning economic resource costs by patient type.

Horizontal Cost Finding

The principal hospital form of cost finding will be referred to here as a "horizontal" system. The primary focus of such a system is on departmental costs.

Because the hospital is typically reimbursed based on the costs a patient incurs in various departments, rather than on the patient type, the costs of intermediate or departmental products are measured. (See Figure 2–2–1.) Even when attempts are made to reimburse hospitals based on patient type, the basis of the reimbursement is some averaging of the costs previously determined by this intermediate, product-oriented method. Thus hospital administrators would know the cost of the radiology or dietary departments or even the cost per X-ray or per meal served, but they do not readily know the total cost impact of offering a specific high-cost,

HOSPITAL INDUSTRY

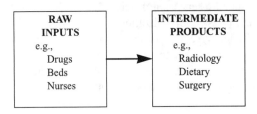

Figure 2–2–1 Horizontal Structure

high-technology service. The administrators have no strong need for that information.

Under the horizontal system the cost for a final product (i.e., the patient treated) is derived by adding charges from each department for units of service the patient consumed from each department. Thus a typical chest X-ray would be charged at the same rate to a pneumonia, lung cancer, or heart surgery patient, assuming the procedures required are the same in each case. No accounting is made of the fact that the addition of a heart surgery program may have increased X-ray volume to the point that an additional X-ray machine was purchased. The fixed cost of the additional machine is charged in equal shares to all patients having chest X-rays, not simply to the heart surgery patients. This method of cost finding would certainly pose a problem if a hospital must decide whether or not to offer a heart surgery program. That program should bear the cost of the new machine, a cost that would not otherwise have been incurred.

To a physician or hospital administrator, it is logical and natural to think of hospital products in terms of radiology and dietary because they are the traditional "cost centers" of the hospital. However, the physicians and administrators are well aware that they are not attempting to produce X-rays, but rather to treat a patient for an ailment.

Vertical Cost Finding

In contrast to horizontal cost finding, a vertical cost-finding system is oriented toward the cost of the final products or outputs. For example, in an automobile factory, a vertical cost system would center on the car model. Different car models would use different raw material resources or inputs, and different costs would be accumulated for each model or final product. (See Figure 2–2–2.) Thus the auto manufacturer would know the cost of Model A, Model B, and Model C. In the case of the hospital, a vertical orientation would lead to a greater focus on the costs for the type of patient treated.

Consider what the effect of horizontal cost finding would be on the auto manufacturer. It would cause him or her to think of costs in terms of radiator production or fender molding without respect to the car model for which the radiator is produced or the fender molded. The result would be an auto manufacturer well versed in the total cost of all radiators and fenders, and even the average cost of a radiator or fender.

However, the manufacturer would not know the difference in cost between a radiator for the

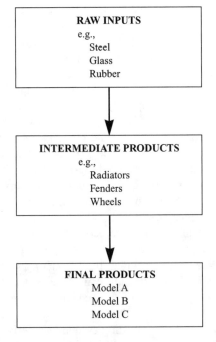

Figure 2–2–2 Vertical Structure

Model A car and one for the Model B car. Such information is more readily provided by vertical cost finding. As a result of the lack of information imposed by the horizontal cost finding system, there would have to be substantial cross-subsidization between the different model cars when their costs were determined.

Comparing Two Cost-Finding Methods

Tables 2–2–1 and 2–2–2 serve to clarify further the distinction between vertical and horizontal cost finding. (All numbers in these and subsequent tables and figures are used for illustrative purposes and are not intended to represent actual costs.) Table 2–2–1 demonstrates the final product orientation of the vertical cost-finding structure. The cost of each final product is determined separately as a sum of the raw inputs utilized in its production. Note that inputs are calculated on a per car or model basis, and differ in cost for each model.

This contrasts with the horizontal cost-finding system depicted in Table 2–2–2. Note that the horizontal orientation is toward the total cost per

month of each revenue center. From this the hospital can calculate an average cost per unit of intermediate product (e.g., cost per meal served). The direct connection between inputs and final outputs or products is lost, although total overall costs of the hospital would be the same whether vertical or horizontal cost finding is used.

The examples posed by Tables 2–2–1 and 2–2–2 represent two hypothetical extremes. The vertical system is not likely to be able to give complete information about each car model. Allocations of joint costs may still be made in some arbitrary fashion. Similarly, the horizontal system will likely be adjusted for products that consume an inordinately weighted share of a department's economic resources.

However, these examples are not without some relevance. Consider the method by which operating room (surgery cost center) costs are assigned to patients. Total costs and total operating minutes are determined for the surgery center and an average cost per minute is calculated. Any procedure requiring 60 minutes is considered to be twice as expensive as a 30-minute procedure. Such a method ignores the possibility that there

Table 2–2–1 Vertical Cost Finding

	Auto Industry		
	Final Products		
Intermediate Products and Raw Inputs per Car	**Model A**	**Model B**	**Model C**
Radiator			
Labor	$ 20	$ 15	$ 30
Steel	20	18	33
Hoses	3	2	4
Total	$ 43	$ 35	$ 67
Engine			
Labor	300	250	500
Steel	860	750	990
Spark plugs	5	4	6
Total	1,165	1,004	1,496
Body			
Labor	400	300	600
Plastic	50	40	80
Metal	500	400	700
Total	950	740	1,380
Total Cost by Model	$2,158	$1,779	$2,943

Table 2–2–2 Horizontal Cost Finding

	Hospital Industry				
Intermediate Products	Raw Inputs for Month				Intermediate Product Total Monthly Cost
	Labor	Equipment	Supplies	Allocation*	
Radiology	$40,000	$20,000	$ 5,000	$3,000	$ 68,000
Dietary	10,000	2,000	60,000	4,000	$ 76,000
Surgery	80,000	30,000	10,000	8,000	$128,000

*Cost allocation from nonrevenue cost centers.

may be short procedures requiring expensive, sophisticated equipment and long procedures that use much less costly resources. The horizontal cost-finding system cannot eliminate cross-subsidization because of the general averaging procedures that are used to find intermediate product costs, such as surgery minutes. An alternative cost-finding system, such as vertical cost-finding, would be needed to uncover the hospital's cost of offering the high-technology, high-cost service.

VERTICAL COST FINDING FOR A NEW PROGRAM

Vertical cost finding can be used for calculating the cost to the hospital of a specific new program or a specialized elective service, such as open heart surgery. Open heart surgery is used as the example here for two reasons. First, it emphasizes that the point of focus in vertical cost finding is the entire service. A hospital administration must decide whether or not to offer heart surgery rather than whether or not to have a heart bypass pump. Traditional hospital cost finding might point out only that the heart pump is a major expense of the surgery cost center. However, the surgery department would have neither the knowledge of the overall costs of treating heart surgery patients, nor the authority to make decisions regarding whether or not heart surgery

should be performed. By looking at the costs of the entire heart surgery program, the administration can make a decision regarding the cost effectiveness of offering heart surgery based on the knowledge of its economic effect on the entire hospital.

The second reason that open heart surgery is used as an example is that a new program or service is the prime target for an early battle between regulators and health care providers over appropriate cost data. Replacement of a worn-out X-ray machine is likely to receive rapid regulatory approval, since all short-term acute-care hospitals need a radiology department. Offering a new program, such as open heart surgery, is likely to draw much greater public scrutiny regarding its cost-effectiveness. Offering all elective services is not essential for the short-term, acute-care hospital to fulfill its basic role.

Note, however, that there are three major uses for the information that cost accounting can provide: (1) decision making, (2) budgeting, and (3) control. The information needed for each of these tasks differs. In the open heart surgery example only information needed for decision making is provided.

Furthermore, the value of the open heart surgery program is not assessed, but its cost-effectiveness for a given hospital is. Thus it may be found in the following example that any given number of heart surgeries should be produced at more or fewer hospitals. This article does not deal with the preferability of medical versus surgical treatment for heart disease.

Preliminary Steps of Vertical Cost Finding

Stated briefly, the problem is—What costs would a hospital incur if it has a program such as open heart surgery, which it would not incur if it did not offer that service? In economic terms, what is needed is the marginal cost to the hospital of the entire heart surgery program and the cost for the specific volume of patients expected. Thus vertical cost finding will provide cost information appropriate to the anticipated utilization of heart surgery facilities.

The first step in vertical cost finding is to determine the exact production process for the program under consideration. The costs for a specific volume can be determined once the production process and input requirements are fully understood. It is possible, however, that the hospital will not know the exact volume of heart surgery procedures it will perform each year. It may want to know the costs for a wide range of volumes, in order to see at what level of utilization it becomes economical to offer a service. Governmental regulations, medical standards, experience of administrators, and sampling techniques must be used to determine an estimate of input requirements at differing volumes.

To find the resource requirements of a program, the hospital must determine which departments come into direct contact with the program's patients. The flowchart in Figure 2–2–3 follows the patient through the hospital from admission to discharge. The flowchart serves as a basis to ensure inclusion of all costs. It includes patient movement, patient contact with hospital personnel, and indirect inputs such as various overhead cost centers. Note that the latter is referred to as days of hospitalization or "routine care." This category includes a variety of items from heat and light to secretarial pools, record-keeping, and parking lot maintenance. All factors of hospital operation must be considered for the effect the program would have on them.

Based on the flowchart, the cost elements of offering heart surgery might be broken down into the following groups: anesthesia, blood processing, cardiac catheterization, cardiac surgery intensive care unit, dietary, ECG [electrocardiogram], inhalation therapy, laboratory, linens, medications, medical/surgical hospital beds, operating room equipment and supplies, operating room personnel, overhead, and radiology.

Identification of Input Factors

Once such groupings are identified for which the addition, deletion, or change in volume of the elective program would affect factors of production (resource utilization), all such input factors are identified. This identification of input requirement variation with volume is a crucial phase of the data collection. The input-output relationships for hospital programs are not well known. Ultimately, however, each input is the responsibility of some individual. These individuals should be called upon to identify the inputs that are required for each heart surgery patient and the amount of each input needed at different volumes.

The inputs must be identified as fixed or variable. As discussed earlier, this is a crucial factor in cost finding. Fixed inputs will typically be the physical environment (hospital rooms and surgery suites, etc.) and equipment required. Variable inputs will be supplies consumed by each patient, such as meals and medications. Some inputs will be semifixed. That is, they will be fixed for a given range of output, but when that range is exceeded, more of the input is needed.

It is relatively simple to calculate the program costs for an ongoing program at a specific volume because all inputs can be observed. In planning a new program or considering volume changes in an ongoing program, hospitals must estimate semifixed costs because the actual range for an input may not be known. While in some cases these inputs have a well-known, technologically fixed capacity, in other cases individuals will have to assess the capacity of inputs based on their experience and expertise.

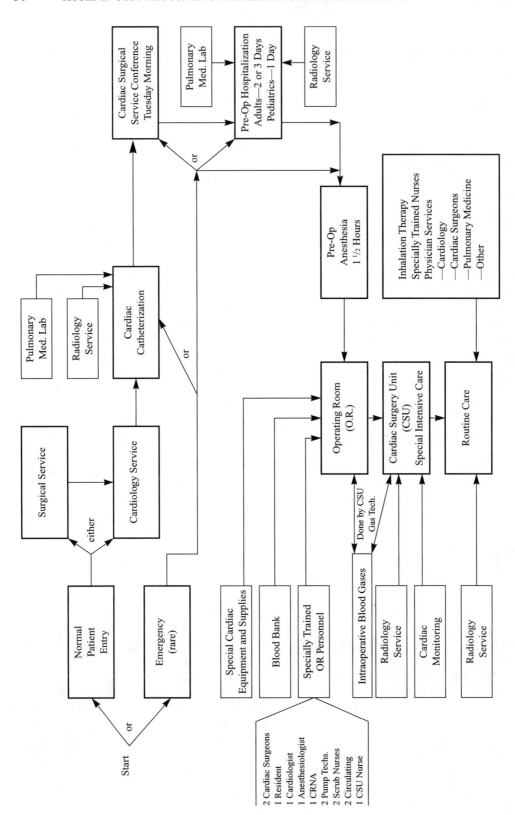

Figure 2–2–3 Cardiac Surgery Patient Flowchart

For example, the head of the linen department can assess the effect of a new program or a volume change in an existing program on the capacity of autoclave (linen sterilization) machines and the head of inhalation therapy can determine the capacity of respirator equipment.

Using the flowchart in Figure 2–2–3, the hospital administration can break the problem into manageable segments. For each cost element, the administration must determine what input requirements the addition of open heart surgery places upon it. These input requirements should be divided into fixed, variable, and semifixed resources. The semifixed inputs must be identified for the volumes at which new increments are needed.

When the hospital administration determines input requirements, it is important that a systems approach be taken. That is, the administration should consider all inputs throughout the entire hospital system that might be affected by the program. These are called "relevant" costs. For instance, if offering heart surgery causes the capacity of the hospital's X-ray machine to be exceeded, then heart surgery must bear the entire cost of a new X-ray machine. Similarly, if the heart surgery program uses facilities that would otherwise be unused, there should be no cost associated with that use, since it is not a relevant cost for the analysis.

Once the input requirements are determined, their cost can be measured and the cost of heart surgery determined. However, the cost measurement can only be made after many conceptual issues are resolved. These issues include the distinction between use of long-run and short-run costs, historical versus replacement costs, treatment of overhead costs, and discrete versus divisible labor inputs.

Cost Concepts

Long Run versus Short Run

The long run is defined as that period during which all factors of production can be adjusted for the desired volume of output. In the short

run, plant and equipment are assumed to be set at a given level, and only certain operating expenses are assumed to be variable. (Actually, there is a continuum of intermediate "runs.")

For example, suppose a hospital decides to provide a program that requires 20 beds, and at the moment there are excess beds. In the short run, the extra cost of the service will include the staffing, but not the construction of the 20 beds. In the long run, new beds will have to be built if the hospital's overall volume for all services is growing. So the long-run cost of the elective product would have to include the entire cost of building the beds, because if the optional program were not offered, 20 fewer beds would have had to be constructed.

When a hospital determines whether long-run costs, short-run costs, or those of some intermediate run are appropriate for use in an analysis, the key criterion is the time horizon of the decision's impact. If the decision is one that is expected to come up for review at frequent short-run intervals, an analysis of short-run costs may be adequate. Thus if a hospital is deciding the hours that a clinic should be open during the next month, the hospital would desire short-run costs. On the other hand, if the decision requires major capital expenditures and is the type that will only be made at long-term intervals, long-run costs are appropriate.

In the case of cost analysis regarding whether to add or delete a program such as heart surgery, major changes within the hospital are required to implement the decision. Once the decision is made, it is unlikely to be changed in the short run; it is intended to be a permanent decision. Thus the hospital considering offering heart surgery is interested in long-run costs.

Historical versus Replacement Costs

The accounting system records costs on a historical purchase price basis. Historical costs are generally used for reporting purposes outside of the hospital industry because such costs are considered to be objective and verifiable. Their use reduces the chance of tampering with data, and the user of the financial statements is thus protected from intentional misleading information about asset values. In periods of stable technology and no inflation, this would not result in serious distortions. However, in recent years there has been neither stable technology nor stable price levels.

Replacement cost tells what it would cost today to replace a building or a piece of equipment. If one views a program as a permanent part of the hospital product mix, then it is expected that equipment and buildings will have to be replaced as they wear out. Historical costs do not give information regarding how much it will cost to replace such facilities. While it is true that in the short run the hospital might be interested in only the cost of items to be replaced currently, for a long-run analysis the hospital must consider the cost of all assets utilized by a program since they will all have to be replaced at some time. Replacement costs are therefore more appropriate than historical costs for the open heart surgery analysis.

Treatment of Joint or Overhead Costs

Joint costs represent a significant measurement problem. The current accounting techniques for hospitals treat this problem by allocating all overhead costs into the revenue-producing centers. Since such allocation procedures are arbitrary at best, they do not provide a good measure of the resources consumed by a specific program.

Fisher has noted that costs that are truly joint cannot be separated and assigned to the activities from which they arise. Since the hospital is interested in the economic cost consequences, arbitrary accounting allocations are inappropriate. Fisher gives an example of the joint cost problem when trying to assess the cost of a weapons system for the Defense Department:

> The operating costs of Headquarters, United States Air Force; the Air Force Academy; the Air Force Accounting and Finance Center; Headquarters, Air

Force Systems Command; and the like, usually should not be allocated to Air Force weapon systems. These support activities are essentially independent of the Air Force's combat force mix. On the other hand, the costs of certain depot maintenance activities in the Air Force Logistics Command and of certain courses in the Air Training Command may be, and often are, appropriately identified as part of the incremental cost of a proposed weapon system.[3]

Similarly, for hospitals it is assumed that there is a basic mix of hospital products that require certain support facilities and personnel. None of these joint costs should be allocated to open heart surgery in the sample analysis unless the amount of cost incurred changes because the heart surgery program is offered. This approach, if used for pricing all hospital products, would not allocate all costs and a loss would result. Here, however, the goal is not rate setting, but rather the determination of the incremental cost incurred by the hospital because it offers heart surgery. Thus for purposes of the vertical cost analysis, costs that would be incurred even if the service were not offered should not be considered part of the cost of the service under investigation, no matter how much the service utilizes those resources.

Divisibility of Labor Inputs

In general, personnel—including technicians, assistants, and nurses—are cross-trained and can perform a number of functions. They can be shifted between tasks as needed. Labor inputs can generally be added or deleted in continuous increments as volume changes. Even though in fact there may be some discrete changes, one can gain a sufficiently close approximation using a smooth-change assumption.

In some cases, this is clearly inappropriate. For example, a heart-lung pump technician is a specialist whose duties may very well be clearly specified in a union contract. Such a technician might be idle when not assisting in open heart surgeries, but will have to be paid during idle hours. In such cases, the technician is a dedicated resource and must be included as a large, discrete increment to costs. The same might be true to some extent for X-ray and medical supervisors, nurses, therapists, orderlies, and some maintenance staff, because some of their functions do not change as volume increases. For example, the catheterization supervisor must regularly check the inventory of catheters regardless of annual patient volume.

Data Accumulation

Once the cost concepts are understood, the accumulation of data requires only a series of worksheets. Figure 2–2–4 presents the flow of such worksheets for open heart surgery. For an understanding of the worksheets, follow Figure 2–2–4 starting with Worksheet A. Shown in Figure 2–2–5, this first worksheet is a diagram that

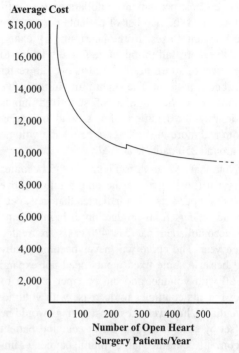

Figure 2–2–5 Worksheet A—Open Heart Surgery, Cost per Patient at Different Volumes

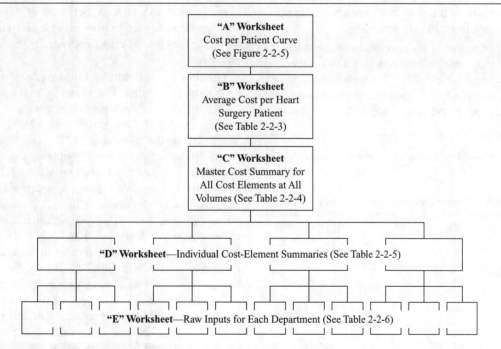

Figure 2–2–4 Data Accumulation Worksheets

plots the cost per patient in dollars on the vertical axis and the number of patients per year on the horizontal axes. In the heart surgery example, the sharp fall in the curve initially is due to the effect of spreading fixed costs over a greater number of patients. The slight jump in the curve results from the addition of semifixed inputs (primarily the addition of a second operating room and more intensive-care beds) at a volume of around 250 patients annually.

Note that the curve in Figure 2–2–5 becomes very flat (horizontal) in the output range above 400 cases per year. This indicates that most economic savings from production at high volume are accomplished if at least 400 cases are treated each year. The curve will never become totally flat because some fixed inputs need not expand at all with volume, and the cost per patient of those inputs continues to decrease with volume. Eventually, however, these cost savings would be offset by such factors as travel cost and patient inconvenience, since large volume per center implies that fewer facilities at greater distances from each other would be needed to perform the heart surgery procedures. Patients would therefore have to travel farther to reach a center performing heart surgery procedures.

The source of the curve in Worksheet A is the average cost information from Worksheet B shown in Table 2–2–3. This worksheet is merely a summary table showing annual volumes and the average costs associated with those volumes.

Table 2–2–3 Worksheet B—Average Cost per Heart Surgery Patient

Annual Patient Volume	Average Cost per Patient
50	$21,133
100	13,775
150	11,546
200	10,429
250	10,495
300	9,906
350	9,470
400	9,177
450	8,943
500	8,740

This information is taken directly from the last row in Worksheet C shown in Table 2–2–4. This worksheet is a summary by cost element and volume. For each possible volume of procedures, this worksheet records the cost from each cost element. These costs can be summed to give the total cost per heart surgery patient, given that a particular volume of such surgeries will take place.

The cost elements in Worksheet C are similar to currently used revenue centers. However, Worksheets D and E (Tables 2–2–5 and 2–2–6) have accumulated data in such a way that each element's costs are related specifically to heart surgery. Furthermore, those costs are given for any desired volume of heart surgery.

Each row in Worksheet C comes from a cost-element summary in Worksheet D. Worksheet D cost-element summaries include equipment, nurses, supplies, and construction costs. These costs are taken from individual Worksheet E tables. That is, there would be one Worksheet E table for each cost element's labor, another for each cost element's supplies, etc. The role of Worksheet E is to determine what raw inputs are needed, what the cost is per unit of input, whether the inputs are fixed or variable in nature, and what the costs of those inputs are at various volumes.

The flow of costs can be followed from one worksheet to another. For example, in Figure 2–2–5 the cost for each patient at a volume of 400 per year is slightly greater than $9,000. In Table 2–2–3 the cost is $9,177. This figure comes from the total of the 400 volume column in Table 2–2–4. And any cost element from Table 2–2–4, for example, operating room equipment and supplies, can be traced to Table 2–2–5. At a volume of 400, the cost per patient for this element is shown in Table 2–2–4 as being $935. In Table 2–2–5 this number is located in the totals column at a volume of 400. Note also in the totals column that costs do not consistently fall per patient as volume increases because of the addition of semifixed inputs at a volume of 250 patients. The supplies cost from Table 2–2–5 can similarly be traced from Table 2–2–6.

Table 2-2-4 Worksheet C—Master Cost Summary

Cost Element	Average Cost Annual Cardiac Surgery Patient Volume									
	50	100	150	200	250	300	350	400	450	500
Anesthesia equipment	$ 47	$ 33	$ 29	$ 25	$ 30	$ 28	$ 26	$ 25	$ 25	$ 24
Blood processing charges	325	325	325	325	325	325	325	325	325	325
Cardiac catheterization	1,813	1,242	1,074	994	943	908	880	857	842	826
Cardiac surgery unit	6,004	3,725	3,060	2,727	2,527	2,406	2,309	2,257	2,197	2,150
Dietary	96	96	96	96	96	96	96	96	96	96
ECG	5	5	5	5	5	5	5	5	5	5
Inhalation therapy	1,364	711	494	384	319	275	247	223	207	192
Laboratory	150	150	150	150	150	150	150	150	150	150
Linens	168	168	168	168	168	168	168	168	168	168
Medications	497	497	497	497	497	497	497	497	497	497
Med/surg hospital beds	1,116	1,116	1,116	1,116	1,116	1,116	1,116	1,116	1,116	1,116
Operating room equipment and supplies	1,374	1,083	985	935	1,020	983	956	935	919	906
Operating room personnel	6,923	3,840	2,880	2,412	2,691	2,380	2,156	2,001	1,891	1,792
Overhead	1,247	780	663	591	604	565	535	518	501	489
Radiology	4	4	4	4	4	4	4	4	4	4
Total	$21,133	$13,775	$11,546	$10,429	$10,495	$9,906	$9,470	$9,177	$8,943	$8,740

Table 2–2–5 Worksheet D—Operating Room Equipment and Supplies Cost Summary

Annual Patient Volume	Average Cost		
	Equip-ment	Supplies	Total
50	$584	$790	$1,374
100	293	790	1,083
150	195	790	985
200	145	790	935
250	230	790	1,020
300	193	790	983
350	166	790	956
400	145	790	935
450	129	790	919
500	116	790	906

NEW PROBLEMS AND A NEW APPROACH

The currently practiced horizontal system of hospital cost finding has developed gradually over many years. Until now it has served as an adequate tool for the cost information needs that existed prior to the relatively recent severe inflation. But the continued rise of hospital costs, persistently greater than the rate of inflation, has created a need for a greater amount of cost finding based on program or product costs. To meet the demands of health systems agencies and to make cost-effective decisions regarding whether it is socially desirable to offer a program or product, today's hospital administrator needs a more vertically or program-oriented cost system than is currently in use.

Table 2–2–6 Worksheet E—Operating Room Supplies

Item	Unit Cost	Quantity	Cost
Sm. steri-drape	$ .66	3	$ 1.98
Lg. steri-drape	1.02	4	4.08
2 oz. irrig. bulb syringe	.46	3	1.38
Urine-meter	1.93	1	1.93
Foley	3.50	1	3.50
5 cc syringes	.08	3	.24
10 cc syringes	.09	3	.27
Needles—18 regular	.43	3	1.29
22 regular	.43	1	.43
22 spinal	.60	1	.60
19 spinal	.60	1	.60
Under H_2O drainage set	6.51	2	13.02
Magnet needle mat	.49	4	1.96
5705-36 argyle chest tubes	2.80	2	5.60
Curity pack	1.40	1	1.40
K 75 threeway stop cock	.20	2	.40
V-5404 McGan IV extension tubing	1.07	2	2.14
Salem sump tube	.98	1	.98
W1990 McGan additive cap	.23	2	.46
Surgical patties (cotton-aids)	26.00	1	26.00
Urine bag 950-18-19 cystie set	1.22	1	1.22
Etc.			720.52
Total			$790.00

NOTES

1. Gibson, R.M. and Fisher, C.R. "National Health Expenditures, Fiscal Year 1977." *Social Security Bulletin* 41:7 (July 1978) p. 7.

2. Demski, J.S. and Feltham, G.A. *Cost Determination: A Conceptual Approach* (Ames, Iowa: Iowa State University Press, 1976).

3. Fisher, G.H. *Cost Considerations in Systems Analysis* (New York: American Elsevier, 1971) p. 73.

Reading 2–3

Horizontal Accounting Considered
for the Hospital Setting

Steven A. Finkler

The last 10 years have seen tremendous tur-moil in the foundations of cost accounting. Start-ing in 1987 with Johnson and Kaplan's seminal book, *Relevance Lost: The Rise and Fall of Man-agement Accounting*,[1] there has been a search for methods of determining costs that would provide the essential information needed to run organiza-tions in an optimal manner. One of the latest de-velopments in the evolutionary process toward improved accounting systems is that of horizon-tal accounting.

The notion of horizontal accounting is that the way to improve the bottom line is by focusing on quality and service rather than control and prof-its. A paradoxical approach, horizontal account-ing argues that profits are improved when you look at other things rather than looking at profits themselves. This is based on the philosophy that no matter how well we keep our eye on our prof-its, that focus alone will not change profits.

The horizontal approach requires a new focus by internal accountants on things that we really haven't spent much time measuring. It requires measuring the value added by our hospital in terms of things that are both relevant to patients and provided in a high quality fashion.

Source: Reprinted from Steven A. Finkler, "Hori-zontal Accounting Considered for the Hospital Set-ting," *Hospital Cost Management and Accounting,* Vol. 8, No. 12, March 1997, pp. 1–7. Copyright 1997, Aspen Publishers, Inc.

The basic concepts of horizontal accounting are quite radical. As such, they are also quite hard to accept. Some of the arguments to be pre-sented in this article are controversial. Will they work? Can they be done? Some argue that they are possible. Many are likely to be skeptical. We would contend that they are a long shot. Many hospitals will never try to adopt horizontal ac-counting as it is described below. And some of those that do will fail to achieve great benefits.

On the other hand, it would be foolish to ig-nore the approach, because it holds the potential for enormous cost savings. If we can figure out a way to measure activities and their relevance and quality—instead of, or in addition to, budgets and variances—we may be able to save substan-tial amounts of money.

We suspect that this topic is worth some thought, and that we are likely to hear more and more about it in various forms over the last few remaining years of this decade.

HORIZONTAL ACCOUNTING AS A COMPENDIUM

A recent book focuses on horizontal account-ing. The book, *Transforming the Bottom Line* by Hope and Hope,[2] presents a model that incorpo-rates many of the elements of change that we have been hearing about for the last 5 to 10 years.

The book presents a heavy dose of reengi-neering, total quality management (TQM), and activity-based costing (ABC). The dichotomy between value-added and nonvalue-added work is a central issue throughout.

Horizontal accounting doesn't throw away any of the valuable elements of the work done in recent years. Rather, it incorporates those concepts and builds upon them.

THE PHILOSOPHY

Our perspectives are changing, but the underlying philosophy of horizontal accounting is still somewhat hard for many of us to swallow. The problem with traditional accounting, as seen by proponents of horizontal accounting, can be succinctly stated as "systems that emphasize control rather than improvement, and low cost rather than high quality and good service."[3] What is wrong with control and low cost?

Accountants who have been trained in the value and importance of control and who can see the benefits of low cost find this different philosophy confusing. Of course we want to show improvement and provide high quality and good service. But how can accountants do that? That is the job of the line staff. Accountants want to provide the information to allow improvement and quality. The contention of proponents of horizontal accounting, however, is that accounting information systems could better assist in that effort by redesigning the very fundamentals of the type of information collected and disseminated throughout the organization.

The recent emphasis in hospitals and industry alike has been on customers. How can we do the best by our customers, so that they will be supportive of our organization? Horizontal accounting argues that the entire accounting process should be considered from the point of view of the customers. We should measure what we are doing that our customers would perceive as valuable and be willing to pay for.

Philosophically, then, we need accounting reports that measure satisfied customers. However, traditional variance reports do not focus on the quality of the product or service, or the amount of work done that is not productive in the traditional sense, but productive in that it really makes a difference to the customer. Designing new reports to capture elements that are important to the long-term profitability of the organization is the challenge of horizontal accounting.

According to the Hope and Hope view, the new accounting that is needed should be based on Theory Y rather than Theory X. Theory X is the view of people that believes they inherently hate work and will slack off unless closely monitored and disciplined. Theory Y proposes that people work for their own satisfaction and are self-motivated. The new approach must be founded in team-based structures, and "will only succeed if it is based on notions of responsibility and trust."[4] Additionally, Hope and Hope note that, "A horizontal information system is rooted in the recognition that *work* is the primary cause of costs, and that the only work worth doing is that which the satisfied customer needs."[5]

It is not clear that these two arguments necessarily go hand in hand. The philosophy that accounting should measure whether activities are really value-added *does* seem to be fundamental to the notion of a new type of accounting information system. If we can figure out a way to do that, we can move hospitals forward in their efforts to maximize their capabilities within their available resources.

Hospitals have been trying to reengineer—work smarter, not harder. They have been trying to eliminate unneeded functions. They have aggressively joined the TQM bandwagon. One of the major limitations in how far this can go is our limited accounting systems, which have trouble measuring quality improvements, the financial impact of customer satisfaction, and the cost of nonvalue-added work.

While some believe there is strong support for Theory Y, others may believe that there are instances where Theory X has some merit as well. It is not clear that one must fully embrace Theory Y in order to realize the potential benefits from a refocus of the things that should be subject to accounting measurement.

DOWNSIZING

Many, if not most, hospitals have gone through recent downsizings. Horizontal accounting argues that downsizings are generally the result of budget cuts. However, budgets focus on inputs, rather than why we need those inputs. Therefore, these downsizings may eliminate vital activities—causing losses rather than savings.

One of the things we must determine when using a new approach to accounting is what it is that each person at the hospital does. Across-the-board layoffs often eliminate important value-added work, as well as the nonvalue-added activities.

The problem of layoffs, therefore, becomes one of the chicken and the egg. Which comes first—the layoffs, or the work reduction? In a horizontal approach, layoffs may still occur. However, first one must measure what each individual does. Then, nonvalue-added activities must be eliminated.

Once we eliminate unnecessary work, one choice is to keep the same workforce and have staff increase the amount of productive work they do. This will increase revenues and profits. Alternatively, we can choose to lay people off because we need fewer people since there is less work to do.

The key to all of this is to avoid the initial focus on layoffs as a cost-cutting tool. Such an approach is often self-defeating, with gradual rehiring and substantial amounts of outsourcing. The essence becomes designing an accounting information system that can actually track what people are doing with their time—and determine why they are doing those things, and whether it makes sense to do so.

NONVALUE-ADDED WORK

According to Hope and Hope:

> Managers are running their businesses with numbers designed for financial reporting and controlling budgets—purposes that have little to do with

questions of adding value or customer satisfaction. But it is these questions that have everything to do with long-term success.... When work audits have been undertaken, results consistently show that most organizations generate huge amounts of work for which the customer receives no benefit. The percentages of "wasted" work vary with each particular audit, but rarely are figures less than 20 percent quoted.[6]

If a hospital has a $200 million total budget for the year, a 20 percent nonvalue-added amount would mean that $40 million is being wasted. Many would argue that in most organizations, substantially more than 20 percent of all work is nonvalue-added. The hospital that can uncover the key to finding that work and eliminating both the work and the costs that are generated by the work stands to gain a significant competitive advantage.

But do hospitals really have that much nonvalue-added work? No one knows. Even more significantly, can they really eliminate that work? Certainly, many would argue that much of the regulation that affects hospitals does not really result in efforts that patients would see as value-added. But the hospital is not at liberty to ignore legal compliance with the regulations.

TQM has taught us that having to redo work means that there was initially nonvalue-added work. But how many accounting systems track such extra effort? Horizontal accounting calls for keeping track of all efforts that are done because something wasn't initially done right.

Some would argue that all meetings are a waste of time. Clearly, that is probably not completely true. But how many hospitals have accounting systems that track any of the cost of wasted time in worthless meetings? If we are to truly adopt the notion that there is nonvalue-added work, then we should be willing to make the effort to eliminate it. But you can't do that until you can find it. And for that you need accounting measurement.

It may not be pleasant at first to start tracking the cost of worthless meetings. Yet how can we assess how far we've come and how far we have yet to go unless we adopt some measurement tools? In the long run, we have the potential to eliminate many of those meetings. That will free up time for managers and staff to do the important parts of their job.

A half-decade ago, Drucker noted that:

> Nurses, every attitude survey shows, bitterly resent not being able to spend more time caring for patients. They also believe, understandably, that they are grossly underpaid for what they are capable of doing, while the hospital administrator, equally understandably, believes that they are grossly overpaid for the unskilled clerical work they are actually doing.[7]

Most hospitals have not ignored this problem. They have tried to find ways to keep nursing doing nursing value-added functions. Ironically, there is not always universal support from nursing when 20 percent of the RNs in a hospital are replaced by clerical workers, aides, and unit hosts or hostesses.

RELEVANCE AND QUALITY

The challenge of today is to design measurement tools to assess the relevance and impact on quality of all of our various efforts or activities. Of course, assessing relevance is a highly subjective task. Such subjectivity immediately raises concerns by accountants who have long tried to rely on verifiable, objective evidence.

Objectivity, however, has its own drawbacks. Balance sheets report assets at historical cost. Internal accountants have not made all of their decisions based on those objective costs. They have taken the next step and insured fixed assets based on their replacement value, even though that value is clearly highly subjective. We do use subjective information when we make decisions. Horizontal accounting only pushes us slightly further in that direction.

ONE VIEW OF THE HORIZONTAL APPROACH

In their book, Hope and Hope put forth a detailed description of a horizontal model.[8]

The essence of their model is that time spent by workers is considered to be the key cost driver. Time spent causes activities to have cost. This is a reversal of the ABC concept that activities drive cost.

To implement horizontal accounting, one must develop a value-adding work index. That index is the product of a quality index and a relevance index.

The index is calculated by gathering data about time spent doing things that are *not* value-added. "By borrowing a well-worn management concept—*exception reporting*—a horizontal information system can record when a person spends time working on non-core activities. In other words, *by recording what people are not supposed to be doing* (correcting work caused by others, revisiting customers, chasing, changing, and generally solving problems), a picture can be painted by the information system of those costs that add no value to the customer."[9]

The horizontal system is similar in some respects to the outcome budgeting approach discussed in the August 1996 issue of *Hospital Cost Management and Accounting (HCMA)*.[10] It shifts the focus from inputs—such as salary, benefits, supplies, and telephone—to activities such as providing care, stocking carts, completing reports, and attending meetings.

Thus, we can redevelop the budget for any department based on the amount allocated to each major activity. For example, a purchasing department budget might change from the following simplified approach:

Staff salaries	$500,000
Inservice education	20,000
Supplies	30,000
Telephone	20,000
Total	$570,000

to a revised budget that appears as follows:

Processing purchase orders	$270,000
Negotiating with vendors	50,000
Updating vendor records	30,000
Reconciling invoice discrepancies	120,000
Attending meetings	40,000
Attending inservice education	60,000
Total	**$570,000**

Now that we can more clearly identify activities, that does not mean that certain activities are worthless and others are completely valuable. Within any activity category, it is possible that nonvalue-added work is taking place.

For example, the purchasing department must process purchase orders, but it is possible that a substantial part of the effort devoted to that activity is irrelevant. Perhaps we always seek out bids from high-priced vendors that we never place orders with. We do it so that we can show that we placed the order at a much lower price than other vendors were quoting.

Consider a situation in which a hospital requires three bids for any outside printing job. One printer in the city is consistently the low bidder and wins every contract. Yet job after job, a bidding process is undertaken before the job is placed with the one printer who is the consistent winner.

As a result of the time-consuming bidding process, there are times that the final print job arrives too late to be of any value. The bidding process is cumbersome and time-consuming—and little wonder. Who rushes to take care of a bidding process that is going to have no impact on who gets the job? How does any of this benefit the ultimate customer?

Is it possible to evaluate the relevance of each area of cost? How can we judge relevance?

If a bidding process has a good chance of lowering the cost for the customer—even an in-house customer who will be charged for the print job—it is value-added.

If there is virtually no chance the customer will benefit or would be willing to pay for that process, then there is little relevance to it. For example, suppose that the hospital's materials man-

ager and buyers judged the relevance of their activities as follows:

	Cost	Relevance	Value-Added
Processing purchase orders	$270,000	90%	$243,000
Negotiating with vendors	50,000	50%	25,000
Updating vendor records	30,000	25%	7,500
Reconciling invoice discrepancies	120,000	0%	0
Attending meetings	40,000	40%	16,000
Attending inservice education	60,000	90%	54,000
Total	**$570,000**		**$345,500**

One of the interesting points of the process is that it is not a critical problem if the estimates are not very accurate. For example, different people might argue over the estimate that negotiating with vendors is only 50 percent relevant to the customer. Perhaps it should be 75 percent. Perhaps 90 percent. The exact number used is not critical, because we are developing a baseline.

Over time, the relevance index is re-estimated periodically to examine whether we are removing the irrelevant work from the process. Therefore, the accuracy of the starting point is not as critical as the measurement of the direction of movement in the index over time. Still, one should try to make as reasonable an estimate as possible.

Lack of relevance of work is only one major problem to be measured by horizontal accounting. The other is the quality of work. While we often note our inability to get a good handle on quality, the Hope and Hope alternative is to measure the amount of poor quality. This can be accomplished by having everyone estimate how much of their cost is incurred correcting things that were not done properly in the first place.

We can see from the quality index in the hypothetical example in Table 2–3–1 that attending meetings in this department is not a result of poor quality. The quality index for meetings is 100 percent. However, much of what goes on at the meetings is irrelevant from the customer's perspective: The relevance index is only 40 percent.

In the example, reconciling invoice discrepancies is both the result of poor quality and also irrelevant to the customer. If we were dealing with an operating room situation, all of the costs of procedures would likely be relevant to the customer, but some of them might be the result of poor quality. In other words, any activity can have both high relevance and high quality, or low relevance and low quality, or a high level of one and low level of the other. For any activity, there is no reason to believe that relevance and quality go hand in hand.

However, together, relevance and quality are essential to determining value-added costs. Readers of *HCMA* will not have much trouble identifying why this approach is called horizontal accounting. Net value-added is determined by taking the total cost of an activity and factoring out the nonvalue-added relevance and quality costs. All that remains in the extreme right-hand column for each activity on each *horizontal line* is the value-added component.

In this example, the total cost of the activities is $570,000. Of that total, only $320,825 is value-added. If we divide the value-added component by the total, we find that a little over 56 percent of the cost is value-added. That 56 percent is the value-adding work index. About 44 percent of the costs of this department are nonvalue-added.

Can we eliminate that 44 percent in one fell swoop? That would be highly unlikely. However, the horizontal analysis points the way for the manager. We can now begin to work to eliminate the nonvalue-added elements, because we have a good idea of what they are and where they are. Further, as we start to eliminate the nonvalue-added elements, we will be able to recalculate the value-adding work index and track our improvement.

COST-BENEFIT TRADEOFFS

All of this may be well and good, but is it worthwhile? Before we completely condemn and discard our existing accounting structure, one must ask how it came to be. Budgets and other elements of control were not implemented in hospitals or other organizations as a way to throw money away, but rather as a way to save money.

The reason forms are filled out and control processes are in place is because, at least at some point in time, an assessment was made that the extra "nonvalue-added" effort was worthwhile. Were we wrong in our initial calculations, or have things changed making the activities no longer valuable enough to justify themselves, or is the whole new movement in accounting just the "emperor's new clothes"?

Table 2–3–1 Determining Net Value-Added Using Horizontal Accounting Method

	Cost	Relevance Index	Value-Added	Quality Index	Net Value-Added
Processing purchase orders	$270,000	90%	$243,000	90%	$218,700
Negotiating with vendors	50,000	50%	25,000	100%	25,000
Updating vendor records	30,000	25%	7,500	95%	7,125
Reconciling invoice discrepancies	120,000	0%	0	0%	0
Attending meetings	40,000	40%	16,000	100%	16,000
Attending inservice education	60,000	90%	54,000	100%	54,000
Total	$570,000		$345,500		$320,825

There is always room for improvement and innovation. Some might condemn horizontal accounting as just the latest fad. However, there is at least an element of sense in its desire to focus on quality and relevance. Others may fully embrace the new approach and be quick to condemn the present accounting structure.

It pays to bear in mind that when reengineering came along, it seemed to be the ultimate solution. Then came TQM, followed before long by ABC. Before most hospitals could even fully embrace ABC, we learned that activity-based management was much more sophisticated, and was really the ultimate solution. Now it is posited that the key is to measure a value-adding work index.

The view here is that there is value to much of the existing accounting structure. Theory Y is a nice ideal, but few organizations can realistically run totally based on such an approach. Some elements of budget and control will remain in nearly all organizations. Yet some evolution is clearly necessary to find a better way.

Horizontal accounting encompasses much of what came before it, and it may eventually be incorporated as a critical element of what comes after it. One would be foolish to throw away every element of accounting that has already been established.

However, one might be just as foolish to ignore the potential benefits of adapting one's system to improve its measurement of activities, the activities' cost, and the portion of that cost that is really value-added.

REFERENCES

1. H. Thomas Johnson and Robert S. Kaplan. *Relevance Lost: The Rise and Fall of Management Accounting.* Boston: Harvard Business School Press, 1987.

2. Tony Hope and Jeremy Hope. *Transforming the Bottom Line.* Boston: Harvard Business School Press, 1996.

3. *Ibid.,* p. 1.

4. *Ibid.,* p. 11.

5. *Ibid.,* p. 12.

6. *Ibid.,* pp. 44–45.

7. Peter F. Drucker. "The New Productivity Challenge." *Harvard Business Review,* November–December 1991, p. 74.

8. Hope and Hope, *op. cit.,* pp. 62–69.

9. *Ibid.,* p. 63.

10. Steven A. Finkler. "Outcome Budgeting Shifts Focus to Meeting Objectives." *Hospital Cost Management and Accounting,* Vol. 8, No. 6, August 1996.

Reading 2–4

Costing Out Nursing Services

Steven A. Finkler

As the nursing shortage has continued to persist, growing attention has been focused on the issue of the cost to provide nursing services to hospital patients.

The nursing shortage itself is curious in that it is not caused by a decrease in the number of available nurses. Actually there are more, not fewer, nurses working in hospitals than there were 5 or 10 years ago. However, during that time period the demand for nursing care hours per patient day has increased—an increase that is not particularly surprising. One factor leading us in this direction is diagnosis-related groups (DRGs). With DRGs having the impact of shortening length of stay, each day patients are in hospitals they tend to be sicker and require more care.

However, the nursing shortage has created havoc in many hospitals. There are instances in which the use of agency nurses has caused nursing departments to exceed their budgets by 20, 50, or even 100 percent. In this environment, there is clearly a need for improved approaches to finding the cost of nursing care for different types of patients.

Source: Reprinted from Steven A. Finkler, "Costing Out Nursing Services," *Hospital Cost Management and Accounting,* Vol. 1, No. 12, March 1990, pp. 1–5. Copyright 1990, Aspen Publishers, Inc.

WHY ARE CURRENT COSTING APPROACHES WEAK?

The essence of the problem requiring some special attention in the area of costing is that nursing costs are currently averaged into the per diem in most hospitals. As a result, all patients in a given unit of the hospital will receive the same daily charge for nursing care services, built into the per diem rate.

In terms of providing management with an understanding of the cost implications of different patients, this provides extremely poor information. It assumes that all patients consume exactly the same amount of nursing care, when we clearly know that different patients have different nursing requirements.

Why has costing for nursing care taken this direction to begin with? In order to charge different amounts to different patients, we must be able to determine different amounts of resource consumption. In some areas of the hospital, it would be virtually impossible to measure differential consumption. For example, how much of the chief financial officer's (CFO's) time is consumed by each patient? One would be hard pressed to show that different patients receive different amounts of benefit from the CFO. Even if they did, it would be impossible to measure.

In the case of nursing, however, different patients do consume different amounts of nursing resources. Nevertheless, until the decade of the 1980s, measurement of differential consumption was, if not impossible, at least too costly to consider. What hospital could assign an accountant to each nurse to observe how much of his or her time was being devoted to each patient?

Today, however, most hospitals have in place a working patient classification system. Such systems are required for hospital accreditation. Patient classification systems require rating patients based on their likely nursing resource requirements. Such systems will not be precisely accurate for each patient. Some patients will require more or less care than would be expected, based on their classification. However, if the system is functioning reasonably well, patient resource consumption will generally match that which is expected based on the classification system.

Patient classification systems can be the basis for a system that allows us to more accurately estimate the cost a hospital incurs for nursing care for different types of patients.

WHY CHANGE THE COSTING APPROACH?

The mere fact that we now have the ability to improve costing does not in itself explain why we would want to improve costing. What is to be gained from having a more accurate measure of the different costs of nursing care for different types of patients?

One argument that is sometimes offered is that separate costing for different types of patients will allow for variable billing. Instead of simply charging all patients the same amount per day for their nursing care, different patients will be charged different amounts, based on their resource consumption.

To the extent that all patients are paid on a prospective payment basis, such as DRGs, variable billing holds little appeal. Thus, for states such as New York and New Jersey, where every

patient is paid on a DRG basis, improving billing systems provides little support for refined costing. On the other hand, hospitals in most states still do charge at least some patients on a non-prospective payment basis. In those cases, variable billing may be a way to better justify hospital bills, and in some cases increase overall revenues to the hospital.

However, care must be exercised if the main focus of improved nurse costing is to change the billing system. On one hand, such a system is beneficial to nursing because it shows in a dramatic way the specific contribution that nursing makes to the overall revenue structure of the hospital. On the other hand, as many states move toward all payer DRG systems, variable billing for nursing services is a step in the wrong direction.

Revenue centers inherently give a department an incentive to generate more revenue by producing more output. Radiology departments have an incentive to take X-rays and lab departments have an incentive to perform lab tests. For prospective payment patients, however, extra services don't result in extra revenues. Thus we must exercise care not to create nursing as a new revenue center with an incentive to overprovide services.

However, the main benefit to improved costing for nursing services is that we can generate information for better management decisions. Is a particular service too costly? What price can be bid for an HMO or PPO contract? These are just a few examples of the types of questions that cannot be answered without reasonably accurate costing information.

Hospital costing has long been based on averages and cross-subsidizations. In the current environment, errors in our calculations of costs become more serious as negotiations for discounted prices become more intense. Thus, if we are mistaken about the resources that a particular class of patient consumes, the ramifications can be quite serious. Averaging of costs is less acceptable than it was in the past.

In addition, as costing becomes more specific and more accurate, not only are we able to deal better with our pricing problems, but we can be more efficient in our management of costs as well. Flexible budget systems can provide better analysis and control of costs, and productivity can be monitored better if we know more about our costs. Since nursing represents such a major component of overall costs, more accurate costing is clearly beneficial to improved management of the hospital.

SHOULD COSTING BE LINKED TO DRGs?

If hospitals are going to move in the direction of more accurate costing of nursing services, one of the critical questions is the determination of the categories for cost. Should we have one nursing cost for medical patients and another for surgical patients? Should we determine the cost for men as opposed to women, or for young people as opposed to old people? Should we have one nursing cost for each type of patient based on ICD code? Should we find the cost by DRG?

Currently we treat all patients as if they were the same for nursing care. If we change this, there is no inherent logical approach to take. The operating room charges patients based on the type of surgery. The lab charges are based on the type of lab test. For nursing there is no easy equivalent. We will have to do our costing based on the type of patient. The question is, how do we categorize patients into different types?

The nursing profession has argued against DRGs. Their contention is that DRGs are not natural groupings based on consumption of nursing resources. Several attempts have been made at such groupings. None of these groupings has been flawless or widely accepted. DRGs are a system for grouping patients that is in use nationwide. And, although not all patients within a specific DRG will consume the same nursing resources, we can find an average amount of nursing resources for each type of DRG.

For example, if our hospital uses a nursing patient classification system that has a scale from one to five, we can sample a group of patients

from each DRG and find out, on average, how many days of the patients' stays were at level one, how many at level two, etc.

Thus, it seems that DRGs, although perhaps not ideal for this purpose in the eyes of the nursing profession, are an adequate categorization for the assignment of differential nursing costs. Many decisions are based on particular DRGs or clusters of DRGs, so DRG-based cost information is valuable. Of course, in a particular hospital, an alternative choice may be made, if it provides information that is more useful for decision making.

AN APPROACH TO COSTING NURSING SERVICES

Nursing care costs consist of the staff costs of direct patient care, the staff costs of indirect patient care (supervisors, secretaries, etc.), patient care related costs (e.g., patient and unit supplies), and overhead (allocated from other departments).

We could try to determine the costs of each of these elements separately for each category of patient, or we can do the costing in some more aggregate fashion. Compromises between accuracy and the cost of refining cost information are always made. The challenge is to decide in any given environment which compromises are reasonable and which are not. We will start with the assumption that all nursing department costs are lumped together (substantial compromise), and later discuss possible refinements.

The key element that allows for improved costing of nursing services is the fact that nursing patient classification systems are currently in place in almost every hospital. Without such systems we know that different patients consume different amounts of resources, but we have no way to measure the differential consumption. With a classification system, once we have classified a patient, we have some idea about the nursing resources he or she consumes.

For example, suppose that we have the following patient classification resource guidelines:

Acuity Level	Hours of Care
1	2.8
2	3.5
3	4.5
4	5.9
5	8.4

In developing the patient classification system, various indicators are used to determine if a patient should be classified as a 1, 2, 3, 4, or 5. Once the patient has been classified, the classification system tells you how many hours of nursing care should be required to treat that patient in your hospital. In the above example, a patient classified as a 4 would typically require on average 5.9 hours of care.

Note that the scale is not linear. A patient classified as a 2 does not require exactly twice as many hours as a 1. A patient classified as a 4 does not consume twice as many hours as a 2. This complicates the calculation of cost somewhat. If the scale was strictly linear, we could add up all of the values and divide into total nursing cost to get a cost per unit of patient classification. That is, suppose we had one patient day that was a 1, one patient day that was a 3, and one patient day that was a 4. The total of 1 + 3 + 4 is 8. If total nursing costs were $1,000, then the cost per patient classification unit would be $125 (i.e., $1,000/8). The cost for a patient day classified as a 4 would be $500 (4 × $125).

However, since the scale is not linear, it is necessary to use a relative value unit (RVU) scale. We can let a patient classified as a 1 have a value of 1 on the relative value scale. Each other classification level would then be calculated in relative proportion to get a set of relative values. For instance:

$$\frac{\text{Level 2}}{\text{Level 1}} = \frac{3.5 \text{ hours}}{2.8 \text{ hours}} = 1.25$$

Therefore the RVU for patient classification level 2 is 1.25, since that patient would consume 25 percent more nursing re-sources than a pa-

tient with classification level 1. Continuing for all classification (acuity) levels:

Acuity Level	Hours of Care	RVU
1	2.8	1.00
2	3.5	1.25
3	4.5	1.61
4	5.9	2.14
5	8.4	3.04

If we were to assume the following information, we can apply this RVU system to develop cost information:

Total nursing costs: $129,548

# of Patient Days at each acuity level:	Level 1	100 days
	2	220 days
	3	350 days
	4	110 days
	5	40 days

The first step is to determine the total amount of work performed by the nursing department. This is done by multiplying the RVUs for each acuity classification level times the number of days at that level.

Acuity Level	Patient Days	× RVUs	=	Total RVUs
1	100	× 1.00	=	100.00
2	220	× 1.25	=	275.00
3	350	× 1.61	=	563.50
4	110	× 2.14	=	235.40
5	40	× 3.04	=	121.60
	820			1,295.50

There were 1,295.5 units of nursing work performed. We can divide this into the total nursing cost to find the cost for each RVU of nursing work:

$$\frac{\text{Total Nursing Costs}}{\text{Total RVUs}} = \text{Cost per RVU}$$

$$\frac{\$129,548}{1,295.50} = \$99.99 \text{ per RVU}$$

Here we can see that the cost for a patient for one day with classification 1 would be $99.99. The cost for a patient with classification 4 would be $99.99 multiplied by 2.14 (the RVU for classification level 4).

How would you calculate the nursing cost for a patient from admission to discharge? Suppose that the average DRG 128 patient had a length of stay of 7 days, with two days classed as a 1, four days classed as a 2, and one day classed as a 4. The nursing cost for DRG 128 would then be:

Acuity Level	Patient Days	× RVUs ×	Cost/ RVU	=	Total Cost
1	2	× 1.00 ×	$99.99	=	$199.98
2	4	× 1.25 ×	99.99	=	499.95
3	0	× 1.61 ×	99.99	=	0.00
4	1	× 2.14 ×	99.99	=	213.98
5	0	× 3.04 ×	99.99	=	0.00
	7				$913.91

Would all patients in a given DRG be expected to consume the same resources? Not really, but we can still be confident that an approach such as this, on average, for any given DRG will give a much more accurate assignment of cost than simply assigning to every patient in a nursing unit the same per diem cost for nursing care.

Have we made any compromises in the costing? Yes. For example, we are implicitly assuming that all nursing costs vary in proportion to the patient classification system. Does that make sense? For example, will a sicker patient who requires more direct nursing care also require more indirect nursing care? More supplies? More overhead? These are empirical questions. The answer to them depends on the specific situation of your hospital.

It may well be that a simple per diem allocation is appropriate for costs such as overhead. Some costs such as unit supplies might also be best allocated on a per diem basis, while other costs such as patient-specific supplies might well be best allocated using the RVU scale. How complex are we willing to make our costing system?

Obviously the best costing of nursing services requires direct continuous observation of each patient and assignment of actual resources consumed. We obviously are not going to go that far in our costing scheme. Patient classification systems, however, have placed us in a position to be able to substantially improve the assignment of nursing costs to patients in an economical way. The RVU system is quite simple and inexpensive, assuming that your hospital has a patient classification system. Whether it pays to go beyond that level of detail will vary from hospital to hospital.

Reading 2–5

Cost Accounting for Emergency Services

John Moorhead

This article outlines an alternative approach to cost accounting in the emergency department. The system described provides a basis for product costing and management control to be used in the context of the overall planning strategy for the department.

The implementation of prospective payment systems has resulted in greater emphasis on planning and financial analysis at the hospital department level. Emergency departments have traditionally been viewed as loss leaders for hospitals, with operating losses balanced by the department's role as an admitting channel that provides opportunities for profits in other departments.

Financial management in any hospital department requires an initial statement of the goals and objectives of the unit, which are usually assigned to the department as part of the hospitalwide planning strategy. Although the emergency department appears to have the ability to attract patients autonomously, marketing plans—including pricing strategies—must support these assigned objectives.

Competition, particularly from freestanding clinics, has forced hospital managers to rethink

their pricing strategies for emergency departments. The resulting management decision-making process for planning, budgeting, and control requires more specific cost information.

Cost accounting requires a definition of the product. It seems appropriate to consider the patient as the product in the emergency department, with the individual services provided (such as triage, nursing care, and ancillary tests) considered as intermediate products or, as Cleverley has defined them, service units.[1] The variety of products (combinations of service units) provided in the emergency department makes the process of determining service level costs potentially complex.

COST ELEMENTS

Managers must determine how many cost elements will make up the costed product. Costs that are generally of interest in this approach are the "direct" costs of providing care.[2] They are costs that can be traced to an individual patient's care and would not be incurred if the patient were not treated. Direct costs can be either fixed or variable, depending on the variability of expenses with relation to changes in volume. Due to the stand-by function of the emergency department, many of the costs are fixed.

Source: Reprinted from John Moorhead, "Cost Accounting for Emergency Services," *Hospital Cost Management and Accounting,* Vol. 1, No. 2, May 1989, pp. 1–7. Copyright 1989, Aspen Publishers, Inc.

The following cost elements are selected for this system:

1. direct labor: salaries and fringe benefits of direct care providers
2. indirect labor: salaries and fringes of administrative and support personnel, such as managers, clerical, and orderlies/aides
3. supplies: categorized as "major" or "minor"
4. department overhead: including capital, teaching, and support services
5. institutional overhead: administrative and support costs, such as plant operation, housekeeping, and laundry

Department managers must assign costs in each of these categories on the basis of volume (the same amount assigned to each patient) or acuity (patient-specific charges) using a criterion of fairness or usefulness in decision making. The total dollar volume is also an important consideration, because it would not be cost efficient to devote significant resources to the identification of patient-specific costs for line items with only a few dollars value, even if the information were potentially useful.

PATIENT CLASSIFICATION

One existing approach to the determination of emergency department patient-specific costs has focused on costing by diagnosis. This method utilizes average labor times per diagnosis to assign diagnoses to one of six or seven service levels, each of which represents a range of standard times. Thus the product is the patient with a specific diagnosis, and is assumed to comprise a relatively constant number of service units. As Dieter has pointed out, "[T]his approach will work, yet accuracy is lost when diagnoses are grouped."[3] He proposes a system for determining a separate cost for each diagnosis. This approach is appealing because of the similarity to DRG concepts, but fails for the same reasons. Providers have questioned the assumption of the constant profile of resources (by service units)

required to produce a given product (patients with the same diagnosis) and thus cast doubt on the accuracy of this methodology.

This approach also lacks accuracy because it is based on the premise that making a diagnosis is the primary goal for providers in the emergency department. However, the main clinical objective for emergency department personnel is timely identification of problems and providing life-saving acute care. Thus when patients leave the department, at which time patients are classified and charges assessed, most patients do not have an accurate diagnosis, but simply a problem list and acuity rating. Patients with a headache, for example, may range from those with a simple tension headache, which is easily relieved in the department, to a patient with acute cerebral infarction who is unconscious and is admitted to an intensive care unit after multiple procedures. Attempting to account for this wide range of acuity by expanding the list of secondary characteristics (admitted vs. not admitted, etc.) makes the process too complicated.

A simpler approach allocates costs to nursing procedures by assigning a relative value to each task. By compiling a summation of relative values for a particular patient, an assignment can be made to a level of service. As labor-related costs account for the majority of the department's operating expenses, this process more accurately reflects the intensity of service provided to an individual patient and thus would appear to be a fair basis for charging. This system is a form of customizing the charges for individual patients by job order costing. As Horngren states, "job order costing is used by organizations whose products or services are readily identified by individual batches, each of which receives varying inputs of direct materials, direct labor, and factory overhead."[4] The emergency department is such an organization.

This system recognizes that intensity of direct service is the best measure of acuity and thus the most valid basis for differential charges. It is also most consistent with the objectives and process of providing emergency care (as outlined above). A further advantage is that the basis for the assignment of direct labor and some overhead costs is a classification (acuity) system based on resource utilization that can also form the basis for staffing needs and productivity assessment in the department.

THE NURSING ACUITY SYSTEM

The purpose of nursing acuity systems is to identify "by task the time required to provide care for the patients."[5] The most accurate method would be to measure the actual time spent with each patient. This is totally impractical in the emergency department. However, each nursing procedure can be assigned a predetermined relative value based on the time taken to perform that task. Initially the relative value might be assigned by the unit manager based on experience in that particular unit. A similar method is to poll each full-time staff nurse on the amount of time it takes him/her to complete each procedure. One factor that has been found to influence these times is experience in the department. Units with quite low turnover have disregarded the lowest and highest times for each procedure (similar to the scoring system used to judge figure skating) when averaging the results from the survey. The most simple method would be to assign one relative value unit for each minute the procedure takes to perform. Like diagnosis costing, this method loses accuracy by averaging, but we feel it has a much narrower range than the diagnosis-based values.

The number of procedures performed in an emergency department makes this task initially appear complex and arduous. However, Baptist[6] has described a procedural costing method that can be used to "allocate the actual direct and indirect costs incurred by each revenue-producing cost center to the services it produced during a given base period." In this method only high-volume procedures were selected for detailed cost analysis. The Pareto principle would support such a strategy, in that generally 20 percent of a department's procedures account for 80 percent of its output or costs.[7] The remaining procedures could be assigned an average relative value.

Identification of these procedures can be accomplished from a review of historical billing data.

Cost information is of value only in that it helps in the decision-making process, and therefore the system should be as simple as possible. Thus, procedures that are identified as those provided to all patients are nondiscriminating and their costs should be allocated to overhead, which is assigned on a per patient basis.

Nursing procedures are particularly well documented in department procedure manuals and reviewed for all incoming staff as part of their orientation process. These form a standard treatment protocol for each service unit. Using time, or assigned relative value, and the nursing cost per minute or relative value, a standard cost is assigned to each procedure.

Table 2–5–1 is a sample of activities and their assigned relative values. Procedure times include preparation of equipment.

At this point there is a basis for cost determination and charge assignment. However, the basis for reimbursement from third party carriers is service levels. It is for this reason that the relative values need to be allotted to service levels. Department managers must determine how many levels of service will be needed to account for the variety of services provided in their particular department. A basic package of services could be bundled to make up the lowest level of service, with a corresponding time total and relative value units (RVUs). This might consist of triage, initial nursing assessment, obtaining vital signs, patient teaching, and discharge instructions. If we use Table 2–5–1, this would be (2.8 + 5.5 + 3.1 + 6.4) = 17.8 minutes and a relative value of 18 units. However, these services are provided to all patients and thus this information is of very little value in decision making. Thus, these procedures might more appropriately be assigned to overhead.

It is important to emphasize that these time ranges and relative values are subject to regular auditing procedures. The assigned times could vary by patient diagnosis or depend on how busy the department happens to be. For example, does the initiation of an intravenous line take the same

Table 2–5–1 Sample of Activities and Assigned Relative Values

Activity	Definition	Time Allotted	Relative Value
Triage	Elicit the patient's chief complaint, complete triage form and turn into admitting	2.8 min.	3
Initial Assessment	Complete a brief history and physical to assess patient's chief complaint	5.5 min.	6
Vital signs	Take one set of vital signs	3.1 min.	3
I.V. start	Preparation and insertion of a peripheral I.V.	8.0 min.	8
Patient teaching/ discharge instructions	Review discharge instructions with patient	6.4 min.	6
EKG	Completion and transmission of an EKG	7.4 min.	7
Administration of medications (includes preparation)	po, ophthal, topical, rectal IM, SQ I.V. push, piggyback	3.2 min. 5.6 min. 6.2 min.	3 6 6
Venipuncture	Drawing labs by venipuncture	4.8 min.	5
Insertion of NG tube		8.7 min.	9
Gastric lavage for O.D.	Assisting M.D. with the insertion of the lavage tube, irrigation of the stomach, instilling the charcoal, removing the tube	36.8 min.	37

amount of time in a busy department for a patient who is the victim of a major traumatic event as for the administration of cryoprecipitate for a young hemophiliac with a hemarthrosis when the department is relatively quiet? The managers of each department will have to validate these times depending on the volume and kinds of patients that are treated there. This process should begin with the high priority procedures mentioned above.

A range of relative values will have to be assigned to each service level. Although most departments might have data showing historical volumes by service levels, the information will not provide enough detail for this system. Knowledge of the volume of patients treated at each relative value total will be necessary for department managers to determine a total of RVUs provided. To account for the effects of seasonality it is necessary to collect these data for a period of one year. It might suffice to collect information for one month each quarter but of

course this method would lose accuracy. One might expect a bell-shaped distribution curve for relative value totals within and between levels.

DIRECT NURSING COSTS

Once the volume of patients treated at each total relative value level is known, it is simply a matter of multiplying the volume times the RVUs and adding to get a total number of RVUs provided in the year. Dividing budgeted annual costs for that category by the number of RVUs gives a cost per RVU. Adding all the costs assigned by acuity to the costs assigned from overhead by volume will give a basis for pricing. Table 2–5–2 provides a structure for determination of total annual RVUs. However, the annual RVUs for each service level have not been calculated.

Each of the seven service levels in Table 2–5–2 has a range of RVUs. A study of the average

Table 2–5–2 Structure for Determining Total Annual RVUs

Service Level	RVUs	Annual Volume	Annual RVUs
1. Minimal	0	3000	0
2. Brief	1–3	5600	?
3. Limited	3–15	6500	?
4. Intermediate	16–30	7800	?
5. Extensive	31–45	4500	?
6. Comprehensive	46–60	930	?
7. Critical Care	over 60	170	?
Total Relative Value Units			?

number of RVUs per patient in each service level must be undertaken. It is too simplistic to assume that the midpoint number of RVUs would accurately reflect the weighted average consumption. For example, in each sservice category, there might be a disproportionate share of patients near either the high or low end of the RVU scale for that service level.

To see this more clearly, consider a hypothetical example for service level 2, "Brief." The 5,600 annual cases for this service level could be composed of 1,000 patients consuming 1 RVU; 2,000 consuming 2 RVUs; and 2,600 consuming 3 RVUs—an average of 2.3 RVUs per patient. Alternatively, it might consist of the reverse: 2,600 with 1 RVU; 2,000 with 2 RVUs; and 1,000 with 3 RVUs—an average of 1.7 RVUs per patient. In neither case would an assumption of 2 RVUs per patient be accurate. The inaccuracy would be even more pronounced at higher service levels, which have broader RVU ranges.

INDIRECT NURSING COSTS

Using a "fairness" criterion, it might be decided that costs will be determined by time for only direct patient functions (easily identified as benefiting an individual patient). It might be argued that indirect nursing activities benefit all patients and therefore could be assigned to overhead. Similar allocation is necessary for nonproductive time (meals, breaks, and personal activities), and time spent on unit-related activities that are necessary for the general management, coordination, and organization of the unit. Examples of these broad activity categories are published elsewhere,[8] but need local modification.

Engineering studies are therefore necessary to identify how much nursing time is devoted on average to each of these activity categories. Although formal time-motion studies are the most accurate determination, work sampling as described by Hagerty[9] has been found adequate to analyze these times.

Table 2–5–3 shows results from one department.[10]

Department managers will now have the necessary information on which to allocate direct labor costs to each service level. Total direct nursing costs are multiplied by the percent direct care and the resulting dollar amount is divided by the total number of RVUs produced annually.

For example,

budgeted direct nursing salaries	$796,374
multiply by 32.8%	$261,210
divide by RVUs	$x.xx/RVU

Thus, direct nursing care costs would be assigned to each service level on the basis of $x per relative value unit. The cost per RVU multiplied by the number of RVUs assigned to a procedure would determine the direct cost per procedure.

Unit managers will have to determine whether all costs will be allocated on the basis of acuity or just direct nursing costs. As Dieter states, "the allocation of indirect (overhead) costs is almost as important as the identification of the direct cost components. The emphasis is on determin-

Table 2–5–3 Percentage of Time Spent in Various Activity Categories

Activity Category	Percentage of Time
Direct care	32.8
Indirect care	26.9
Unit related	20.3
Personal	20.0

ing whether a direct cost/benefit relationship can be determined between each chargeable and every direct and indirect cost, and if so, to quantify that relationship."[3] He continues, "[M]ost of the other expenses within the department can be directly related to the acuity of the patient." The total dollar amount in each category will determine the effect on patient charges if assigned to overhead or by RVUs. Allocation of categories with costs of $1 to $2 is less important than those with costs of $10 to $15. This assignment is arbitrary and should be made on the basis of fairness.

Nursing indirect and unit related costs would seem to vary by acuity and thus should be assigned on the basis of RVUs. Personal time is much less clear but the absolute dollar amount makes us favor including it with acuity-based costs.

OTHER LABOR

Assignment of the costs associated with support staff on an acuity basis seems logical as are costs of managers allocated to overhead. The need for support staff is somewhat dependent on absolute volume but clearly determined by intensity of service provided. Managers' costs are fixed and assigning them on a relative value basis would not contribute to the decision-making processes within the department. Management is perceived as a service from which all patients benefit. Physician services are required by Medicare regulations to be priced and costed separately, and are therefore not included in these discussions.

MATERIALS

Most department charging structures are designed to capture material resource consumption through individual supply charges at least for "significant" items. "Significant" is usually defined on the basis of cost and thus would again be a direct variable expense to an individual patient. Examples of significant supply items are individual procedure trays. By definition these

supplies would only be used in the care of service levels 4–7. This limited number of items can be listed on the billing form with charges passed through to the individual patient on the basis of the cost incurred to the department.

"Minor" supplies are a relatively small cost in actual dollars and are easily assigned to the acuity category. As Dieter explains, "[I]n studies I have completed, a direct correlation has consistently been identified between a procedure's acuity level and length and its utilization of nonchargeable supplies."[3]

DEPARTMENT AND INSTITUTIONAL OVERHEAD

Total costs assigned to the overhead category are divided by budgeted volume for the department to provide the basis for the basic charge per patient.

PRICING DECISIONS

Setting prices for services begins with a basic fee that encompasses a share of all costs assigned to overhead and thus is the same for each patient. The other component is a charge based on the assigned service level, which is determined by the total relative value of the procedures provided to that patient. It is this component that is of value in making a decision as to whether the department is better off with that particular category of patient. Of course, the costs only provide a basis for the prices. The goals, objectives, and philosophy of the department will also help to determine the absolute charge levels. For example department managers must consider the competitive nature of the local health care system. If competition from local free-standing urgency centers and prevalence of ED deductibles means that service levels 1–3 are price-sensitive, then charges in those levels must correspond to basic urgency care charges. However, price must be set at greater than variable costs so that the contribution margin is greater than zero. Some costs might be shifted to other service levels that are less price-sensitive.

Charge assignment using this system requires that individual procedures must be identified for each patient. This is usually done at the time of treatment. This form of charging has been criticized as being too complicated and time-consuming for nurses. However, I believe that this system reinforces the nurses' sense of accomplishment. It also allows nurses to look at these charges as more like professional fees, as the process identifies all services provided to individual patients. The development of this system is also facilitated by active involvement by the entire nursing staff. This kind of system has been well accepted by nursing units.

PRODUCTIVITY

Cost information is of value only as it aids in the management decision-making process.[2] Productivity is one parameter upon which decisions regarding the number and skill level of staff for hospital units are based. There is a very close tie between the cost accounting and the productivity management systems. "Ideally," according to Dieter, "these two systems share the same data base of standards for the labor components of cost per procedure."[3] With hospitals' market share of health services in decline, "the challenge for hospitals is to keep costs low while continuing to provide high quality patient care," argues Minyard, who goes on to say that some "argue that reducing the skill level may reduce the quality of care, which is likely to be any hospital's competitive edge in the future."[10] The system

described above will provide the foundations for a productivity monitoring system and will allow managers to evaluate productivity as one basis for these staffing and pricing decisions.[11]

NOTES

1. Cleverley, W., "Product Costing for Health Care Firms," *Health Care Management Review,* 1987, 12(4), pp. 39–48.

2. Finkler, S., "A Microcosting Approach," *Hospital Cost Accounting Advisor,* 2(12), May 1987, pp. 1–4.

3. Dieter, B., "Determining the Cost of Emergency Department Services," *Hospital Cost Accounting Advisor,* 2(1), April 1987, pp. 1, 5–6.

4. Horngren, C., and Foster G., *Cost Accounting: A Managerial Emphasis,* 6th ed. Englewood Cliffs, N.J.: Prentice Hall, 1987, chapter 4.

5. Dieter, B., "Determining the Cost of Nursing Services," *Hospital Cost Accounting Advisor,* 2(9), February 1987, pp. 1, 5–7.

6. Baptist, A., et al., "Developing a Solid Base for a Cost Accounting System," *Healthcare Financial Management,* January 1987, pp. 42–48.

7. Keegan, A., "Saving Money throughout the Cost Accounting Installation Cycle," *Hospital Cost Accounting Advisor,* 2(10), March 1987, pp. 1–7.

8. Hallstrom, B.J., "Utilization of Nursing Personnel: A Task-specific Approach," *Nursing Outlook,* 19(10), 664–667.

9. Hagerty, B., et al., "Work Sampling: Analyzing Nursing Staff Productivity," *JONA,* 15(9), September 1985.

10. Minyard, K., et al., "RNs May Cost Less Than You Think," *JONA,* 16(5), May 1986.

11. Nauert, L., et al., "Finding the Productivity Standard in Your Acuity System," *JONA,* 18(1), January 1988.

3

Product Costing

Reading 3–1

Job-Order Costing in Physician Practice

Lorelei S. Cheli

Changes in the reimbursement system for physicians' services, like those for hospitals, require the physician in private practice to examine cost issues. Traditionally, the physician in private practice has used a competition-oriented pricing called "going-rate" or "imitative pricing."[1] There is no rigid relationship between price, costs, or demand. Since costs have been difficult to measure, the going-price methodology has been thought to yield a price that is considered fair. A going-rate competition-oriented pricing strategy has been fostered by Medicare and private insurers whose reimbursement rate is based on usual, customary, and reasonable fees. This type of costing can no longer be used exclusively. Pressures from several different forces necessitate a more exacting means to measure costs in private practice.

Maximum allowable actual charges (MAACs) regulate the fee for services and procedures a nonparticipating physician can charge Medicare patients. These fees are considerably lower than those for non-Medicare patients. A focus on cost containment will continue and a physician who has a choice of serving Medicare or other patient types can make a practical decision only if some form of cost information is available.

Current findings show that HMOs that have signed up Medicare patients have difficulty meeting their obligations. Costs have created problems for smaller HMOs. During 1987, 29 of the 159 HMOs (more than 18 percent) that contracted with Medicare later decided to get out of the Medicare market.[2] Some health plans still providing Medicare coverage are losing money, while others are reluctant to get involved. Economies of scale are an important factor in the success or failure of a group in the Medicare market. Smaller operations account for half of the HMOs that have withdrawn from Medicare. Location is an important factor, since Medicare payment rates tend to be lower in rural areas. Similarly, a physician contracting for a prospective payment with an HMO or Medicare through the MAAC reimbursement system encounters cost issues.

The nursing shortage is another factor in rising costs in private practice. In the past, many nurses chose office work and accepted lower pay scales to avoid hospital shifts and weekend rotation. Hospitals have taken several steps to lure nurses back to hospital nursing. Flexible scheduling and higher pay scales have created more competition for skilled office nurses. As a result, higher hourly rates are being demanded by nurses employed in private practice settings.

A final area of concern is growing competition among physicians. Health care organiza-

Source: Reprinted from Lorelei S. Cheli, "Job-Order Costing in Physician Practice," *Hospital Cost Accounting Advisor,* Vol. 4, No. 10, March 1989, pp. 1–6. Copyright 1989, Aspen Publishers, Inc.

tions now engage in competitive pricing by offering lower than average prices for certain services (e.g., "St. Louis Hospital guarantees lower rates for outpatient surgery"). Price advertising for private physicians is moving in a similar direction (e.g., cataract procedures). Physicians allocating funds for marketing and advertising need cost information to establish which market segments to target. A choice of patient type may be limited in certain specialties, but the location where services are performed should be considered.

Costs of personnel and overhead are important considerations when opting to perform procedures (e.g., flexible sigmoidoscopy) in the private office setting. The choice is often available to the physician and patient to use a hospital procedure room. The costs incurred by the private physician practice in offering the convenience of an in-office procedure should be carefully evaluated.

With the past payment structure, profits were large enough that no benefits were seen to measuring costs. A much simpler structure, with fewer alternatives for providing care and services, meant fewer choices on how to deliver care. This simplified system no longer exists. Physicians who do not examine the alternatives cannot satisfy patient needs as cost efficiently as possible and, in turn, meet their own financial goals.

Historical costs provide the basis for a framework for responsibility accounting that should be formulated for private practice. Historical cost records of any particular service or office procedure are rarely maintained. However, past material costs are easily obtained, and can be used in the process of establishing actual costs of any procedure or service.

In most private practice situations the person ordering supplies can pinpoint volume that was purchased on a monthly basis. Care must be taken in choosing a material purchase as a basis for measuring volume. For example, the number of throat culture media used per month would not be a good indicator of sore throat visits if the physician does not culture every sore throat.

Each material must be viewed in relation to the practitioner's usual practicing habits.

Examining a material order for EKG mounts, where only one per cardiogram is used regardless of the practitioner, is a quick way to judge volume performed with no considerable error. Other services are not isolated as simply. To count these requires examining daily ledgers. One method would be to have the office person who gives the final bill to the patient, itemizing procedures and services, begin to maintain daily accounts.

Knowing volume of procedure types in itself is a valuable tool that private practices should have. Some practitioners can estimate the volume of some procedures. If the practice is highly specialized, this is obvious. Other more varied practices (e.g., internal medicine, general surgery, family practice) have less definitive information. Volume records enable the provider to predict employee needs and measure increases or decreases in demand. Volume records are a form of control on the physicians' habits for specific procedures. Variations in volume of any standard procedure performed per volume of patients can be reviewed. Volume also indicates which procedures or services a practice would most want to know costs for. Costs of other less frequently performed services could also be valuable, since these can incur greater costs because of their low volume.

To establish costs, a job-order costing system can be used to identify materials that are easily linked to a procedure. Different patient types typically require different materials and consume varying amounts of physician and nursing time. The job-order cost record will also serve a control function. Deviations can be investigated to determine underlying causes.

In a medical setting, as in industry, equipment and labor can cause deviations in standards. Patient type can also be isolated as a cause for deviation once standards are established. Medicare patients typically require more assistance from personnel and occupy examining rooms for longer periods of time than younger patients.

EKG JOB-ORDER COSTING EXAMPLE

Materials and labor can be directly isolated as elements of a specific treatment. For example, the direct materials and labor for an EKG might be

EKG Direct Materials

$ .09	Sigma Pads
.13	Mounts
.40	Pillowcase
.47	Gown
.40	Drape
.20	EKG Machine Paper
.13	Table Paper
$1.82	Direct Material Cost

EKG Direct Labor Cost

$2.26	Technician: 17 minutes @ $8.00 per hour (perform and mount EKG)
3.20	MD: 4 minutes @ $48.00 per hour (interpretation and report to patient). See appendix, p. 100.
$5.46	Direct Labor Cost

Overhead must also be allocated to each procedure to determine a close approximation of costs of different procedures. A medical practice incurs a substantial amount of fixed overhead independent of the type of procedures it performs. For a family practice these might include the following per year:

Fixed Overhead

$ 8,000	Malpractice and Other Insurances
36,000	Rent
1,668	Utilities
34,400	RN/Manager and Secretary
21,000	Benefits (Pension, Health Ins., SS)
	Office Equipment Depreciation
250	Reception Area $2,500/10 years
300	Clerical Equipment $6,000/20 years
250	Telephone $5,000/20 years
500	Copy Machine $3,000/6 years
1,300	Other
$101,868	Total Cost (approximately $102,000)

To apply this overhead, an application base must be selected to serve as a common denominator for all procedures. Each procedure is considered a cost objective that shares overhead expenses. The above costs are incurred on an annual basis independent of volume of procedures performed or hours of operation. If hours of operation are used as an application base, then for each hour of operation the overhead rate is $102,000/2,200 expected hours, or $46 per hour.

Increasing expected hours of operation would decrease the fixed overhead application rate, but would not necessarily generate the procedure volume needed to increase profits.

If volume of procedures is used as an application base, then for each procedure the overhead rate is $102,000/7,000 expected procedures, or $14.57 per procedure.

This volume is based on historical demand. If the practice is able to see greater volume within its current hours of operation, the fixed overhead per procedure can decrease.

EKG Fixed General and Direct Overhead

$14.57	Total budgeted overhead ($102,000/ 7,000 total budgeted procedures)
.33	EKG machine depreciation (Cost $2,000/10-year life = $200 per year divided by 600 budgeted EKGs)
$14.90	Overhead Cost
1.82	Direct Material Cost
5.46	Direct Labor Cost
$22.18	Total EKG Cost (materials + labor + overhead)

Medicare Patient EKG Profit

$29.80	Medicare MAAC reimbursement (as of January 1988)
−22.18	Costs (from above)
$ 7.62	Medicare Patient Profit

Non-Medicare Patient EKG Profit

$35.00	Charge to non-Medicare and other insurers BC/BS
−22.18	Costs
$12.82	Non-Medicare Patient Profit

SIGMOIDOSCOPY JOB-ORDER COSTING EXAMPLE

Materials

$1.16	Cidex ($6.95/6 current demand monthly)	
.30	Gauze	
.42	Gloves	
.13	Table Paper	
.42	Gown	
.40	Drape	
.40	Pillowcase	
$3.23	Material Cost	

Direct Labor Costs

$ 8.00	Technician Time (1 hour @ $8.00 per hour set up, assist procedure, clean equipment)
16.00	MD Time (20 minutes @ $48 per hour)
$24.00	Labor Cost

Fixed General and Direct Overhead

$14.57	Per Procedure
2.31	Sigmoidoscope Depreciation ($5,000 cost/5 years = $1,000/432 budgeted procedures)
$16.88	Overhead Cost
3.23	Material Cost
24.00	Labor Cost
$44.11	Total Sigmoidoscopy Cost

Medicare Patient Profit

$111.73	Medicare MAAC as of January 1988
–44.11	Costs
$ 67.62	Medicare Patient Profit

Non-Medicare Patient Profit

$130.00	Charge to non-Medicare patients, other insurers BC/BS
–44.11	Costs
$ 85.89	Non-Medicare Patient Profit

OFFICE VISIT INTERMEDIATE COST EXAMPLE

Direct material costs are usually minimal.

$ .83	Nurse Time (5 minutes @ 10.00 per hour)
12.00	MD Time (15 minutes @ $48 per hour)
$12.83	Direct Labor Cost
14.57	Fixed General Overhead per Procedure
$27.40	Total Cost

Medicare Patient Profit

$ 25.00	Medicare MAAC as of January 1988
–27.40	Total Cost
$ –2.40	Medicare Patient Loss

Non-Medicare Patient Profit

$ 33.00	Charge to other non-Medicare patients as of January 1988
–27.40	Total Cost
$ 5.60	Non-Medicare Patient Profit

ALLERGY IMMUNIZATION COST EXAMPLE

Material, Labor, and Overhead

$ .19	Syringe
.13	Table Paper
16.00	MD Time (20 minutes @ $48.00 per hour)
.83	Nurse Time (5 minutes @ $10 per hour)
14.57	General Overhead
$ 31.72	Total Cost

Medicare Patient Profit

$ 7.00	MAAC
–31.72	Cost
$ –24.72	Loss

Non-Medicare Patient Profit

$	10.00	Other Non-Medicare
	−31.72	Cost
$	−21.72	Loss

Allergy Immunization Costs without Physician Labor Costs:

$	.19	Syringe
	.13	Table Paper
	.83	Nurse
	14.57	General Overhead
$	15.72	Total Cost

Medicare Patient Profit

$	7.00	MAAC
	−15.72	Cost
$	−8.72	Loss

Non-Medicare Patient Profit

$	10.00	Other Non-Medicare
	−15.72	Cost
$	−5.72	Loss

Clearly some procedures are distinguished as profit makers and others as losers. In each practice these can be isolated. Decisions as to which patient types and procedures to encourage cannot be based on profit motives alone. Certain services (e.g., allergy injections) cannot be labeled as procedures in the sense that they should be allocated the same overhead rate. An allergy injection requires that a physician be physically present in the facility should an emergency arise during the 20 minutes a patient is required to wait for a reaction. Rarely is the physician needed. To charge an allergy injection cost with 20 minutes of physician time along with overhead would result in a cost of $31.72 for an allergy injection. This is clearly not reasonable, since the physician during that 20-minute time period is seeing other patients.

USE VARIANCES

Job-order costing has its limitations in health care. While the concept is simple, complexities develop, and the demands on staff time to keep track of cost in itself must be considered. However, by initiating job-order costing, standards for direct labor and material or supply costs can be developed on appropriate procedures.

For example, an efficiency or use variance could be developed for Medicare patients versus the standard of non-Medicare patients. From job-order costing it is determined that, on average, Medicare patients will require two to three minutes more time with technicians to undress and receive the explanation of the procedure.

Time spent with physicians is usually two to five minutes longer for an EKG interpretation. There are several valid reasons for these unfavorable use variances. The elderly usually have a more complicated medical history, which in turn generates questions regarding medication and general condition. Often information must be given to a family member who coordinates the patient's care as well as to the patient. As the elderly in almost all health situations require more time from expensive personnel, Medicare should consider this as a real-cost item in setting their regulated reimbursement rates.

Whether Medicare allows for these differences or not, they are informative for the provider and should be calculated. For example, suppose that an EKG has a standard requirement of 17 technician minutes and 4 MD minutes. However, suppose that for Medicare patients, the actual average is 19 and 6 minutes, respectively. The following variances may be calculated.

Technician Time Use Variance

Actual Inputs × Std. Prices	Std. Allowed × Std. Prices
19 min × $.133	17 min × $.133
$2.53 —	$2.26 = $.27 U

MD Time Use Variance

6 min × $.80	4 min × $.80
$4.80 —	$3.20 = $1.60 U

Staff performance can be compared with coworkers in regard to use variance. The employee who spends more time than the standard should be evaluated to uncover the reasons. Motivation and competition among employees is an additional benefit to job-order costing. As staff members were asked to log their time for specific procedures, comparisons resulted. Who performed the fastest EKG, who disinfected and cleaned the sigmoidoscope the quickest, and who spent the most time talking to patients?

The dominant means of control in most private practice settings historically has been personal observation. The manager's perceptions of the relationship of inputs to outputs without any analysis of cost and benefits has guided decision making. With cost information on specific procedures acquired through job-order costing, performance of personnel, volume of procedures, and costs can be evaluated. Comparisons of performance from year to year through a budget system can evolve. Summarizing the past performance forces a budget-type planning of the future.

With every appointment scheduled, the future of a practice is being planned or budgeted. That budget must reflect a desirable mix of procedures or services to ensure a profitable outcome. With job-order costing the manager has a more accurate cost basis on which to budget patient types.

Appendix: Analysis of Physician Wage

Annual Salary Desired $105,600

Fees from hospital patients:

$	200	per day (5 patient visits at $40.00 per visit)
or	1,400	per week (7 days per week)
or	70,000	annually (50 weeks per year)
	−20,000	(estimated uncollected)
$	50,000	Total from hospital patients

$105,600	total income desired
−50,000	hospital income
$55,600	office income desired

Fees from office income:
28 office hours per week × 48 weeks =

1,344	hours per year
−192	(4 hours per week reading, education)
1,152	hours available

$55,600	income ÷ 1,152 hours per year = $48.26/hour
$ 48.00	approximate hourly rate

NOTES

1. P. Kotler and R. Clark, *Marketing for Health Care Organizations* (Prentice-Hall, Inc., New Jersey, 1987, p. 362).
2. "HMOs Hit Medicare Snags," *Physician's Washington Report*, March, 1988, p. 3.

Reading 3–2

Product Cost Analysis in the Clinical Laboratory

Leonard D. Scinto

Cost accounting systems in health care organizations are primarily designed to provide organizationwide cost data to senior administration. A high tech department such as the clinical laboratory requires a different cost system: one that produces accurate data at the production cost level. It is important to recognize that neither system is superior to the other. Each system is necessary for effective and efficient management. They each provide different cost information since their products are different. The health care organization's products are discharged patients; a laboratory's products are test results.[1] The two cost systems are in reality one system, as shown in Figure 3–2–1. They should fit together well in order to derive the maximum information at all levels. The cost elements at the lowest level drive the system. It is at this level that laboratory managers manage production costs. A special cost model must be developed for this purpose.

The major controlling influence on costs produced within the clinical laboratory is the choice of laboratory instrumentation used at the workstation level. Laboratory instruments influence the two largest and important expenses in any laboratory budget: labor and reagent test supplies. To determine the cost of a laboratory test on a specific instrument, a product costing method must be used. One such method in use has been named the instrument cost accounting technique (ICAT).[2] This is the major method emphasized in the cost accounting guidelines devel-

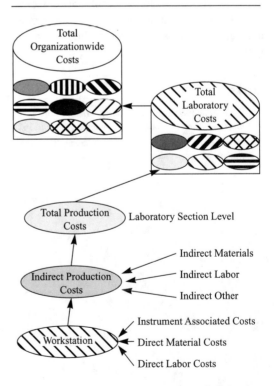

Figure 3–2–1 Organizationwide Costs and Laboratory Costs

Source: Reprinted from Leonard D. Scinto, "Product Cost Analysis in the Clinical Laboratory," *Hospital Cost Management and Accounting,* Vol. 1, No. 7, October 1989, pp. 1–8. Copyright 1989, Aspen Publishers, Inc.

oped by the National Committee for Clinical Laboratory Standards.[3] ICAT, which is based on standard cost accounting principles, examines the costs that are directly linked to the production of a laboratory test.

LABORATORY TEST COST CONSTRUCTION

Green and McSherry cite four major aspects of cost control systems[4]:

- cost data collected at the time the work is performed
- comprehensive cost data obtained from all inputs of the work process
- establishment of standard costs for these inputs
- monthly variance investigation of all relevant standard costs

Product cost analysis is the basic starting point for any cost accounting approach in the clinical laboratory. Figure 3–2–2 outlines the classification of laboratory costs. A microcosting study is first performed to establish the prime cost of each laboratory test at the workstation level.

This part of the analysis deals with three prime cost aspects of laboratory analysis: instrument associated costs, direct material costs, and direct labor costs. Next, indirect production costs are determined for each test. These are specific for each laboratory section (chemistry, immunology, etc.), leading to a total production cost. Finally, general laboratory operating overhead costs are allocated to each test. The resulting product is the total laboratory cost for a particular test. This bottom-up cost analysis approach is illustrated in Figure 3–2–3.

To simplify the analysis of the three prime cost calculations, a PC-based worksheet (such as Lotus 123 or Microsoft Excel) is extremely helpful. An example of such a worksheet is shown in Exhibit 3–2–1. The worksheet should be generically designed, so it can be used in any laboratory section to determine the costs associated with any instrument or test method.[5]

Instrument Associated Cost Analysis

The various entries on Part 1 of the test cost worksheet provide the basis for instrument associated cost calculations. This information is used in two equations to calculate the instrument's depreciation and maintenance costs per test. It is important not to overlook either of these items in any laboratory test cost analysis. Depreciation costs represent the reduction in value of the instrument as it ages and becomes obsolete. The method of depreciation I have used here is straight-line (the method in use at my hospital) although accelerated depreciation methods can be employed.[6] Maintenance costs involve the expense of cleaning, adjusting, and repairing an instrument in order to provide optimal performance.

Test Material Cost Analysis

After each analyte under study has been listed on the worksheet, direct test costs are divided into four segments[7]:

1. the total number of patient tests performed
2. the cost of reagents per test
3. the cost of the test-associated disposables per test
4. the cost of any other instrument-related disposables per test

Laboratory activities and consumables to be considered in test performance analysis include some or all of the following[7]:

1. price per test kit or total reagent costs
2. number of tests per kit or total reagent volume
3. number of controls run per test
4. number of calibrators run per test
5. single or replicate analysis per test
6. cost of disposable items used to perform the test
7. cost of specimen collection and processing
8. total number of tests performed during the study period.

LABORATORY TOTAL
TEST COST

$\parallel$

| COLLECTION AND REPORTING COSTS | + | LABORATORY ADMINISTRATIVE COSTS | = | GENERAL LABORATORY OVERHEAD |

include
• specimen collection and
  processing
• report delivery
• interpretive reporting
• data processing

include
• management salaries
• continuing education
• allocated hospital overhead
• quality assurance
• safety and infection control
• marketing
• communications (phones/fax/
  modem)

+

TOTAL PRODUCTION
COST
(LAB SECTION LEVEL)

$\parallel$

| INDIRECT MATERIAL COSTS | + | INDIRECT LABOR COSTS | + | OTHER INDIRECT COSTS | = | INDIRECT PRODUCTION COSTS |

include
• general lab supplies

include
• supervision
• staff training
• overtime

include
• test method research
  and evaluation

+

| INSTRUMENT COSTS | + | DIRECT MATERIAL COSTS | + | DIRECT LABOR COSTS | = | PRIME COST |

include
• maintenance
• repairs

include
• reagents
• calibration

include
• pre-analytical,
  analytical, and
  post-analytical
  time

Figure 3-2-2 An Analysis and Classification of Laboratory Costs

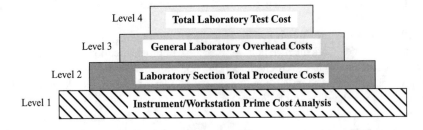

Figure 3-2-3 Laboratory Test Cost Tower: A Bottom-Up Approach. Laboratory test cost analysis is developed by tracing laboratory costs through each level in the tower from bottom to top.

Exhibit 3–2–1 Laboratory Test Prime Cost Worksheet

PART 1: TEST INSTRUMENT RELATED COSTS

Name: Ektachem-700 Chemistry Analyzer
Manufacturer: Eastman-Kodak
Purchase Price: $121,000
Life Expectancy (Years): 10
Annual Calibration Cost: $3,849
Total Tests: 75,851

Annual Quality Control Cost: $12,228
Annual Maintenance Cost: $14,300
Study Period (Days): 60
Starting Date: 1/3/99
Completion Date: 3/3/99

Instrument Cost Calculations (Per Test)

A. **Depreciation Costs (Straight-Line)** =

$$\frac{\text{Purchase Cost}}{\text{Life Span}} \times \frac{1 \text{ Year}}{365 \text{ Days}} \times \frac{\text{Study Period (Days)}}{\text{Total Tests}}$$

Calculation $0.03 Per Test

B. **Maintenance Cost** =

$$\frac{\text{Annual Maintenance Cost}}{365 \text{ Days}} \times \frac{\text{Study Period (Days)}}{\text{Total Tests}}$$

Calculation $0.03 Per Test

C. **Calibration Costs** =

$$\frac{\text{Annual Calibration Cost}}{365 \text{ Days}} \times \frac{\text{Study Period (Days)}}{\text{Total Tests}}$$

Calculation $0.01 Per Test

D. **Quality Control Costs** =

$$\frac{\text{Annual QC Cost}}{365 \text{ Days}} \times \frac{\text{Study Period (Days)}}{\text{Total Tests}}$$

Calculation $0.03 Per Test

TOTAL INSTRUMENT COSTS $0.10 Per Test

PART 2: DIRECT TEST MATERIALS COSTS

Test Name	Reagents	Test- Related Disposables	Instrument- Related Disposables	Total Tests	Material Cost (Per Test)
Glucose	$ 2,924.36	$100.84	$ 302.52	10,084	$0.33
BUN	2,709.28	96.76	290.28	9,676	0.32
Sodium	2,412.54	92.79	278.37	9,279	0.30
Potassium	2,558.92	98.42	295.26	9,842	0.30
Chloride	2,680.47	92.43	277.29	9,243	0.33
CO_2	2,244.24	93.51	280.53	9,351	0.28
Creatinine	2,090.66	95.03	285.09	9,503	0.26
Cholesterol	2,750.63	88.73	266.19	8,873	0.35
TOTALS	$20,371.10 +	$758.51 +	$2,275.53 ÷	75,851 =	$0.31

Direct Material Costs Calculation (Per Test) = $\dfrac{\text{Reagents Costs + Test Disposables + Instrument Disposables}}{\text{Number of Tests}}$

continues

Exhibit 3–2–1 continued

PART 3: DIRECT TEST LABOR

Time Segment	FTE Minute/Test	Annual Salary	Time Segment Labor Cost
Pre-Analytical	1.5	$27,740.00	$0.41
Analytical	1.0	$27,740.00	0.27
Post-Analytical	2.0	$27,740.00	0.55
Totals	4.5		$1.23

Direct Labor Cost Per Test Calculations:

Step One:

$$\frac{\text{Annual Salary}}{\text{2,080 Paid Hours/Year}} \div 60 \text{ Minutes} = \text{Salary Cost/Minute}$$

Step Two:

Salary Cost/Minute × Minutes To Perform Test = Salary Cost/Test

Step Three:

Salary Cost/Test × 1.23 Fringe Benefit Factor = Total Labor Cost/Test

Calculations:

	Pre-Analytical	Analytical	Post-Analytical	Total
Step 1	$0.22	$0.22	$0.22	
Step 2	$0.33	$0.22	$0.44	
Step 3	$0.41	$0.27	$0.55	$1.23

PART 4: TOTALS

Test Name	Instrument Costs	Material Costs	Labor Costs	Test Prime Costs
Glucose	$0.10	$0.33	$1.23	$1.66
BUN	0.10	0.32	1.23	1.65
Sodium	0.10	0.30	1.23	1.63
Potassium	0.10	0.30	1.23	1.63
Chloride	0.10	0.33	1.23	1.66
CO_2	0.10	0.28	1.23	1.61
Creatinine	0.10	0.26	1.23	1.59
Cholesterol	0.10	0.35	1.23	1.68

The formula for direct materials per test is shown in Part 2 of the worksheet. The number of tests are divided into the cost of reagents, test associated disposables, and instrument related disposables.

Direct Labor Cost

This is the total compensation required for personnel to perform all of the pre-analytical, analytical, and post-analytical steps of a test. The College of American Pathologists (CAP) Workload Recording Method, the only nationally recognized workload accounting system for clinical laboratories, was not developed for the purpose of test cost analysis, although many clinical laboratories use it for this purpose for lack of a better system. It was intended to be used to determine staffing needs as well as to measure productivity.[8] Consequently, it overlooks most (if not all) of the pre- and post-analytical steps in laboratory test production. These two steps are important labor intensive aspects of test analysis. They provide far more information on labor costs than a time study method that uses just the analytical phase in test production, as is the case in the CAP method.

Pre-analytical Time

This begins when the specimen arrives in the laboratory and continues up until the start of analysis. It involves activities such as specimen centrifugation, separation, and preparation. Since different staff members may be involved with various pre-analytical aspects, it is important to accurately record the time and labor rate of each staff member.

Analytical Time

This is the analysis time required to perform all required procedures up to reporting of results. This is usually the least labor-intensive phase, since most testing done in the clinical laboratory today is performed on microcomputer-directed high speed automated analyzers. Operation intervention in this phase is usually minimal.

Post-analytical Time

This accounts for the labor required to report results. This includes entering and verifying results in a computer, sorting, filing, and telephoning reports. Time spent daily, weekly, and monthly performing instrument maintenance should be recorded in this phase.

The ICAT method calculates the full fiscal burden, not just productivity of a laboratory instrument or test method. The total number of full-time equivalents (FTEs) per minute required to produce a test and the total labor cost (annual salary plus fringe benefits) of personnel performing the work are determined for each of the three analytical time segments, as shown in Part 3 of the worksheet.

INDIRECT COSTS OF TEST PRODUCTION

These are costs that cannot be directly related to a test or the instrument required to produce the test. As illustrated in Figure 3–2–2, they include the cost of indirect labor, materials, and other items that cannot be directly charged to the laboratory test. These costs are commonly added on as a proportionate share to the direct costs associated with a particular test. Indirect production costs at the lab section level can be calculated out to a single per-test cost by dividing the section level's total indirect cost by the total number of tests performed in the section. This single per test cost when added to the prime cost will give the full production cost at the laboratory section level. Another tier of indirect costs is incurred at the department level. These costs include the collection and reporting of all laboratory tests as well as the allocated hospital overhead costs assigned to the laboratory department. Other indirect cost items that are important to consider in overall operations are listed in Figure 3–2–2.

These are related to the nontechnical aspects of the production process: marketing, administration, and maintaining a safe and adequate work environment.

The general laboratory overhead can be converted to a per-test unit cost by dividing the total overhead cost by the total number of tests produced in all laboratory sections. The general laboratory overhead per test added to the full production cost (at the section level) ultimately yields the total laboratory cost per test.

TEST COST ANALYSIS AS A MANAGEMENT TOOL

Test cost analysis provides important financial information to laboratory managers. It can identify proper batch sizes to minimize waste, analyze the fiscal impact of a new proposed equipment purchase, and analyze the cost efficiency of existing instrumentation. Cost analysis provides managers with a rational mechanism for selecting the most cost-effective testing method among several new laboratory procedures, all claiming to be the least expensive to use. Laboratory budgeting becomes more effective with a cost analysis system in place. Managers who have accurate and timely test cost and workload information at their disposal are able to accurately project the effects of adding new or increased testing on staffing requirements, inventory, revenues, and expenditures.

Many laboratories have set testing charges based on a comparison with other laboratories in their market area. This method is highly unreliable. Total laboratory test cost can vary widely from laboratory to laboratory due to different methods, instruments, labor costs, and operating overhead. Laboratories using test cost analysis can identify actual direct supply and reagent costs, instrument costs, labor costs, and indirect overhead costs. Using total laboratory test cost, laboratory managers can assign a realistic charge for a test and method.

The establishment of the Prospective Payment System has given clinical laboratories a strong motivation for establishing true laboratory test costs. It has become increasingly important for clinical laboratories to focus on the actual costs of tests used to diagnose and monitor patients who are classified by DRGs. Clinical laboratory scientists and administrators working with various medical specialists are selecting the most sensitive and specific tests required to identify and monitor disease conditions within selected DRGs. Test choices are then grouped together to form a unique DRG-focused test panel. The test costs associated with this test panel are then calculated and can be rolled into other organization-wide costs to determine the fully loaded cost of a particular DRG category. Exhibit 3–2–2 shows the results of laboratory test costs for a new admission with diabetes.[9]

CONCLUSION

Every laboratory has a unique cost profile for the tests it performs. This is the result of different instruments, wage and benefit packages, employee productivity levels, and various costs associated with reagents, supplies, and overhead in a particular laboratory. Laboratories using idealized test cost data provided by a diagnostic manufacturer, which only include reagent and supply costs, will underestimate actual laboratory test costs by the exclusion of labor costs and other indirect expenses. The use of product cost analysis leads to improved management control by allowing laboratory managers to identify the optimal frequency and size of test runs, and efficient staffing for each workstation, as well as identifying and choosing economical reagents and testing supplies.

The laboratory product cost analysis I have outlined here provides test costs and operation costs at various levels, beginning at the instrument/workstation, moving up to the section level, and ending at the laboratory department as a whole. The full laboratory test cost can then be used to determine the combined cost of a test profile for a specific DRG category. This laboratory DRG cost can then be used directly in the health care organizationwide cost system to monitor a full cost per patient admission.

Exhibit 3-2-2 Laboratory Cost Analysis Worksheet for a Diabetes Admission

DRG 294, Diabetes ≥ 36 Years Old
Principal Diagnosis:
Type 2 Diabetes Mellitus with Renal Manifestations
Non-Insulin Dependent

Test	Direct Cost Per Test			Indirect Costs	
	Instrument Cost	Materials Cost	Labor Cost	Production Cost	Laboratory Overhead
Chemistry Profile					
Glucose	$0.10	$0.33	$11.01	$1.98	$4.06
BUN	0.10	0.32			
Sodium	0.10	0.30			
Potassium	0.10	0.30			
CO_2	0.10	0.28			
Chloride	0.10	0.33			
Creatinine	0.10	0.26			
Albumin	0.10	0.26			
Cholesterol	0.10	0.35			
Urine Creatinine	0.10	0.97	1.53	0.44	
Urine Microscopic	Manual	0.26	2.35	0.37	
Hemoglobin	0.15	0.14	1.10	0.75	
Hematocrit	0.15	0.14	1.10	0.75	
TOTALS	$1.30	$4.24	$17.09	$4.29	$4.06

DRG 294: LABORATORY TOTAL COST $30.98

In today's rapidly changing health care environment, clinical laboratory managers must be able to measure the actual cost of laboratory operations in order to make informed decisions and provide effective financial management of the clinical laboratory department.

NOTES

1. Patterson, P.P. Cost Accounting in Hospitals and Clinical Laboratories: Part 1, *Clinical Laboratory Management Review* 1988, 2(6):345.

2. Travers, E.M. and Krochmal, C.F. A New Way to Determine Test Cost Per Instrument, Part 1, *Medical Laboratory Observer* 1988, 20(10): 25.

3. National Committee for Clinical Laboratory Standards. *Draft Guidelines on Laboratory Cost Accounting.* Villanova, Pa.: NCCLS, 1987.

4. Green, H.H. and McSherry, E. New case mix management tool for the DRG era, *VA Practitioner* 1985, 2:64.

5. Travers and Krochmal, p. 28.

6. Weston, J.F. and Copeland, T.E. "Managerial Finance," pp. 63–66.

7. Travers and Krochmal, p. 27.

8. College of American Pathologists, *Manual for Laboratory Workload Recording Method,* pp. 1–2, 1985.

9. Travers and Krochmal, p. 60.

BIBLIOGRAPHY

Dominiak, G.F. and Louderback, J.G., *Managerial Accounting.* Boston, Mass.: PWS-Kent Publishing, 1988.

Finkler, S.A., *Budgeting Concepts for Nurse Managers.* New York, N.Y.: Grune and Stratton, 1984.

Gore, M.J., Financial Management of the Clinical Laboratory: How To Improve Present Systems. *Medical Laboratory Observer,* 1988, 20(3):37–40.

Horngren, C.T., *Cost Accounting: A Managerial Emphasis,* sixth edition. Englewood Cliffs, N.J.: Prentice-Hall, 1986.

Horngren, C.T. and Sundem, G.L., *Introduction to Financial Accounting,* third edition. Englewood Cliffs, N.J.: Prentice-Hall, 1987.

Matz, A. and Usry, M.F., *Cost Accounting: Planning and Control,* seventh edition. Cincinnati, Ohio: Southwestern Publishing, 1980.

Sattler, J. and Smith, A., *Financial Management of the Clinical Laboratory.* Oradell, N.J.: Medical Economics, 1986.

Suver, J.D. and Neumann, B.R., *Management Accounting for Healthcare Organizations.* Chicago, Healthcare Financial Management Association, 1985.

Reading 3–3

Product Costing for Health Care Firms

William O. Cleverley

The implementation of the prospective payment system has brought enormous interest in cost accounting, and this interest is not limited to the hospital industry. The interest in developing sophisticated cost accounting systems is present in all sectors of the health care industry. Most, if not all, of this interest is a reflection of fixed prices for services and increasing economic competition among health care providers.[1]

This article identifies a framework for the discussion and development of cost accounting systems in the health care sector. Great reliance is placed on the similarities rather than the differences in cost accounting systems as they exist in industry. The framework requires two sets of standards, one relating to the production of departmental products, and one relating to the treatment protocol for defined patient categories.

RELATIONSHIP OF COST INFORMATION TO PLANNING, BUDGETING, AND CONTROL

Cost information is of value only as it aids in the management decision-making process.[2] Figure 3–3–1 presents a schematic of the planning, budgeting, and control process in any business. Of special interest is the decision output of the

Source: Reprinted from William O. Cleverley, "Product Costing for Health Care Firms," *Health Care Management Review,* Vol. 12, No. 4, Fall 1987, pp. 39–48. Copyright 1987, Aspen Publishers, Inc.

planning process. This process should detail the products or product lines that the business will produce during the planning period.

Products and Product Lines

The term product or product line seems fairly simple and easy to understand in most business

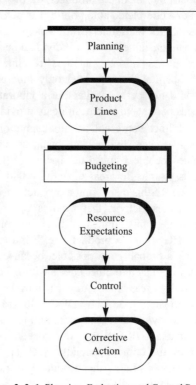

Figure 3–3–1 Planning, Budgeting, and Control Process

firms. For example, an automobile manufacturer produces cars. The finished car is clearly the product of the automobile firm. Individual types of cars may be grouped to form product lines such as the Chevrolet product line of General Motors.

Is the definition of a product as simple in the health care sector? Many individuals feel very strongly that products cannot be defined easily in health care firms. The major dilemma seems to arise in the area of patients versus products. In short, is the patient the product or is the product individual services such as laboratory tests, nursing care, and meals? In most situations the patient is the basic product of health care firms. This means that the wide range of services provided to patients, such as nursing, prescriptions, and tests, should be viewed as intermediate products and not final products. There is little difference between this situation and that in most manufacturing settings. For example, fenders are on one hand a product but they are really nothing more than intermediate products to the final product of a completed automobile. The automobile is sold, not the fenders. In the same vein, a treated patient, rather than an individual service provided in isolation, generates revenue. In short, a hospital that provided only laboratory tests would not be a hospital but a laboratory. One needs patients to be a health care provider.

Product lines represent an amalgamation of patients in a way that makes business sense. Sometimes people use the term strategic business units to refer to areas of activity that may stand alone. In this discussion a product line is a unit of business activity that requires a go or no go decision. In this context, a diagnosis-related group (DRG) is not a product line. Eliminating one DRG is probably not possible, because that DRG may be linked to other DRGs within a clinical specialty area. For example, it may be impossible to stop producing DRG #36 (retinal procedures) without also eliminating other DRGs such as DRG #39 (lens procedure). In most cases the clinical specialty, such as ophthalmology, constitutes the product line rather than an individual DRG.

Budgeting and Resource Expectations

The budgeting phase of operations involves a translation of the product line decisions reached earlier in the planning phase into a set of resource expectations. The primary purpose of this activity is twofold. First, management must assure itself that there will be sufficient funds to maintain financial solvency. Just as individuals must live within their financial means so must any health care business entity. Second, the resulting budget serves as a basis for management control. If budget expectations are not realized, management must discover why not and take corrective actions. A budget or set of resource expectations can be thought of as a standard costing system. The budget represents management's expectations about how costs should behave given a certain set of volume expectations.

The key aspect of budgeting is the translation of product line decisions into precise and specific sets of resource expectations. Five basic steps are involved:

1. defining volume of patients by case type to be treated in the budget period;
2. defining standard treatment protocol by case type;
3. defining required departmental volumes;
4. defining standard cost profiles for departmental outputs; and
5. defining prices to be paid for resources.

The primary output of the budgeting process is a series of departmental budgets that spell out what costs should be during the coming budget period. In the development of a budget, the establishment of three separate sets of standards is involved.

Control

The control phase of business operations monitors actual cost experience and compares it to budgetary expectations. If there are deviations from expectations, management analyzes the causes for the deviation. If the deviation is favorable, management may seek to make whatever action created the variance a permanent part of operations. If the variance is unfavorable, action will be taken to prevent a recurrence, if possible. Much of the control phase centers around the topic of variance analysis.

COSTING PROCESS

Most firms, whether they are hospitals, nursing homes, or steel manufacturers, have fairly similar costing systems. In fact, the similarities outweigh the differences in most cases. Figure 3–3–2 provides a schematic of the cost measurement process that exists in most business firms.[3] This process consists of three activities: valuation, allocation, and product specification.

Valuation

Valuation has always been a thorny issue for accountants, one that has not been satisfactorily resolved even today. One need only see the current controversy over replacement costs versus historical costs to see the problem in full bloom. For discussion purposes, the valuation process has been split into two areas: basis and assignment over time. To some degree these two areas are not mutually exclusive and overlap with one another. However, both determine the total value of a resource that is used to cost a final product.

The valuation basis is the process whereby a value is assigned to each resource transaction occurring between the entity being accounted for and another entity. In most situations this is historical cost. Once a value for a resource is established, there are many situations where that value will have to be assigned over time. Specifically, there are two major categories of situations. First, in many situations the value is expended prior to the actual reporting of expense. The best example of this is depreciation. Second are situations where expense is recognized prior to an actual expenditure. Normal accruals such as wages and salaries are examples of this category.

Allocation

The end result of the cost allocation process is assignment of all costs or values determined in the valuation phase to direct departments.[4] Two phases of activity are involved in accomplishing this objective. First, all resource values to be recorded as expense in a given period are assigned or allocated to the direct and indirect departments as direct expenses. Second, once the initial cost assignment to individual departments has been made, a further allocation is required. In this phase the expenses of the indirect departments are assigned to the direct departments.

Using this framework for analysis, costing issues may be subcategorized. In the initial cost

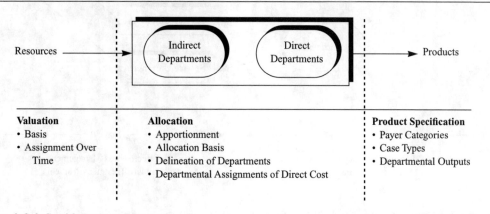

Valuation	Allocation	Product Specification
• Basis	• Apportionment	• Payer Categories
• Assignment Over Time	• Allocation Basis	• Case Types
	• Delineation of Departments	• Departmental Outputs
	• Departmental Assignments of Direct Cost	

Figure 3–3–2 Cost Measurement Process

assignment phase, there appear to be two major areas that relate to the underlying costing process: assigning cost to departments and defining the indirect and direct departments. The first area concerns situations where the departmental structure currently specified is not questioned, but some of the initial value assignments may be. For example, premiums paid for malpractice insurance might be charged to the administration and general department or more directly to the nursing and professional departments that are involved. In the second area, the existing departmental structure may be revised. For example, the administration and general department may be split into several new departments such as nonpatient telephones, data processing, purchasing, admitting, business office, and other.

In the second phase of cost allocation, which consists of reassignment from indirect departments to direct departments, there are also two primary categories: selection of the cost apportionment method and selection of the appropriate allocation basis. Cost apportionment methods such as stepdown, double distribution, or simultaneous equations are simply mathematical algorithms that redistribute cost from existing indirect departments to direct departments given defined allocation bases. An example of the selection of an appropriate allocation basis for an indirect department might be square feet covered or hours worked for housekeeping.

Product Specification

In most health care firms there are two phases to the production (or treatment) process. Figure 3–3–3 provides a schematic of this process and also introduces a few new terms.

In stage one of the production process resources are acquired and consumed within de-

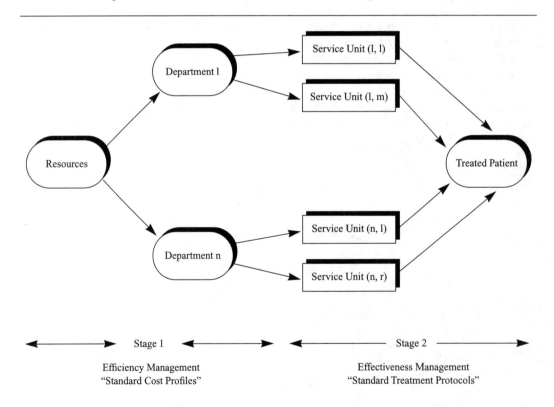

Figure 3–3–3 Production Process for Health Care Firms

partments to produce a product that is defined as a service unit (SU). All departments have SUs but not all departments have the same number of SUs. For example, the nursing department may provide four levels of care, acuity level 1, 2, 3, or 4. The laboratory may have 100 or more separate SUs related to specific tests they provide. Not all SUs can be directly associated with the delivery of patient care. Some SUs may be indirectly associated with patient treatment. For example, the housekeeping staff may clean laboratory areas, but there is no direct association of this effort with patient treatment. However, the cleaning of a patient's room is a housekeeping SU that could be associated with a patient.

The second production phase relates to the actual consumption of specific SUs in the treatment of a patient. Much of this production process is actually managed by the physician. This is true irrespective of the setting (e.g., hospital, nursing home, home health care firm, or clinic). The physician will prescribe the specific SUs required to effectively treat a given patient.

The lack of authority in this area complicates management's efforts to budget and control its costs. This is not meant to be a negative reflection of current health care delivery. Everyone would prefer to have a qualified physician directing care as opposed to a lay health care executive. This is perhaps the area of greatest difference between health care firms and other business entities. Management at General Motors can decide which automobiles will have factory-installed air conditioning and tinted glass. A hospital will find it very difficult to direct a physician to prescribe or not prescribe a given procedure when treating a patient.

Products to be costed may vary depending on the specific decision under consideration. At one level, management may be interested in the cost of a specific service unit or departmental output. Prices for some SUs, such as X-ray procedures, may have to be established, and management needs to know their costs. In other situations the cost of a specific treated patient or grouping of treated patients may be desired. For example, management may wish to bid on a contract to provide home health services to a health maintenance organization (HMO). It is important for them to understand what the costs of treating HMO patients are likely to be. Once the contract is signed, management needs to determine the actual costs of treating patients from the HMO in order to measure overall profitability from that segment of the business. Alternatively, a grouping of patients by specialty may also be necessary. A hospital may wish to know if it is losing money from treating a particular DRG entity or some grouping of DRGs, such as obstetrics.

STANDARDS DEVELOPMENT

The key to successful product costing systems is fairly simple to identify. Management must be able to develop and maintain two systems: standard cost profiles (SCPs) and standard treatment protocols (STPs).

Figure 3–3–3 illustrates the relationship between these two systems. The linking pin between the systems is the SU concept. In the simplest language, management must be able to know what it costs to produce an SU. It must also know what SUs are needed to treat a given patient.

Standard Cost Profiles

An SCP is not a new concept. It has been used in cost accounting systems in manufacturing for many years. There are two key elements to an SCP: the defined SU being costed and the profile of resources required to produce the SU.

As mentioned, the number of SUs in a given department may vary. Some departments may have one while others may have 100 or more. If the number of SUs is large, there may be an unacceptable level of costing detail involved to make the system feasible. In these situations it may be useful to aggregate some of the different SUs. For example, the laboratory may have 1,000 or more tests to perform. It may make sense in this situation to develop cost profiles for only the most commonly performed tests and use some arbitrary assignment method for the remaining tests.

The SU does not have to be a product or service that is directly performed for a patient. Many of the so-called indirect departments do not provide services or products to the patient. Instead, their products or services are consumed by other departments, both direct and indirect.

It is also important to note that many indirect departments may have SUs that are directly provided for the patient. For example, the dietary department is often considered to be indirect because no revenue is billed for its product to the patient. However, a meal furnished to a patient is an SU that is just as direct as a laboratory test or a chest X-ray. Similarly, the housekeeping staff may provide cleaning services to a patient's room, and that cleaning service is a direct service consumed by the patient.

SUs may also be categorized as direct or indirect. A direct SU is one that may be associated with a given patient. An indirect SU is a service or product provided to another department as opposed to a patient. The differentiation between direct and indirect SUs is important not only in the development of SCPs but also in the development of STPs. Direct SUs must be identified when STPs are defined while indirect SUs need not be specifically identified, although some estimate of allocated cost is often required.

An SCP for a given SU should list the resource expense categories[5] of direct expenses, such as labor, materials, and departmental overhead, and allocated overhead. In addition, the SCP should ideally categorize the expense as variable or fixed. This separation is important to many areas of management decision making. Specifically, variable and fixed cost differentiation is critical to many incremental pricing and volume decisions. Variable and fixed cost differentiation is also important to flexible budgeting systems and management control.

Table 3–3–1 presents an SCP that will be used for discussion purposes. In the table, the SU being profiled is a regular patient meal provided by the dietary department. The total cost of providing one regular patient meal or SU #181 is $2.50. Variable cost per meal is $1.30 and average fixed cost per meal is $1.20.

In most situations direct labor will be the largest single expense category. In this example, this is not true because the direct material cost, mostly raw food, is larger. It would be possible, and in many cases desirable, to define direct labor costs by labor category. For example, in this case cooks, dietary aides, and dishwashers could be listed separately.

An important point to resolve is the division of cost into fixed and variable quantities. Table 3–3–1 indicates that .05 units of variable labor time are required per meal and .05 units of fixed labor are required per meal. A variety of methods that might be useful in splitting costs into fixed and variable elements is discussed in the literature.

Table 3–3–1 Standard Cost Profile for Dietary Department, Regular Patient Meal*

| Cost Category | Quantity Required | | Unit Cost | Variable Cost | Average Fixed Cost | Average Total Cost |
	Variable	Fixed				
Direct labor	.05	.05	$ 6.00	$ .30	$ .30	$ .60
Direct materials	1	0	1.00	1.00	0	1.00
Departmental overhead	0	1	.50	0	.50	.50
Allocated costs						
Housekeeping	0	.1	1.00	0	.10	.10
Plant operation	0	1	.10	0	.10	.10
Administration	0	.02	10.00	0	.20	.20
Total				$1.30	$1.20	$2.50

* Expected volume = 1,600 SU #181

The fixed cost assignment is an average that is based on some expected level of volume. It is important to remember this point when developing SCPs. A decline in volume below expected levels will raise the average cost of production.

The third column in Table 3–3–1 is unit cost. This value represents management's best guess as to the cost or price of the resources to be used in the production process. For example, the dietary SCP indicates a price of six dollars per unit of direct labor. This value reflects the expected wage per hour to be paid for direct labor in the dietary department. Again, it might be possible and desirable to further break out direct labor into specific job classifications. This will usually permit better costing but it does require more effort.

Any fringe benefit costs associated with labor should be included in the unit cost. For example, the average direct hourly wage in the dietary department might be five dollars per hour, but fringe benefits may average 20 percent. In this case the effective wage would be six dollars per hour.

Departmental overhead consists of expenses directly charged to a department that do not represent labor or materials. Common examples might be equipment costs, travel allowances, outside purchased services, publications, and other small items. Usually these items do not vary with level of activity or volume but remain fixed for the budgetary period. If this is the case, assignment to an SCP can be based on a simple average. For example, assume that the dietary department expects to provide 200,000 regular patient meals next year. Furthermore, assume that the department has been authorized to spend $100,000 in discretionary areas that constitute departmental overhead. The average cost per meal for these discretionary costs would be $.50 and would be fixed.

Allocated costs are probably the most difficult to assign in most situations. In the dietary example only three areas are included, which is probably an understatement. A number of other departments would most likely provide service to the dietary department and would be included in the SCP.

There are two major alternatives to provide estimates of allocated costs in an SCP. First, individual costing studies could be performed and services from one department to others could be recorded. This process may be expensive and not worth the effort. For example, utility costs could be associated with each department if separate meters were installed. But the installation of these meters would probably not be an effective expenditure of funds, because costing accuracy would not be improved enough to justify the extra expense.

The second approach to allocating overhead costs would be a simple averaging method. All overhead costs might be aggregated and apportioned to other departments using direct expenses, full-time equivalents, or some other basis. This method is relatively simple, but its accuracy is suspect if significant variation in departmental utilization exists.

The best approach to costing is to identify as many direct SUs as possible. These SUs can be directly associated with a patient, and there are far more of these SUs than most people believe. For example, a meal provided to a patient is a direct SU that is currently treated as an indirect product in most costing systems. Laundry and linen departments have certain SUs that are directly associated with a patient, such as clean sheets and gowns. Housekeeping departments provide direct services to patients when they clean rooms. Administration and medical records departments also provide specific services to patients in the form of processed paperwork and insurance forms. When many of these costs that are currently regarded as indirect are reclassified as direct, there will be a substantially lower level of indirect costs requiring allocation. This system would improve the costing of patients, who are considered the product, and make the allocation of indirect costs less critical. Currently, indirect costs in many health care settings may be in excess of 50 percent of total cost. With better identification of services provided or SUs, the actual percentage could be reduced to 25 percent or lower.

Standard Treatment Protocols

There is an analogy between an STP and a job order cost sheet used in industrial cost accounting. In a job order cost system, a separate cost sheet is completed for each specific job, because each job may be different from jobs performed in the past and jobs to be performed in the future. Automobile repairs are an excellent example of a job order cost system. A separate cost sheet is prepared for each job. The cost sheet also serves as the bill or invoice to the customer.

Health care firms operate in a job cost setting. A patient's treatment may vary significantly across patients. The patient's bill may be thought of as a job order cost sheet. The bill reflects the actual services provided during the course of the patient's treatment. Of course, not all of the services provided are reflected in the patient's bill. For example, meals provided are rarely charged as a separate item.

In a typical job order cost setting, standards may not always be developed. When someone drops a car off for service, the dealer does not prepare a standard job order cost sheet. He or she has no incentive to do so because he or she expects the person to pay the actual costs of the service when he or she picks up the car. Otherwise, the dealer may retain the car as collateral.

A similar situation used to exist in health care firms. The client or patient would pay for the actual cost of services provided. Today this situation does not exist for many products. Health care firms are often paid a fixed fee or price irrespective of the range of services provided. Medicare's DRG payment system is an example of this type of payment philosophy.

Because the majority of revenue may be derived from fixed price payers, it is necessary to define STPs where possible. Table 3–3–2 provides an STP for DRG #208. This STP is intended to be used as an illustration only and should not be considered a realistic STP for DRG #208.

An examination of Table 3–3–2 shows that costs are again split into fixed and variable components. For example, this STP requires 25 patient meals at a variable cost of $1.30 per meal and a fixed cost of $1.20 per meal. The basis for these data would be the SCPs. In the dietary example, the split between variable and fixed cost is reflected in Table 3–3–1.

This separation of fixed and variable costs is extremely valuable for management in planning and control decisions. For example, if Medicare paid the hospital $1,400 for every DRG #208 treated, in the short run it would be financially wise to continue treating DRG #208 cases, because the payment of $1,400 exceeds the variable cost of $1,014.50 and therefore contributes to fixed costs.

Table 3–3–2 Standard Treatment Protocol, DRG #208, Disorder of Biliary Tract

SU No.	SU Name	Quantity	Variable Cost/Unit	Fixed Cost/Unit	Total Cost/Unit	Total Variable Cost	Total Fixed Cost	Total Cost
1	Admission process	1	$48.00	$52.00	$100.00	$ 48.00	$ 52.00	$ 100.00
7	Nursing care level 1	1	80.00	40.00	120.00	80.00	40.00	120.00
8	Nursing care level 2	7	85.00	45.00	130.00	595.00	315.00	910.00
9	Nursing care level 3	1	110.00	45.00	155.00	110.00	45.00	155.00
29	Pharmacy prescriptions		38.00	19.00	57.00	38.00	19.00	57.00
38	Chest X-ray	1	12.00	8.00	20.00	12.00	8.00	20.00
46	Laboratory CBC	1	4.00	3.50	7.50	4.00	3.50	7.50
49	Other laboratory tests		85.00	55.00	140.00	85.00	55.00	140.00
57	Patient meals	25	1.30	1.20	2.50	32.50	30.00	62.50
65	Clean linen changes	5	.60	.50	1.10	3.00	2.50	5.50
93	Room preparation	1	7.00	3.00	10.00	7.00	3.00	10.00
						$1,014.50	$573.00	$1,587.50

Table 3–3–2 also depicts two areas where no actual quantity is specified. Pharmacy prescriptions and other laboratory tests are not individually identified. Instead the total cost of the services is shown with a separation into fixed and variable costs. Because of the large number of products provided in each of these areas, it would be impossible to develop an SCP for every possible laboratory test or pharmacy prescription. Some of the heavier volume laboratory tests or pharmacy prescriptions may be separately identified and costed. Table 3–3–2 indicates that a complete blood cell count (CBC) is a separate SU in the laboratory department.

Some of the items shown in Table 3–3–2 may not be reflected in a patient's bill. Patient meals, clean linen changes, room preparation, and admission paperwork processed would not usually be reflected in the patient's bill. In addition, separation of nursing care by acuity level may not be identified in the bill. Many hospitals do not distinguish between levels of nursing in their pricing structures.

The final point to emphasize is that not all SUs will show up in an STP. Only those SUs that are classified as direct will be listed. A direct SU is one that can be directly traced or associated with patient care. The costs associated with the provision of indirect SUs will be allocated to the direct SUs. The objective, however, is to create as many direct SUs as possible.

VARIANCE ANALYSIS

Variance analysis provides a useful summary of the health care production process. In general there are four types of variances that will be identified in the variance analysis phase of control given earlier systems of standards.[6] The four variances are price (rate), efficiency, volume, and intensity. The first three variances are a direct result of the development of the SCPs and result from departmental activity. A rate or price variance reflects the difference between the price actually paid and the standard price multiplied by the actual quantity used and may be expressed in the following way:

$$\left(\begin{array}{c} \text{Actual} \\ \text{price} \end{array} - \begin{array}{c} \text{Standard} \\ \text{price} \end{array} \right) \times \begin{array}{c} \text{Actual} \\ \text{quantity} \end{array}$$

For example, assume that the dietary department in Table 3–3–1 actually produced 1,500 patient meals for the period in question. To produce these meals it used 180 hours of labor and paid $6.25 per hour. The price or rate variance would be $45.00, expressed as ($6.25 – $6.00) × 180 hours. This variance would be unfavorable because the department paid $6.25 per hour when the expected rate was $6.00. The actual quantity of labor used was 180 hours.

An efficiency variance reflects productivity in the production process. It is derived by multiplying the difference between actual quantity used and standard quantity by the standard price and may be expressed in the following way:

$$\left(\begin{array}{c} \text{Actual} \\ \text{quantity} \end{array} - \begin{array}{c} \text{Standard} \\ \text{quantity} \end{array} \right) \times \begin{array}{c} \text{Standard} \\ \text{price} \end{array}$$

In the example above, the efficiency variance would be $150 unfavorable, expressed as (180 hours – 155 hours) × $6.00. Standard labor is derived by multiplying the variable labor requirement of .05 by the number of meals produced, 1,500, to get 75 hours. The budgeted fixed labor requirement of 80 hours (.05 × 1,600 meals) is added to this figure. During the period 25 hours more labor than expected were used, resulting in the unfavorable efficiency variance of $150.

The volume variance reflects differences between expected output and actual output. Volume variances exist in situations where fixed costs are present. If no fixed costs existed, resources required per unit would be constant. This would mean that the cost per unit of production should be constant. For most situations this is not a reasonable expectation, because fixed costs do exist. The volume variance is derived by multiplying the expected average fixed cost per unit by the difference between budgeted volume and actual volume and may be expressed in the following way:

$$\left(\begin{array}{c} \text{Budgeted} \\ \text{volume} \end{array} - \begin{array}{c} \text{Actual} \\ \text{volume} \end{array}\right) \times \begin{array}{c} \text{Average fixed} \\ \text{cost per unit} \end{array}$$

In the case of direct labor for the dietary department, the volume variance would be an unfavorable $30, expressed as (1,600 meals – 1,500 meals) × $.30.

The total of these variances equals the difference between actual costs incurred for direct labor and the standard cost of direct labor assigned to the SU, a patient meal in this example.

Actual direct labor ($6.25 × 180 hours)	$ 1,125
– **Standard cost** ($0.60 × 1,500 meals)	900
= **Total variance**	$ 225
Price variance	$ 45
Efficiency variance	150
Volume variance	30
Total variance	$225

The intensity variance results from the difference between the quantity of SUs actually required in treating a patient and the quantity called for in the STP. For example, if 20 meals were provided a patient categorized as DRG #208, there would be a favorable variance of five meals given the STP data in Table 3–3–2.

Intensity variances are generically defined in the following way:

$$\left(\begin{array}{c} \text{Actual} \\ \text{SUs} \end{array} - \begin{array}{c} \text{Standard} \\ \text{SUs} \end{array}\right) \times \text{Price per SU}$$

The intensity variance for this patient with respect to meals would be a favorable $12.50, expressed as (20 meals – 25 meals) × $2.50.

It may be useful to split intensity variances into fixed and variable elements. In this example, it is probably not fair to say that $12.50 was realized in savings because five fewer meals were delivered. Five times $1.30, the variable cost, may be a better reflection of short-term realized savings.

In addition to determining variances, it is important to specify the party responsible for the variances. After all, this is part of the basis for standard costing—being able to take action through individuals to correct unfavorable variances. It is clear that three variances—price, efficiency, and volume—will be isolated in the department accounts. However, the departmental manager may not be responsible for all variation, especially in the volume area. Usually, most departmental managers have little control over volume. They merely react to the services required from their departments.

The intensity variance can be largely associated with a given physician. Most of the SUs are of a medical nature and result from physician decisions regarding testing or length of stay. It may be very useful, therefore, to accumulate intensity variances by physicians. Periodic discussions regarding these variations can be most useful to both the health care executive and the physician. Ideally, physicians should take an active role in developing the STPs.

Using a standard costing approach based on SCPs and STPs is an effective way to assess planning decisions. It is also useful in control decisions. As prospective pricing and competitive discounting take on greater importance, so will standard costing in the increasing effort to contain health care costs while providing quality care.

NOTES

1. Cleverley, W. "Cost Accounting Pins a Value to DRGs." *Modern Healthcare* 14 (April 1984): 172–179.

2. Horngren, C. *Cost Accounting: A Managerial Emphasis.* 4th ed. Englewood Cliffs, N.J.: Prentice-Hall, 1977.

3. Cleverley, W. "Reimbursement Management." *Topics In Health Care Financing* 4 (Fall 1977): 13–28.

4. American Hospital Association. *Cost Finding and Rate Setting for Hospitals.* Financial Management Series. Chicago: AHA, 1968.

5. Lerner, W., Wellman, W., and Burik, D. "Pricing Hospital Units of Service Using Microcosting Techniques." *Hospital and Health Services Administration* 30 (January–February 1985): 7–28.

6. Suver, J., and Neumann, B. *Management Accounting for Health Care Organizations.* Chicago: Hospital Financial Management Association, 1981.

Reading 3–4

A Microcosting Approach

Steven A. Finkler

In the current financial environment for hospitals, there has been general dissatisfaction with the cost accounting information traditionally available. This has led many hospitals to seek out new, computerized cost accounting systems. One approach that has been receiving growing attention in the research literature is the use of microcosting on either a regular or a special study basis.

Microcosting, sometimes referred to as component enumeration, is the process of closely examining the actual resources consumed by a particular patient or service. This may be done on an ongoing basis, either manually or by computer, or on a one-shot basis, typically manually.

The main thrust of a microcosting effort is to avoid arbitrary allocations as much as possible in collecting cost information for some particular purpose. In that way, the information generated is far superior for decision-making purposes. However, hospitals have traditionally relied to a great extent on such allocations, which save a great amount of accounting time and effort although they generate less informative data.

DIRECT COSTS

The costs that are generally of interest in microcosting used for special studies are the "direct

Source: Reprinted from Steven A. Finkler, "A Microcosting Approach," *Health Care Management Review,* Vol. 12, No. 4, Fall 1987, pp. 39–48. Copyright © 1987, Aspen Publishers, Inc.

costs" of providing care. They are costs that are incurred in order to provide the care but that would not be incurred if the patient were not treated. This type of cost is often called the "relevant cost" or "incremental cost."

The classification of a cost as direct or indirect for a microcosting study depends to some degree on the number of patients. For example, one lab test can be performed with no addition of equipment, so equipment is not a cost of treating the patient in a special-purpose microcosting study. However, if the volume of patients and lab tests per patient rises beyond some level, additional equipment will be needed, and it becomes a direct cost.

Similarly, five minutes of extra nursing time for one patient will not have any impact on costs. On the other hand, one or two hours of extra nursing time per patient day for a number of patients will generate substantial additional costs. Those costs can be identified only by microcosting studies.

Suppose, for example, that two different types of patients are both classified by a patient acuity system as being at the most costly level for the unit, perhaps a 5 on a scale of 1 to 5. One type of patient might well consistently require a half hour or an hour more of care per patient day, unless we happen to have a really outstanding patient acuity system.

Note also that direct costs may be either variable or fixed. For example, suppose that we wanted to microcost the impact of AIDS patients' outpatient visits on the hospital. If the hospital has a clinic, labor costs (staff, physicians and nurses) may vary with volume, while space and equipment would not. In that situation, labor is a variable cost that is a direct increment resulting from patients' visits. If the clinic is already fully equipped and has sufficient capacity for the AIDS patients, then the depreciation and other fixed costs of the clinic would not be increased by visits by AIDS patients, at least in the short run.

However, if the volume of AIDS patients is so great that an additional clinic area must be added, the cost of acquiring the space and equipping it becomes a direct cost relevant to the AIDS patients, even though these items are fixed rather than variable costs.

The microcosting would have to include such fixed costs. To find the cost per AIDS patient visit, those fixed costs would have to be allocated. However, because the fixed costs were incurred specifically because of the extra patient volume due to the AIDS patients, the allocation is not an arbitrary allocation of a preexisting joint cost.

Certainly, in setting a price for services, the hospital may choose to include a share of general overhead costs. However, since the same amount of joint costs would be incurred regardless of whether we choose to treat these additional AIDS patients or not, they are inappropriate information for making a decision as to whether we are better off with or without the AIDS patients.

COST MEASUREMENT

We frequently talk of using direct or incremental or relevant costs (see for example, "Cost Information for Nonroutine Decisions," *Hospital Cost Accounting Advisor,* Vol. 1, No. 3), but relatively little is written about how to obtain them.

The microcosting method calls for the development of a flowchart that identifies all of the activities that constitute the productive process of providing the care under investigation. Once the flowchart is developed, the direct variable and fixed costs are identified. The amount of re-

sources consumed by each workstep in the process of providing the care is measured, and the costs of the components are determined.

Time and motion studies and work-sampling are often employed to determine the personnel time consumed by each workstep or element. This approach to costing is time consuming and therefore costly. However, it provides a very accurate measure of resources actually consumed and their cost.

The steps involved in microcosting are (a) preparation of detailed flowcharts, (b) description of the worksteps involved in each flowchart step, (c) development of data collection instruments and a sampling plan, (d) measurement of personnel time, disposables, and depreciation for each workstep, and (e) assignment of dollar costs for the resources consumed in each of the worksteps.

Preparation of Detailed Flowcharts

In order to identify the resources consumed during a patient stay or visit, it is first necessary to make a flowchart of the patient stay or visit. First a generic flowchart documents the range of possible reasons for hospitalization. For each of those reasons, a separate flowchart must be created tracing the patient from admission to discharge. For each part of each of these flowcharts, the specific ancillaries consumed and other major resources utilized must be determined.

Staff in each of the various departments affected should be interviewed to verify the accuracy of the flowcharts.

Description of the Flowchart Worksteps

To measure the cost of the resources, it is necessary to detail the worksteps that make up each major step in treating the patient. Again, clinical staff should be interviewed to check the accuracy of the workstep definitions.

The resources consumed at each workstep must be analyzed to determine whether they are direct costs for the study patient group. For example, blood storage facilities are probably an indirect overhead cost that will not change because of the transfusions for any specific type of patient. On the other hand, the cost of intravenous lines is directly associated with the patient receiving blood.

Development of Data Collection Instruments

After the relevant worksteps have been identified, a set of data collection instruments should be developed. An instrument that divides each workstep into segmented, measurable units or work elements should be developed for each procedure. Each of these instruments will provide a structured record of the consumption of personnel time and supplies for each work element within the workstep. The level of detail of the worksteps can vary depending on the desired level of accuracy and detail in the microcosting results.

Measurement of Time, Supplies, and Depreciation

A cost-finding team should observe the various worksteps for which costs are to be estimated. Time and motion studies should be conducted of hospital personnel carrying out each step. Personnel should also be asked to estimate the length of time it takes them to carry out each task and then to monitor and record their own performance times. These data sources can then be used for cross-validation purposes.

At the same time observations must be made of the various supplies, equipment, and facilities that are used for each step of the process.

Assignment of Dollar Costs

Using the information obtained from the purchasing, payroll, and accounting departments, one can associate the costs of labor, supplies, and equipment with the amount consumed, as recorded in the data collection instruments discussed above. Costs are first determined on a per-unit basis. Costs for each workstep can then

be determined by accumulating the cost of the units consumed in that workstep. All of the worksteps can be accumulated to determine the total costs of treating a patient in one hospitalization or clinic visit.

A MATTER OF DEGREE

The practical use of microcosting is a matter of degree. It is not simply a case of whether or not to microcost, but of how far to carry the microcosting process.

Microcosting is generally applied in rather limited situations, such as determining the cost of administering a particular drug or the cost of some other clinical intervention. This is because the required level of data collection detail for microcosting is substantial. In limited situations, microcosting can be carried out in great detail. Such detail may not always be necessary.

At the other extreme, aggregation of cost information may yield too little information to be of much use in making decisions, such as whether to try to attract a particular type of patient. For example, to assume, as many hospital cost accounting systems do, that all patients receive an equal amount of nursing care per day, is far removed from microcosting. We obtain very little information about the true cost of nursing resources for any particular type of patient.

However, if we were to study patient care for a particular type of patient, such as an AIDS patient, and determine that AIDS patients actually consumed 12 hours of nursing care per patient day in an ICU, while other patients with the same DRG received only six hours, we would be making a movement toward microcosting.

To determine whether the 12 hours of care for an AIDS patient day in an ICU are all RN care or are split in a measured proportion between RN and LPN would be a movement toward greater accuracy. To determine whether the RN care received by a patient was from a senior experienced nurse or a newly licensed RN would be a movement further along the microcosting continuum. To determine exactly which nurse delivered the care and what her hourly rate is would be a further movement. To determine how much time was spent by each specific nurse on each general type of activity (such as giving medication, bathing the patient, etc.) would be a further movement.

To determine the amount of time spent on each element of each activity would be a further movement along the microcosting continuum. For example, we could determine how long it takes to prepare a medication, how long to carry the medication to the patient's bedside, how long to insert an IV, and so on.

The more detailed we get in the microcosting process, the more expensive the costing effort. As a result, microcosting tends to be a matter of degree. One must use judgment in making the trade-off between the value of more precise information and the cost of obtaining it. It is inappropriate to use resources to gain a greater level of detail than is needed to adequately answer the questions that have been posed.

WHO SHOULD MICROCOST?

In some microcosting studies, a large accounting firm or other firm with expertise in industrial engineering techniques is hired to perform the time and motion studies and the remainder of the data collection. However, this is an expertise that will become more and more important to hospitals over time, and in the long run it is probably cheaper and more efficient for hospitals to develop a microcosting capability internally.

4

Cost Allocation

Reading 4–1

The Distinction between Cost and Charges

Steven A. Finkler

A popular topic recently has been the assessment of the economic efficiency with which hospital services are provided. For example, the literature on the economic effects of regionalization has been increasing.[1–4] More studies of economic impact have been appearing in medical journals as society's concern over health care costs has increased. Which services will be provided and where they will be provided are receiving greater scrutiny, and cost has become a major issue. Because the results of scrutiny, such as decisions regarding capital investment, have a direct impact on the medical community, medical researchers are taking an active part in assessing the economic efficiency of services and procedures, and practitioners are becoming concerned with the results of those studies. The medical researcher assessing financial information is entering the complex area of financial management. It is important that both the researcher and the practitioner be aware of some of the complications of hospital financial management.

Most studies of economic efficiency attempt to examine costs incurred under different situations.

Source: Reprinted from Steven A. Finkler, "The Distinction between Costs and Charges," *Annals of Internal Medicine,* Vol. 96, No. 1, January 1982, pp. 102–109. Copyright 1982, American College of Physicians.

If a large number of hospitals with a wide range of volume for a particular service all have approximately the same cost per unit, one may conclude that volume does not have a significant impact on cost. However, these studies often use the charges that appear on patient bills as a proxy for cost. The terms cost and charges are used interchangeably in such studies, creating a serious problem in evaluating results because charges typically vary from actual costs. This article traces the process by which hospitals find their costs and set their rates that determine charges so that readers of research on medical economic efficiency can determine whether charge information was used in studies where cost information would have been more appropriate, or vice versa.

THE ROOTS OF THE MISUNDERSTANDING

It is not surprising that many members of the medical community assume there is a close relation between costs and charges. Since most health organizations are nonprofit, it is logical to assume that price is set to be equal to cost. Furthermore, there has been substantial focus on the ills of cost-reimbursement systems such as Blue Cross, Medicare, and Medicaid because of the direct relation between cost and reimbursement.

As costs rise, reimbursement rises automatically. There is minimal incentive to be efficient and control costs if all cost increases are automatically passed to Blue Cross or the government.

This example of passing on costs is an oversimplification of the cost-reimbursement mechanism, but is basically correct. Costs, after disallowance of specific items, are the amount that Blue Cross, Medicare, and Medicaid pay. However, none of those three groups pays the amount that is known as charges. Charges are list prices. The power of Blue Cross' size and the legal clout of the government entitle them to demand discounts off the list price. In fact, the discounts are so great that often Blue Cross, Medicare, and Medicaid pay less than the average cost.[5]

On the other hand, self-pay patients and private insurance companies other than Blue Cross have significantly less clout, and pay not only the costs they have incurred, but also make up any loss the hospital incurs when it gives substantial discounts to Blue Cross, Medicare, and Medicaid. Charges must be set high enough to make sure this compensation occurs.

Before getting into the specifics of the cost-finding and rate-setting process, an example may elucidate the basic distinction between cost and charges. Consider two automobile manufacturers with a similar line of cars. The first manufacturer, JM, is huge, selling 10 million cars. The second manufacturer, Kryler, is smaller, selling only 1 million cars. Both had been producing their cars for a cost of $4,200 each. Then the government introduced a law stating that a pollution control system must be developed. Each firm invested $1 billion to solve the pollution problem. To JM, this resulted in a cost increase of $100 per car ($1 billion ÷ 10 million cars). To Kryler, with its smaller volume of cars to absorb the development costs, this increased costs by $1,000 per car ($1 billion ÷ 1 million cars). JM cars then cost $4,300 to produce and Kryler cars cost $5,200 to produce. JM sold its new cars for $5,000. At this price they made a $700 profit per car.

If one asked a buyer of a JM car, "What did it cost?" the buyer would undoubtedly say, "$5,000." However, we wouldn't expect the buyer to use the $5,000 price interchangeably with cost when cost was meant in the economic sense of the cost of production. Although we would never assume the purchase price to be equal to the production cost, we often make that assumption with respect to hospital services.

The Kryler car, which is virtually identical to the JM car, also had a price of $5,000. At this price they will lose $200 per car. Why didn't Kryler charge the production cost for the cars? At a $5,200 Kryler price, all customers would have purchased cars from JM. So Kryler was forced to charge only $5,000 and incur a loss.

One can think of Kryler as a low-volume producer of a medical service such as open heart surgery, and JM as a high-volume producer of open heart surgery. Kryler's cost per unit is much higher because of the need to spread fixed costs over fewer units. Examination of the price charged by the two gives no clue to the differences in production cost. Yet, while we wouldn't assume that the same selling price of two manufacturers means they have the same cost of production, we do make that assumption about hospitals.

This doesn't imply that hospitals are just like automobile makers. JM and Kryler are openly in competition. One earns a profit, the other loses money. Yet non-profit hospitals have been known to compete with each other. Furthermore, while some hospitals lose money, others (even if not making a net profit) must profit enough on the self-pay patients to make up for losses on Medicaid patients.

Unit costs are not always an inverse function of volume. Economic theory generally predicts that economies of scale will exist over a certain range of volume, but above that range diseconomies are expected. For example, in health care the regionalization process would at some point result in travel costs exceeding the savings of further regionalization. We neither support nor deny the existence of scale economies in the production of specialized health services; however, information about the price charged at medical centers with different volumes is inadequate to assess whether scale economies exist.

THE COST-FINDING PROCESS

In an economic sense, cost is represented by foregone opportunities. If we use a resource for one purpose, it cannot be used for another. We can think of cost in terms of the resources consumed. If one patient consumes more resources than another, we would say that the patient causes the health care institution to incur more cost.

For most studies of economic efficiency, the costs in question may be thought of as marginal costs. A marginal cost is the extra amount of resource consumption incurred for providing a service as compared to the costs of not providing the same service. For instance, how much more will a hospital consume if it has a neonatal intensive care unit than if it does not? We can think of the marginal cost for an entire service, such as neonatal intensive care, or for an extra patient in neonatal intensive care.

The dollar measurement of resource consumption is difficult. Hospital costs are in fact frequently the charge of a producer from whom the hospital has purchased resources. For example, a bypass pump costing the hospital $80,000 to buy may have cost the vendor only $60,000 to produce. The vendor in turn has purchased the components elsewhere, so the pump cost includes charges of its vendors. Thus, the dollar measurement of actual resource consumption cost is quite complicated. However, we can distinguish between the cost to the hospital and the charges by that hospital. Economic cost will be used to refer to the price paid by the health care institution for the resources it consumes. It is conceivable that for some studies a researcher might wish to add to this other cost, such as increased travel for patients, visitors, and physicians. In other cases researchers may be more interested in vendor costs than hospital costs. The issue at hand is not what measure is appropriate for any study, but the idea that charges are not equal to, nor necessarily a good approximation of, what a hospital pays for the resources it consumes in providing services.

Studies of economic efficiency usually start with a definition of economic cost as being the price paid for the resources consumed. In comparing the cost of performing 100 open-heart operations at one location to the cost of 50 open-heart operations at each of two locations, the economic issue is whether the one, centralized high-volume location results in less total resource consumption than the total of the resources consumed by the two separate low-volume locations. In economic theory, the consumption would be less if some of the resources are fixed costs. A resource is a fixed cost if the amount consumed does not vary with volume. For example, if a bypass pump can handle up to 250 patients per year, the high-volume center might need one, whereas the low-volume centers would need one each. Total cost would be higher for two centers than for one, since two pumps are used instead of one. This assumes that extra costs of centralization such as increased travel do not more than offset the cost of the additional pump.

However, under the pricing system in health care organizations, the patient charges at both the low- and high-volume centers will not reflect the difference in resource consumption of bypass pumps. The hospital cost accounting systems do not accumulate cost information by patient, but by department instead. In assigning resource consumption costs to departments, a large degree of accuracy is lost. Depending on the specific accounting procedure, costs may not be assigned to the department in which the consumption occurred.

Once the costs have been allocated to the various departments, they are assigned to units of service, which are used to allocate costs to individual patients. At this stage the association of actual resource consumption with the measured accounting cost becomes less precise. Not only may a department be attempting to assign a total amount of cost that is not representative of the resources consumed by that department, but it also may assign its costs to patients in a different proportion than their actual consumption of that department's services. Thus, what the health care organization calls the patient's cost is not the economic cost in the sense of the specific resources the patient consumed. Studies that have recognized this to be the case, either implicitly or explicitly, measured cost by directly examining resource consumption,[2-3, 6] a task that requires more time, effort, and cost than does use of charge data. The costs accumulated by the hospital cost accounting system will be called the accounting cost here.

DETERMINATION OF EACH DEPARTMENT'S COSTS

Most costs incurred by each department can be directly associated with that department. Most salaries and supplies are department specific. However, there is an element of cost that arises because of the services departments provide for each other. It is the cost of these services that is of particular interest.

For example, when a patient has a roentgenogram, all resources consumed in providing that roentgenogram are part of the patient's cost. One of the costs is the laundry expense of the laboratory coat worn by the technician. However, that cost is incurred in the laundry department and must be charged to the X-ray department. In a similar fashion, since patients do not come into direct contact with the laundry department, all of its costs must be charged to the various departments that utilize its services.

Ultimately, all costs must be assigned to the departments that charge the patients directly for their services. In a hospital, departments such as radiology, laboratory, and operating room are known as cost and revenue centers. Departments such as admitting, housekeeping, maintenance, and dietary are cost centers only. All of the expense of the cost centers must be assigned to the revenue centers. This allows the organization to accumulate all costs in the departments for which bills are issued, and determine how much it must charge to recover all of its costs.

To understand fully the problems of equating resource consumption with the patient generating that resource consumption, it is necessary to see how the cost allocation process works.

The commonest method for allocation is the step-down method. This method allocates the costs of one cost center to all other cost centers, both those that are and are not revenue centers. Once the costs have been allocated from a cost center, it is deemed "closed," meaning that no other cost center can assign costs to it. After each cost center is allocated, there remains one center fewer in the analysis.

A "depreciation" cost center might seem reasonable, and depreciation would be the first center allocated. All departments consume some space, yet none provides any services to the building itself. If depreciation is allocated fairly to the departments, there is no problem, but determination of a fair basis is a problem. Should depreciation be based on square feet or cubic feet? Are all areas of the building equally costly to build? Other cost centers cause similar problems. Should laundry department costs be based on pounds or pieces? Although such allocations usually are arbitrary, the process typically is not a major problem in cost determination.

A more serious problem is that of cost centers providing services to each other. The general administration departments service the housekeeping department, which in turn keeps the administrative departments clean. Which department is allocated first? The order of allocation can have a significant impact on which department ultimately bears the costs of the organization.

In Table 4–1–1 four departments are shown, two of which are revenue centers and two of which are not. Cost centers A and B each incur $100 of cost directly. The laboratory incurs $100 directly and medical/surgical incurs $500. Using some relatively fair allocation basis, we determine that 70% of center A's services are provided to center B, 25% to the laboratory, and 5% to medical/surgical. Cost center B does not provide any service to center A and only 20% of its efforts are for the laboratory. Most of center B's services (80%) are provided to medical/surgical. We would expect that most of center A's cost should wind up in medical/surgical, since 5% of center A's cost goes directly to medical/surgical,

Table 4–1–1 Hypothetical Use of Cost Centers

| | Nonrevenue Cost Centers | | Revenue Cost Centers | | |
	A	B	Lab	Med/Surg	Total
Direct department cost	$100	$100	$100	$500	$800
Relative use of center A		70%	25%	5%	
Relative use of center B	0%		20%	80%	

Table 4–1–2 Hypothetical Allocations to Revenue Centers

| | Nonrevenue Cost Centers | | Revenue Cost Centers | | |
	A	B	Lab	Med/Surg	Total
Direct department cost	$100	$100	$100	$500	$800
Distribution of center A	−100	+70	+25	+5	
Subtotal	$ 0	$170	$125	$505	
Distribution of center B		−170	+34	+136	
Total		$ 0	$159	$641	$800

and 70% of center A's cost goes to center B, which allocates 80% of its cost to medical/surgical. Since 70% × 80% = 56%, and we have 5% directly from center A to medical/surgical, 61% or $61 out of center A's $100 should wind up in medical/surgical. Additionally, 80% of center B's cost, or $80, should go to medical/surgical. Altogether, approximately $141 of the $200 total cost of centers A and B should wind up in the medical/surgical revenue center.

Table 4–1–2 shows what happens when we step-down from center A to B to the revenue centers. Center A is allocated in a 70%, 25%, 5% proportion to center B, laboratory, and medical/surgical, respectively. Center B, which then has $170 of cost because of allocations from center A, is allocated to laboratory and medical/surgical in a 20%, 80% proportion, respectively. The outcome is exactly what makes sense from an economic resource consumption perspective; $141 of cost centers A and B winds up in medical/surgical.

However, there may be reasons for an organization to change the allocation order. Suppose for example that due to Medicare ceilings on the medical/surgical per diem reimbursement rate, the hospital cannot receive more than $600 in revenues for the medical/surgical cost center. The hospital will lose $41.

A restatement of the allocation order, going from B to A to the revenue centers, is shown in Table 4–1–3. Center B's cost is allocated to center A, laboratory, and medical/surgical in the 0%, 20%, 80% proportion that it provides service to those departments (Table 4–1–3). However, center A's cost must be allocated solely between laboratory and medical/surgical, since department B is already closed. Because center A provides 25% of its services directly to the laboratory, and only 5% of its services directly to medical/surgical, the allocation is on a proportion of 25 to 5. This result means that five sixths of center A's cost winds up in laboratory and only one sixth in medical/surgical, even though in reality center A pri-

Table 4-1-3 Hypothetical Distribution of Costs

	Nonrevenue Cost Centers		Revenue Cost Centers		
	B	A	Lab	Med/Surg	Total
Direct department cost	$100	$100	$100	$500	$800
Distribution of center B	−100	+0	+20	+80	
Subtotal	$ 0	$100	$120	$580	
Distribution of center A		−100	+83	+17	
Total		$ 0	$203	$597	$800

marily serves B and center B primarily serves medical/surgical. Since Medicare reimburses laboratory without a ceiling, and medical/surgical costs are now only $597, the hospital does not lose the $41 it would have lost by allocating center A to B first instead of center B to A. This process has been referred to as creative accounting.

Although the example presents an extreme case, consider how many departments are in a hospital and that many of these departments provide services to several other departments. Since the hospital or other health care organization is more concerned with recovering its full costs than with assigning each department exactly the costs for which it is responsible, it would be reasonable to expect the organization to order the departments for step-down in an advantageous sequence.

In the management of a health care organization, securing maximum reimbursement is vital. However, researchers must be aware that this effort may result in cross-subsidization among departments. Ultimately, the cost assigned to the patient may be wrong due to allocation methods meant to secure maximum reimbursement rather than to accurately reflect resource consumption on a department-by-department basis. Because departments are closed to allocation progressively, even if there were no attempt to increase reimbursement some departments would not be able to allocate their expenses to the other departments that cause them to consume resources, leading to probable misallocation.

ALLOCATION OF DEPARTMENT COSTS TO UNITS OF SERVICE

Once costs have been assigned to departments, some measure of unit cost must be determined to use as a basis for rate-setting. For example, the laboratory must determine the cost per blood gas test; the radiology department must know the cost per chest roentgenogram; the pharmaceutical department must know the cost per aspirin. These costs must be calculated in such a way that the total costs of the revenue centers (after receiving assigned costs from the nonrevenue cost centers) are allocated to the individual units of service provided. There are four basic methods for this allocation; each hospital will probably use all four, selecting for each department the most applicable method.

The Weighted Procedure Method

For routine tasks, the weighted procedure method is especially useful. Each product of a department is assigned a number of relative units. For example, in the laboratory each test would have a number assigned to it that represents its relative resource consumption. These weightings are based on consumption of supplies, equipment, and personnel. State hospital associations frequently compute a standardized set of relative value units that hospitals may refer to. The process requires evaluating how much time each procedure uses, such as direct production, preparation, evaluation, and supervision time. The cost of this time is based on the hourly rate plus fringe benefits of appropriate personnel. Total personnel cost is added to materials and equipment costs, consisting of overhead, equipment depreciation, and direct materials used. Once a total is determined for each procedure, all procedures are compared. One procedure, twice as costly as another, would be assigned a relative value twice as high as that of the other procedure. In this way a standardized list of relative values may be prepared. Different hospitals can assign their different costs using the standardized list as a basis for the relative resource consumption of each test.

A blood gas test might have a weighting of 40, whereas an acetone test might have a weight of 10. Thus, if a laboratory did 100 blood gas tests and 200 acetone tests, there would be a total of 6,000 relative value units (40 units × 100 tests = 4,000; 10 units × 200 tests = 2,000; 4,000 + 2,000 = 6,000). If the total cost of the laboratory (both direct costs and those assigned through the step-down process) were $1,200, the cost per relative value unit would then be 20 cents ($1,200 ÷ 6,000 total units). Therefore, the cost of a blood gas test would be $8 (40 units at 20 cents apiece) and an acetone test would be $2 (10 units at 20 cents).

The main problem with the weighted procedure method is the expense of performing the necessary observations of each procedure and then converting the various components into units suitable for assessing relative values. This procedure is so costly, in fact, that most hospitals use industry standards rather than computing the relative values themselves.

All institutions do not provide their services in exactly the same manner. In one hospital the pay scale for technicians is higher than another. Different hospitals use different machines for similar tests. Consider an example where a blood gas test is given 40 relative value units based on 10 units for labor, 20 units for equipment, and 10 units for a variety of other factors. If two hospitals have different pay scales, but exactly the same equipment, it is not possible for the labor cost to be exactly half as much as the equipment

cost in both hospitals. However, the use of industry-wide standard relative value units per type of test implies that to be the case.

This problem results because the use of industry-wide relative value unit standards assumes all hospitals to be exactly the same. The resource consumption for each type of test is assumed to be the same in every hospital relative to all other tests in that hospital. That is, if a blood gas test is twice as expensive as an acetone test in one hospital, it is twice as expensive as an acetone test in every hospital. This assumption is highly unlikely given the differences between hospitals. Yet, the cost to calculate the relative values separately in each institution would be excessive. Industry standard relative values are good enough for the main hospital cost accounting purpose, which is to allocate the costs of the departments to the patients. Slight misallocations between patients are tolerable, as long as all costs are distributed to the patients. But a researcher using this information must be aware that the cost for any type of patient, when measured in this way, is one step farther away from economic cost in the sense of resource consumption.

The Hourly Rate Method

The problems of using time as a proxy for resource consumption are even greater. The common approach for assigning costs of departments such as surgery, physiotherapy, inhalation therapy, and anesthesia is to accumulate all costs for the department and then divide by the total amount of service provided, using minutes or hours as a measure of service. If there are 60 hours of inhalation therapy during the month and the total costs of the department are $6,000, there is a cost of $100 per hour ($6,000 ÷ 60 hours).

In general this approach is reasonable if all patients tend to make use of the same resources. The chief problem, however, is when a department has a wide variety of resources available for use, but the patients' consumption of those resources varies widely. For example, a patient having an appendectomy does not require the equipment available in the operating room for use in open-heart surgery. Yet such patients are charged as much on a per-minute basis as the patient having open-heart surgery. Essentially, the operating room is a source of substantial cross-subsidization between patients requiring expensive equipment and those who do not.

Consider the implications of this subsidization in the regionalization debate. If 50 open-heart operations are done in a hospital per year, the hospital must acquire a significant amount of specialized equipment. Assuming that the average length of time of an open-heart procedure is 4 hours, then the 50 patients having heart surgery account for 200 hours of surgery time. If the hospital has three operating rooms, busy on average 8 hours per day, 5 days a week, 50 weeks per year, there are 2,000 hours of surgery. Patients having open-heart surgery are assigned only 10% of the cost for operating-room equipment that had to be added for them. Any estimation of the effects of regionalization on a service such as open-heart surgery is inaccurate if it uses the operating room cost assigned to the patient having heart surgery, instead of estimating the extra resources consumed. Clearly, no one wants to win the debate on regionalization based on misspecification of data. Thus, it is not possible to draw conclusions about cost in the economic sense of resource utilization if one uses cost data assigned on the basis of hourly usage.

The Surcharge Method

The third method for the allocation of department cost to patients also creates a gap between cost assigned and resources used. This method is commonly used by pass-through departments such as central supply or pharmacy. The main cost in these departments is for the supplies that they purchase, stock, and pass-through to the patient. The costs of the department, excluding the purchase price of items, to be passed through, are compared to the direct cost of the items passed through to determine a surcharge rate. For example, if the pharmacy department has a total cost for pharmaceuticals of $100,000,

and has other costs, such as labor and overhead, of $50,000, then the surcharge rate is 50% ($50,000 ÷ $100,000).

The implications of this method are astonishing. A patient consuming an aspirin costing a penny would be assigned a cost of 1.5 cents for the aspirin and its purchase, stocking, and distribution. The patient consuming an expensive drug costing the hospital $10 would be charged $15. The discrepancy between the $1/2$ cent of labor and overhead to process the aspirin and the $5 to process the sophisticated medication may be partly offset by a policy to assign a minimum processing cost for each pill or drug, and then allocate remaining costs on a surcharge basis.

Per Diem

In departments or cost centers where these three methods are deemed inappropriate (such as in the maintenance, housekeeping, nursing, or dietary departments), total costs are divided by total patient days to determine a cost per patient-day, or a per-diem cost. Here the opportunities for cross-subsidization, or averaging across patients, become the greatest. Who pays for the availability of the defibrillator at the end of the hall: the patients who use it, those who are likely to use it, or everyone? If the cost is thrown into the per diem, everyone will pay based on their length of stay. It would seem that the patients highly unlikely to use the defibrillator are having too much cost assigned, whereas those likely to use it or actually using it are assigned too little cost. Nevertheless, such equipment ordinarily is accounted for on a per-diem basis.

SUMMARY OF THE COST-FINDING PROCESS

This entire cost-allocation process derives accounting costs rather than economic costs. In addition to the various issues just discussed, accounting costs differ from economic costs because by their very nature they tend to be average costs. The total cost for a department is divided by the number of units of service, to get an average cost per unit. As discussed earlier, however, economic cost is based on a marginal concept. Thus, if we asked the cost to do an additional roentgenogram, the economic cost would include only the extra or additional resources needed for that additional procedure. This cost would probably include no equipment cost, since the equipment already would be there. The accounting cost of an additional roentgenogram would be the average cost for roentgenograms of that type and would include a share of the cost of the machine. The correct choice depends on whether we are concerned with how many more dollars the hospital spends (economic cost), or with how much the hospital must collect for each roentgenogram if it is to break even (accounting cost). The key issue is awareness that accounting costs are significantly different in many respects from economic costs.

It is inappropriate to use the terms cost and charges interchangeably, and this section has reviewed the cost-finding process in hospitals because charges are not set until accounting costs are determined. As a measure of economic cost, we have used the concept of resource consumption. Studies of economic efficiency or cost-effectiveness take this approach. In assessing alternatives, we must consider the cost of the resources consumed under the various alternatives.

The cost-finding process is difficult. Starting out with a desire to determine the cost of resources consumed by each patient, one finds problems such as the desire to increase reimbursement based on costs, the need for expedient methods that are not costly in themselves, and theoretical problems regarding the actual consumption of services of jointly consumed resources. Of greater importance is the institution's goal of expedient methods for assigning costs to patients. This goal does not necessarily require that costs be assigned based on true resource consumption by the various patients. There is no requirement in health care cost accounting systems that a patient having open-heart surgery should be assigned 100% rather than 10% of the cost of specialized equipment.

Cross-subsidization between expensive and less expensive patients has long been hospital practice. Accounting costs need not represent economic cost.

In light of this fact, we find that costs are not always allocated in line with resource consumption. Cost allocation to departments depends on how good the base is and the order of step-down. Reimbursement can vary greatly with the sequence selected. Allocation by the department to patients depends on the accuracy of the standard relative units used in a particular institution; the cross-subsidization that occurs in assignment of costs on a time basis; how seriously the surcharge method distorts cost allocated from true resource consumption; and how seriously the general averaging to get a per-diem rate biases costs upward or downward from the cost of resources actually consumed by a patient.

Thus, when one contrasts costs and charges, it must be clearly stated whether charges are being compared to the economic costs based on resource consumption or to the accounting costs based on the hospital's cost-finding system. In this paper, as in most research, economic costs are compared with charges. When accounting cost is used, it is only as a proxy for economic cost, and as the reader may have ascertained, a proxy of questionable value due to the potential differences between economic and accounting cost for a specific patient.

Determination of Charges

Charges are based on the rate-setting process. The first part of the rate-setting process, as described above, consists of converting resource consumption to department costs, department costs to a cost per unit of service provided, and assigning units of service to patients. Those costs form the foundation for cost-based reimbursement. With a few adjustments, reimbursers such as Blue Cross, Medicare, and Medicaid will pay those amounts. The cost-based reimbursement process applies to over half of hospital receipts coming from the government alone.[7]

MAKING THE NUMBERS COME OUT RIGHT

The process of setting charges is not complete at that point. What if a patient cannot pay his or her bill? Many patients are too wealthy for government assistance, but not wealthy enough to pay a $30,000 hospital bill, thus creating a "bad debt." If the hospital is not to lose money every year and eventually go out of business, someone must pay that patient's cost. Thus, patients are charged more than their cost, so that those who pay will cover the losses from those who do not.

There are other factors besides bad debts that cause charges to be greater than cost. Hospitals typically provide free service to families of staff physicians. Often educational programs such as preventive care, family planning, and childbirth classes are provided below cost as a community service. Additionally, Blue Cross in various states disallows some additional items. And Medicare and Medicaid sometimes impose maximum reimbursement rates. All of these factors must be compensated for, but government and Blue Cross will not bear a share of these costs. Therefore, less than half[7] of all patients must compensate for all of the debts, free service, community programs, and disallowed costs. The result is that charges may be substantially more than costs.

We have considered only the recovery of past costs. Yet for a hospital to survive, it must acquire equipment representing new technological advances, and it may need to expand services. At the least, it must replace equipment that wears out or becomes obsolete. New machines cost more than the old ones they replace, but accounting rules allow only the original cost of equipment to be included as a factor in cost calculations. If a hospital pays $50,000 for a roentgenographic machine, its cost is spread out over its lifetime, which may be 5 years. The cost of roentgenograms will be based on a machine cost of $50,000. But if we charge for roentgenograms based on that cost, how will the machine be replaced in 5 years when the same model costs

$80,000 or $100,000 because of inflation? Charges must also include an element to cover expansion and replacement, and since only a small fraction of patients pay at the charge rate, the increase of charges over costs is substantial.

Essentially, the first rule of charges is to make the institution solvent. Given the various costs of the institution, including needs for replacement and expansion, and considering the amount to be received by the reimbursers, charges must be set so that those who pay at the charge rate will make up any difference between total costs and reimbursement. Thus, the average charge is substantially higher than hospital measured costs.

GENERAL AGREEMENT ON RATES

The gap between economic cost and charges is great considering the differences between economic cost and accounting cost, and the need to set charges at a level higher than accounting cost, but the greatest factor in the distortion between cost and charges is the last step in the rate-setting process: comparison of costs to the community. Before final determination of rates, hospitals compare themselves to other hospitals to make sure their rates are in line with the general community. Why this process occurs is unclear, but there may be fear that utilization review committees or government regulators will seize price differentials as signs of inefficiency. Comparison may be made simply not to appear out of line or may relate to basic notions of supply and demand. If one hospital charges more for a major procedure than another, private insurance and self-pay patients will want to use the less expensive hospital. The hospital can ill afford to lose the business of the group that carries a substantial burden in ensuring the solvency of the institution.

Whatever the cause, consensus pricing is widely practiced and the implications enormous. Consider a hypothetical example of two hospitals, each offering open heart surgery—one at a volume of 50 patients and another at a volume of 500. The low-volume hospital has a cost per patient of $5,200, and the high-volume hospital has a cost per patient of $4,300. This discrepancy occurs because there are fewer patients at the low-volume hospital to share a variety of equipment and other fixed costs relating to open-heart surgery.

Under a consensus approach to pricing, the low-volume hospital, if it found that the other hospital charged $4,500, would then set its charge at approximately $4,500. The high-volume producer charges $200 more than cost to recover debts and so forth. This rate leads to a loss of $700 per patient at the low-volume hospital, or a total of $35,000 ($700 × 50 patients). However, this loss is easily offset by increasing the charge in some area where the hospital is particularly efficient, or else by spreading the loss out over a very-large-volume service where it will have minimal effect—for example, 7 cents extra per laboratory test over the hospital's 500,000 volume of laboratory tests. Thus, a charge of $30.07 versus $30.00 for a particular laboratory test would cause much less public notice than a charge of $5,200 versus $4,500 for open-heart surgery.

This discussion is not meant to be an argument for or against regionalization. The numbers are hypothetical and do not make a case for the existence of economies of scale, but demonstrate that charge information cannot be used to prove that economies of scale do not exist. The intent is merely to show the fallacy of using charges to determine if regionalization reduces total resource consumption or cost.

This fallacy has sometimes been formally recognized in research, and sometimes ignored. Marty and associates[8] explicitly recognized the problem. However, they used data on charges and concluded from an examination of charge information that greater volume in itself does not lead to greater economy. This is a highly questionable conclusion to draw on the basis of charge information.

Schwartz and Joskow[1] briefly raise the issue that if charges are an accurate reflection of cost, certain results follow. However, their article does not discuss whether charges will bear any resemblance to cost. They support their contention of the relative insignificance of scale economies in open-heart surgery by citing the fact that in a study[1] examining open-heart surgery caseloads ranging from 60 to 600 patients per year, there was no significant difference in the bills. Given the consensus approach to setting charges, one would not expect to find any difference in the bills, regardless of how substantial the underlying cost differences may be.

The study of Hansing[4] has the same problem. He concluded that regression analysis did not show a fall in charges as volume increased. In fact, Hansing uses costs and charges interchangeably throughout his paper. Economic theory predicts a fall in costs as volume increases, spreading fixed costs over more patients. There is no theory to support expectations of a fall in charges as volume increases. Extreme care is required in drawing conclusions and making policy recommendations based on charge information if those policy decisions are to be based on the cost of providing the care, as opposed to the amount charged for the care. Indeed, it is risky to assume that there is a reasonable correlation between charges and economic cost.

Many studies of the economic efficiency of health care institutions take a social perspective.[1,4] What are the potential savings to society from a particular action such as regionalizing tertiary care? In free-market competitive industries we do not worry about efficiency from a societal viewpoint. An inefficient high-cost producer will be driven out of business by efficient competing firms (low-cost producers). However, in health care, reimbursement tends to be largely cost-based. High-cost producers may receive higher reimbursement rather than being forced out of business. Therefore, studies of economic efficiency in health care institutions tend to focus on the costs of that institution and, all things being equal, whether it costs one institution more than another to provide the same service.

The use of charge data as a proxy for cost can lead researchers to draw unwarranted conclusions about economic efficiency, specifically in studies that contend they are comparing cost, when in fact they are comparing charges. In some cases researchers may well be interested in charge information directly. However, the research questions must be clearly delineated. For example, if a medical researcher were concerned with the economic impact of two competing treatments for a disease, he might be interested in the direct economic impact on patients to be treated for that disease. Charge information might be an appropriate measure. However, if a hospital charged substantially less than its economic costs for treating that disease, it would possibly increase charges for other patients. The total economic impact of the two alternative treatments on all patients might be better assessed by analysis of cost information rather than of charges. The researcher should carefully assess the appropriate data for the research question being posed.

SUMMARY OF THE PROCESS OF SETTING CHARGES

Charges are essentially list prices. Any organization has a right to set a price for its product or services. In the health care field, many purchasers of health care services get a substantial discount from the list price. In fact, they pay a cost-based reimbursement price that may be below average cost.

In determining a list price, profit organizations have often used an approach referred to as charging what the market will bear. If product A costs $100 to produce and can be sold for $150, it yields a $50 profit. If product B costs $120 to produce and can be sold for $125, then it yields only a $5 profit. There is no necessary relation between cost and price.

Nor is there a set relation between cost and price (charges) in health care. An initial difference between cost and price is built into charges to allow for expansion, replacement, bad debts, and disallowed (for reimbursement) costs. Then the resulting set of charges, which are already greater than cost, are adjusted to a community norm. This norm may be more or less than the economic cost or even the accounting cost for a specific patient.

CONCLUSION

In a nonprofit organization, how can there be a difference between cost and charges? If there is not going to be a profit, won't prices (charges) be set so that they are exactly equal to cost? The answer is no; charges are not set equal to costs. In fact, they cannot be if the organization is to survive.

On average, charges must exceed costs because of the need for expansion and replacement of equipment and facilities, increasingly expensive due to inflation and technologic improvement. Charges must exceed costs to cover care to the indigent and courtesy care; costs of a community service; and items disallowed by Blue Cross, Medicare, and Medicaid. And, since the self-pay and non-Blue-Cross private reinsurers make up a small percentage of all patients, charges must be substantially above cost for those who do pay at "list price," since they alone must bear all of the costs and expansion and replacement needs not covered by Blue Cross, Medicare, and Medicaid.

Furthermore, charges are adjusted to get a desired rate structure usually based on community norms. The frequently stated Blue Cross position of paying the "lower of cost or charges" is a reflection of how commonly adjustments to the rate structure are made. Even though charges must be high enough to cover bad debts, expansion, replacement, and disallowed cost, Blue Cross's policy points out that there are likely to be situations in which charges are set lower than cost. And the very existence of paying "lower of cost or charges" is likely to lead to some manipulation of costs and charges to maximize reimbursement.

The gap between accounting costs and charges is potentially great, although in some cases it might be relatively small. There is also a gap between economic cost and accounting cost to contend with, whether that gap results from efforts to increase reimbursement or merely to expeditiously allocate cost. That gap is also potentially great, but in some instances might be small. Researchers attempting to assess economic efficiency must clearly defend their reason for believing these gaps are small if they use charges as a proxy for cost; otherwise, they should collect data on resource consumption and directly attempt to measure economic costs. Readers of research on economic efficiency should be aware of the complexity of the problems involved when costs and charges are assumed to be equal, so that they may make an informed evaluation of the results of such studies.

ACKNOWLEDGMENTS

Grant support: from the National Health Care Management Center at the Leonard Davis Institute of Health Economics, University of Pennsylvania; grant HS-02577 from the National Center for Health Services Research, Office of the Assistant Secretary of Health, Department of Health and Human Services; and the Accounting Department of the Wharton School, University of Pennsylvania.

NOTES

1. Schwartz W.B., Joskow P.L. Duplicated hospital facilities. *N Engl J Med.* 1980;303:1449–57.
2. Finkler S.A. Cost-effectiveness of regionalization: the heart surgery example. *Inquiry.* 1979;16:264–70.
3. McGregor M., Pelletier G. Planning of specialized health facilities: size vs. cost and effectiveness in heart surgery. *N Engl J Med.* 1978;299:179–81.
4. Hansing C.E. The risk and cost of coronary angiography: I. Cost of coronary angiography in Washington State. *JAMA.* 1979;242:731–4.
5. Berman H.J., Weeks L.E. *The Financial Management of Hospitals.* 3rd ed. Ann Arbor: Health Administration Press, 1976:61–4.
6. Harper D.R. Disease cost in a surgical ward. *Br Med J.* 1979;1:647–9.
7. Gibson R.M. National health care expenditures, 1978. *Health Care Financing Review.* 1979;1:1–36.
8. Marty A.T., et al. The variation in hospital charges: a problem in determining the cost/benefit for cardiac surgery. *Ann Thor Surg.* 1977;24:409–16.

Reading 4–2

Using Reciprocal Allocation of Service Department Costs for Decision Making

Lawrence M. Metzger

INTRODUCTION

The allocation of service department costs to other service and hospital production departments has long been a standard procedure in hospitals for such purposes as financial reporting, Medicare records, and other third-party reimbursement requirements. Traditionally, the most commonly used allocation method has been the step-down method. The purpose of this article is to describe the use of the reciprocal allocation method as an alternative to the step-down method for cost allocation purposes. The reciprocal method will not only serve financial reporting requirements but will also provide relevant and accurate information for potential decision-making situations.

STEP-DOWN ALLOCATION

Under the step-down method, service department costs are allocated in sequence to the departments they serve. The departments are ranked so that the cost of the one that renders service to the highest number of other departments is allocated first, and the cost of the one rendering service to the lowest number of other departments while receiving benefits from the

Source: Reprinted from Lawrence M. Metzger, "Using Reciprocal Allocation of Service Department Costs for Decision Making," *Hospital Cost Management and Accounting,* Vol. 4, No. 9, December 1992, pp. 1–6. Copyright 1992, Aspen Publishers, Inc.

highest number is allocated last. In essence, the step-down method is a one-way or one-direction allocation method.

This assumption of a one-way service between departments works well enough for financial reporting and in some cases represents the flow of the use of services quite well. For example, consider two service departments: medical records and the hospital cafeteria: While medical records personnel would indeed use the cafeteria to eat, it is unlikely that medical records directly services the cafeteria. In this case the step-down method is quite appropriate as an allocation method.

But there are also numerous situations in which service departments service or interact with each other simultaneously. Maintenance, for example, would service the cafeteria and maintenance personnel would eat in the cafeteria. The hospital power plant would serve the administration department, and the administration department would provide service to the power plant. Cafeteria personnel would also eat in the cafeteria, and the power plant would consume power to run its own operations. In effect these service departments consume part of themselves.

Assigning the costs of support services to production departments can do more than determine costs. The allocation procedure can set up an internal market for the supply and demand of internally produced services. By charging for service departments' output, the hospital can

1. ration demand for user departments
2. provide signals on service department efficiency
3. facilitate comparison of externally supplied services

In general, the step-down method will not compute sufficiently accurate service department cost information for the uses listed above when extensive interactions exist among service departments; this is where the reciprocal method becomes valuable.

RECIPROCAL ALLOCATION

The reciprocal method is conceptually appealing because it recognizes the simultaneous interaction of service departments rather than the somewhat arbitrary, one-directional relationship the step-down method assumes. The accuracy and relevance of the reciprocal method derives from its recognition of the reciprocal relationships of costs among service departments.

Mechanically, the reciprocal method allocates the costs of service departments on a simultaneous basis. The method requires solving a series of simultaneous equations—generally as many equations as there are service departments. The calculations quickly become cumbersome, requiring the use of matrix algebra to solve. Until recently, this method was not practical due to the lack of readily available software to solve the equations.

The reciprocal allocation method can provide useful information for decision making when service departments

1. have variable costs
2. provide service to other service departments or to themselves

A service department's variable costs are those driven in the short run by a specific cost driver. For example, a portion of the power plant costs could be driven by, or variable with respect to, kilowatt hours consumed by the various departments. When there are variable costs in the serv-

ice departments, the relationship between the cost and the other departments—both service and production—is more cause and effect than a pure allocation.

The true variable cost to operate such interacting service departments includes not only the direct variable costs of each department but a portion of the variable costs from the supporting departments.

EXAMPLE

The following example will develop the reciprocal model and show how its output can be used for both financial reporting and decision making. The example illustrates the relationships among four individual service departments in a particular hospital. The four service departments are the hospital's (1) power plant, (2) cafeteria, (3) administration department, and (4) maintenance department.

One advantage of the reciprocal method is that much of the information needed has already been determined for the other allocation procedures. The step-down method requires, at least in one direction, some measure of service department costs and cost drivers for allocation purposes. Statistical analysis—using such techniques as linear regression—can be used at relatively low cost to further refine the data for the reciprocal method.

For this example, statistical analysis has determined the variable costs of the four service departments and the relevant cost drivers for the past year. These data are shown in Table 4–2–1.

RECIPROCAL ALLOCATION PROCEDURE

Matrix algebra will be used to calculate the reciprocal allocation values. (An in-depth discussion of matrix algebra will not be presented here. Refer to a business math book for an explanation of this procedure.) The mechanics of matrix algebra will be handled using the matrix inversion function on Lotus 1-2-3.

Table 4–2–1 Summary of Costs and Cost Drivers

Department	Cost Driver	Cost Driver Level	Variable Cost
Power plant	Kilowatt hours	100,000	$ 600,000
Cafeteria	Number of employees	1,000	160,000
Administration	Payroll dollars	2,000,000	400,000
Maintenance	Number of work orders	100	200,000
Total			$1,360,000

The following steps should be used when applying the reciprocal allocation method with Lotus:

1. Determine the percentage each department uses of the service provided by each service department, including the amount each service department consumes of its own service. These percentages would be based on the volume of the cost driver used by each department. These assumed percents are shown in Table 4–2–2.

For example, of the 100,000 kilowatt hours consumed for the past year, 15 percent was consumed by the power plant itself (S1), 8 percent by the cafeteria (S2), 10 percent by administration (S3), and 12 percent by maintenance (S4). The column labeled "Production" represents the combined percent usage of the cost drivers of all the production departments, examples of which include medical/surgical services, outpatient services, or the nursery. Production departments consumed 55 percent of the total kilowatt hours of power generated by the power plant. In a full allocation situation, the detail of this usage would be broken out by specific production department. Such detail is not necessary for this example.

The amount of the cost driver consumed by each department would be known from the already completed statistical analysis.

2. Set up simultaneous equations for each individual service department to solve for how much cost each service department will ultimately allocate. The equations consist of two parts: the first part is the known variable costs determined from the cost analysis shown above; the second is the percentage of services each service department consumed of itself and the amount of services allocated to it from the other service departments.

This information is provided by the figures in each column of Table 4–2–2. For example, the power plant (S1) allocates its own variable cost of $600,000 plus the amount it consumes of its own service (15 percent of itself) plus the 10 percent of cafeteria cost it consumes plus the 8 percent of administration cost it consumes and finally the 20 percent of maintenance cost it uses. The formulas for the power plant (S1) and the other service departments are as follows:

$S1 = \$600,000 + .15(S1) + .10(S2) + .08(S3) + .20(S4)$
$S2 = \$160,000 + .08(S1) + .05(S2) + .07(S3) + .08(S4)$
$S3 = \$400,000 + .10(S1) + .15(S2) + .08(S3) + .12(S4)$
$S4 = \$200,000 + .12(S1) + .10(S2) + .07(S3) + .05(S4)$

3. Set these equations up into matrix form. To solve them, gather all the unknowns on the left side of the equations and all the known values on

Table 4-2-2 Percent of Total Cost Driver Consumed in Each Department

Department	S1	S2	S3	S4	Production	Total
Power plant (S1)	15%	8%	10%	12%	55%	100%
Cafeteria (S2)	10%	5%	15%	10%	60%	100%
Administration (S3)	8%	7%	8%	7%	70%	100%
Maintenance (S4)	20%	8%	12%	5%	55%	100%

the right side. This procedure would yield the following:

$$+.85(S1) - .10(S2) - .08(S3) - .20(S4) = \$600,000$$
$$-.08(S1) + .95(S2) - .07(S3) - .08(S4) = \$160,000$$
$$-.10(S1) - .15(S2) + .92(S3) - .12(S4) = \$400,000$$
$$-.12(S1) - .10(S2) - .07(S3) + .95(S4) = \$200,000$$

Expressing the above in matrix form yields the following:

$$\begin{array}{ccc} \mathbf{X} & \mathbf{S} & \mathbf{C} \end{array}$$

$$\begin{bmatrix} +.85 & -.10 & -.08 & -.20 \\ -.08 & +.95 & -.07 & -.08 \\ -.10 & -.15 & +.92 & -.12 \\ -.12 & -.10 & -.07 & +.95 \end{bmatrix} \times \begin{bmatrix} S1 \\ S2 \\ S3 \\ S4 \end{bmatrix} \quad \begin{array}{c} \$600,000 \\ \$160,000 \\ \$400,000 \\ \$200,000 \end{array}$$

Expressed in equation form: $X \times S = C$. To solve for the values of S1 through S4, which represents the total costs to allocate for each department, solve for the inverse matrix of X and multiply the inverse matrix by the C matrix.

4. Enter the data shown in Step 3 for both the X matrix and the C matrix into the Lotus spreadsheet. Use the matrix inversion feature in the program to find the inverse of the matrix. The "/ Data Matrix Invert" command calculates the inverse of the X matrix.

The inverse matrix is as follows:

$$\begin{array}{cccc} 1.253 & .186 & .146 & .298 \\ .135 & 1.098 & .105 & .134 \\ .182 & .219 & 1.135 & .200 \\ .186 & .155 & .113 & 1.119 \end{array}$$

5. Use the inverse matrix to calculate the reciprocal cost. This is determined by multiplying the inverse matrix by the matrix, which consists of the variable cost for each department (matrix C). This procedure is also available on Lotus with the "/ Data Matrix Multiply" operation. These amounts will be used for allocating the service department costs for reporting purposes.

The calculated reciprocal costs for each service would be:

S1:	\$899,660
S2:	\$325,374
S3:	\$638,508
S4:	\$405,466

These amounts represent the service department's initial variable cost, plus the amount allocated to each service department from the other service departments.

The allocation of the service department variable costs is shown in Table 4–2–3.

Notice that the total amount of cost allocated to the production departments equals the total original amount of service department variable cost: \$600,000 + \$160,000 + \$400,000 + \$200,000 = \$1,360,000. So the reciprocal method has allocated the correct amount of cost for financial reporting purposes.

DECISION-MAKING ANALYSIS

In addition to the allocation information above, a key advantage to the reciprocal method is the data it can provide for decision making.

Table 4-2-3 Allocation of Service Department Variable Costs*

	S1	S2	S3	S4	Production
Initial cost	\$600,000	\$160,000	\$400,000	\$200,000	N/A
Assigned by S1	134,949	71,973	89,966	107,959	\$ 494,813
Assigned by S2	32,537	16,269	48,806	32,537	195,225
Assigned by S3	51,081	44,696	51,081	44,696	446,956
Assigned by S4	81,093	32,437	48,656	20,273	223,006
Assigned out	(899,660)	(325,374)	(638,508)	(405,466)	0
Net cost assigned					\$1,360,000

*Any small differences in totals are due to rounding.

Refer back to the inverse matrix. The numbers on the main diagonal (the line running from the upper left to the lower right) are called the reciprocal factors for the service departments. The reciprocal factor for S1 is 1.253; for S2, 1.098; for S3, 1.135; and for S4, 1.119. These factors tell us how much the total production of the service department will fall if the external demand (outside the service department) on the service department is reduced by one unit.

For example, a one-kilowatt-hour reduction in demand will reduce kilowatt-hour requirements in the power plant by 1.253 hours.

More information may be taken from this output. The next item that can be calculated is the charge rate. The individual reciprocal costs for each department divided by the total level of the cost driver used for each service will yield the charge rate for that particular service:

S1: $899,660/100,000 kwh   = $9.00/kilowatt hour
S2: $325,374/1,000 employees = $325 per employee
S3: $638,508/200,000 payroll $ = $3.19/payroll dollar
S4: $405,466/100 work orders = $4,055/work order

It turns out that the charge rate (for variable costs) is equivalent to the out-of-pocket or marginal cost of the service. So for the power plant, if the total demand by the production divisions were reduced by one kilowatt hour, the total variable costs in the system would fall by $9.00. This charge rate provides an accurate measure of the marginal cost of providing the service.

The charge rate has various uses. It can be used to help ration demand for user departments by providing relevant and accurate data for setting charge-back prices. Also, it can help measure service department efficiency by providing data that helps set standard costs for these services. In addition, if an outside bid to provide a service—such as power or a contract for maintenance—is received, the charge rate would be compared to the price quoted for the outside service.

More useful information may also be found in the reciprocal output. If a service department with reciprocal relationships is shut down, the number of units of service that would have to be purchased externally would be lower than the current production of the internal service department. When the units of service are purchased outside, the current reciprocal pattern of consumption is altered, because the remaining departments do not have to provide service to the external supplier.

Continuing on, dividing the total level of the service department cost driver by the service department's reciprocal factor provides information about the number of outside units that would have to be purchased if internal production were discontinued. Again using the power plant as the example: 100,000 kwh/1.253 = 79,808 hours. If the hospital discontinued internal production of power, 79,808 kilowatt hours of power would have to be purchased externally. The power plant consumes 20,192 (100,000 – 79,808) units of its own output.

It also turns out that dividing the reciprocal cost by the reciprocal factor will yield the total variable cost saved or avoided if this service is eliminated. This amount can be used along with the charge factor above to compare against alternative sources of this service.

In this example the results would be as follows:

S1: 899,660/1.253   = $718,005
S2: 325,374/1.098   = $296,333
S3: 638,508/1.135   = $562,562
S4: 405,466/1.119   = $362,347

For the power plant (S1), the total variable cost avoided if the power plant were shut down is $718,005.

SUMMARY

This article has provided a look into the use of the reciprocal method as an alternative to more conventional methods of hospital service department cost allocation methods. The reciprocal method can be used with readily available software and with data that are largely already known. This method will provide not only appropriate allocation values for financial reporting but data that can be used for hospital decision making. In the highly competitive and sometimes hostile environment in which hospitals now fight to survive, any additional relevant data—especially that generated at almost no additional cost—should be provided to managers to help in the decision-making process.

BIBLIOGRAPHY

1. Hay, L., Wilson, E. *Accounting for Governmental and Nonprofit Entities,* 9th edition. Boston, Mass.: Irwin, 1992.

2. Kaplan, R., Atkinson, A. *Advanced Managerial Accounting,* 2nd Edition. Englewood Cliffs, NJ: Prentice-Hall, 1989.

Reading 4–3

RVUs: Relative Value Units or Really Very Useful?

Kirk Mahlen

By now, I'm sure that everyone involved in hospital finance has at least heard of the term "RVU." Yet, for many, doubts still exist as to what is actually involved in developing RVUs and effectively utilizing those values for procedure/patient-level costing. The purpose of this article is to provide an easy-to-understand, step-by-step example describing RVU development and use of RVUs in procedure/patient-level costing.

Given that everyone accepts the need to move away from RCCs as a costing method in the current regulatory environment, RVUs are an extremely cost-effective solution for improving the reliability and accuracy of cost data for many hospitals. With assistance from hospital department heads, it is possible to develop and maintain RVU cost information in most hospitals with a minimum of 1 FTE. While limited assistance and/or direction from an outside "expert" is certainly optional, it is strongly suggested in order to avoid certain pitfalls.

In addition to personnel resources, software will be required to facilitate the development and maintenance of procedure-level intermediate product costs. Suitable microcomputer software is available from several vendors at prices ranging from approximately $5–$10,000. This soft-

Source: Reprinted from Kirk Mahlen, "RVUs: Relative Value Units or Really Very Useful?," *Hospital Cost Accounting Advisor,* Vol. 4, No. 8, January 1989, pp. 1–7. Copyright 1989, Aspen Publishers, Inc.

ware should have the ability to convert cost data to RVUs. Ultimately, in order to be of any use in managerial decision-making, the RVUs must be utilized for procedure/patient-level costing and integrated with a comprehensive patient-level database. From this, our goal is reasonably accurate and refined profitability analysis by, but not limited to, physician, specialty, payer, MDC, DRG, and product line. Adjusting for severity level and incorporating standard treatment profiles will further enhance this capability. For a relatively minor investment, RVUs provide a major improvement in the accuracy and thus, usability, of cost information for managerial decision-making.

PERFORMING THE MANAGEMENT STEPDOWN

It is likely that cost information will continue to be recorded in the general ledger (GL) by department and sub-account. Hospitals simply do not maintain procedure-level cost information as they do for gross charges. Under PPS, hospital net revenue is largely dependent on its case mix or DRGs. If we expand our interpretation of the basic accounting principle which maintains that we match revenues with expenses, then, under this new product-driven market, it becomes absolutely essential to accurately determine cost and profitability at the DRG or product level.

Obviously, cost at the DRG or product level should tie-back to the GL costs. This can be accomplished by first performing a management stepdown using existing GL department-level cost information and later allocating stepdown results to the procedure/patient level using RVUs. In order to reduce the potential for bias inherent in performing a single stepdown, the preferred method for performing the cost allocation would be simultaneous equations (provided the capability exists). For purposes of this example, I have chosen to utilize the single stepdown methodology due to relatively universal familiarity with its use.

[Note: Over the years the order of stepdown has been set by hospitals in a manner so as to optimize reimbursement. In the opinion of Hospital Cost Accounting Advisor, use of stepdown for RVU costing is an easy—but unsatisfactory—approach. Much effort and cost will be expended to develop RVUs that are "tainted" right from the start. For a small marginal increase in cost (relative to the costs of installing an RVU system), the reciprocal (or simultaneous equation approach) method of cost allocation can be used. Such a method eliminates all distortions created by the order of the stepdown allocation. Editor.]

1. We begin our simplified example with GL direct cost information for four departments:

Depts	Direct Costs
Hskpg	$ 1,000
Admin	2,000
Lab	5,000
X-ray	4,000
Total	**$12,000**

2. Next, we refine our direct cost information by aggregating GL sub-account costs into specified expense classifications and performing any management-defined adjustments and reclassifications that may be required. Salary, nonsalary, and capital expense classifications are frequently used:

Depts	Sal	Nonsal	Cap	Total
Hskpg	$ 600	$ 300	$ 100	$ 1,000
Admin	1,000	700	300	2,000
Lab	4,000	500	500	5,000
X-ray	3,000	800	200	4,000
Total	**$8,600**	**$2,300**	**$1,100**	**$12,000**

3. Initially, this next step can be very time-consuming. Depending upon technique and the amount of effort expended, it can also be somewhat subjective. Here we identify components of cost and designate either a percentage or dollar amount of our direct costs as either fixed or variable. This is usually done through management consensus by examining GL departmental costs at the subaccount level of detail. Any subjectivity is significantly reduced as the hospital gains experience in using the data and refining fixed/variable assumptions. Unfortunately, in most cases, fixed/variable cost data are unavailable in the GL.

[Note: Although used infrequently by hospitals prior to the initiation of PPSs, techniques such as linear regression can be used to take historical cost patterns (containing no fixed/variable cost distinctions) and estimate fixed and variable costs. There is substantial potential for improvement over subjective management estimates if one uses such techniques. See any currently used cost accounting text for further information. Editor.]

Once the fixed/variable determinations are made, automated systems can be put in place to automatically calculate the fixed/variable cost components.

Depts	Direct Fixed			Direct Variable		
	Sal	Nonsal	Cap	Sal	Nonsal	Total
Hskpg	$ 300	$ 100	$ 100	$ 300	$ 200	$ 1,000
Admin	700	400	300	300	300	2,000
Lab	1,000	100	500	3,000	400	5,000
X-ray	1,000	200	200	2,000	600	4,000
Total	**$3,000**	**$ 800**	**$1,100**	**$5,600**	**$1,500**	**$12,000**

4. In order to determine allocated direct and indirect costs for our two revenue-producing centers, it will be necessary to perform a management-defined cost allocation or stepdown. Before we can do this, it is necessary to develop allocation statistics for each overhead center and its components of direct cost. For obvious reasons, every attempt should be made to use those statistics that are most appropriate for accurate management cost allocation as opposed to Medicare or other third party allocation requirements:

Housekeeping (Sq. Ft. Cleaned)

Depts	Direct Fixed			Direct Variable	
	Sal	Nonsal	Cap	Sal	Nonsal
Hskpg					
Admin	20	20	20	20	20
Lab	40	40	40	40	40
X-ray	40	40	40	40	40
Total	100	100	100	100	100

Administrative (Hours of Support)

Depts	Direct Fixed			Direct Variable	
	Sal	Nonsal	Cap	Sal	Nonsal
Hskpg					
Admin					
Lab	500	500	500	500	500
X-ray	500	500	500	500	500
Total	1,000	1,000	1,000	1,000	1,000

[Note: A separate statistic can be created for each component of cost. The need for this is particularly obvious for capital costs.]

5. With appropriate software, we are now ready to perform the management stepdown for each overhead item and its components of cost from Step 3:

Departments' Housekeeping Allocation

Depts	Direct Fixed			Direct Variable		
	Sal	Nonsal	Cap	Sal	Nonsal	Total
Hskpg						
Admin	$ 760	$ 420	$ 320	$ 360	$ 340	$ 2,200
Lab	1,120	140	540	3,120	480	5,400
X-ray	1,120	240	240	2,120	680	4,400
Total	$3,000	$ 800	$1,100	$5,600	$1,500	$12,000

Departments' Administrative/Final Allocation

Depts	Direct Fixed			Direct Variable		
	Sal	Nonsal	Cap	Sal	Nonsal	Total
Hskpg						
Admin						
Lab	$1,500	$ 350	$ 700	$3,300	$ 650	$ 6,500
X-ray	1,500	450	400	2,300	850	5,500
Total	$3,000	$ 800	$1,100	$5,600	$1,500	$12,000

6. Finally, we are able to summarize allocated direct/indirect, fixed/variable, and salary/nonsalary/capital costs for our revenue producing centers. It is these components of cost that will ultimately be allocated to departmental procedures and patients based on RVUs:

Rev Depts	Direct Fixed			Direct Variable		
	Sal	Nonsal	Cap	Sal	Nonsal	Total
Lab	$1,000	$ 100	$ 500	$3,000	$ 400	$ 5,000
X-ray	1,000	200	200	2,000	600	4,000
Total	$2,000	$ 300	$ 700	$5,000	$1,000	$ 9,000

Rev Depts	Indirect Fixed			Indirect Variable		
	Sal	Nonsal	Cap	Sal	Nonsal	Total
Lab	$ 500	$ 250	$ 200	$ 300	$ 250	$ 1,500
X-ray	500	250	200	300	250	1,500
Total	$1,000	$ 500	$ 400	$ 600	$ 500	$ 3,000

[Note: The Indirect Fixed and Variable are the costs allocated from the nonrevenue departments in Step 5. Editor.]

DEVELOPMENT OF RVUS

1. RVUs are simply an expression of the relative cost of one procedure to another within a given department. As such, the first step in developing RVUs involves performing a cost study to determine variable intermediate product costs for significant procedures in the department to be studied. Most hospitals have chosen to use the 80/20 rule to study the 20% of a department's procedures that account for 80% of its revenues

or units. Since cost per procedure is generally not known prior to performing the cost study, it would not be available as an indicator in determining which procedures should be studied. The 80/20 rule is strictly arbitrary and can be adjusted or applied differently to each department. For example, in departments having a relatively small number of resource intensive procedures, it would be most appropriate to study all procedures. The exact cutoff should be determined based upon an examination and ranking of each department's procedures based upon either charges or units. Of course, there is nothing preventing the hospital from studying any procedure regardless of where it falls using an 80/20, 90/10, or 50/50 rule. The primary issue here involves the trade-off between the amount of resources committed to studying a given procedure and its relative significance.

The cost study is usually performed with short-term but extensive involvement on the part of hospital department heads. A procedure cost profile, similar to the example depicted below, must be developed for all procedures studied. Unstudied procedures are assigned costs using one of several default methods available.

Dept: Laboratory

Procedures	Unit Amt.	×	Unit Cost	Total Cost
CBC				
Technician	10 Mins	×	$.20	$2.00
Total Salary				$2.00
Needles	5 Units	×	$.05	$ .25
Paper	1 Sheet	×	$.25	.25
Test Tubes	2 Units	×	$.50	1.00
Total Supply				$1.50
Strep Screen				
Technician	5 Mins	×	$.20	$1.00
Total Salary				$1.00
Slides	58 Units	×	$.05	$2.90
Swabs	4 Units	×	$.025	.10
Total Supply				$3.00
Urinalysis				
Technician	15 Mins	×	$.20	$3.00
Total Salary				$3.00
Containers	1 Unit	×	$1.00	$1.00
Total Supply				$1.00

Dept: X-ray

Procedures	Unit Amt.	×	Unit Cost	Total Cost
Chest X-ray				
Technician	25 Mins	×	$.20	$ 5.00
Total Salary				$ 5.00
Film A	2 Units	×	$5.00	$10.00
Total Supply				$10.00
Head X-ray				
Technician	60 Mins	×	$.20	$12.00
Total Salary				$12.00
Film B	1 Unit	×	$8.00	$8.00
Total Supply				$8.00

[Note: Even with RVUs some degree of cost inaccuracy will exist. For example, a chest X-ray is shown as taking 25 minutes in the example in this article. However, chest X-rays for some types of patients may usually take 10 minutes while chest X-rays for another type of patient may typically take 40 minutes. Use of the 25-minute RVU measure for all chest X-rays therefore creates its own distortion. Editor.]

2. We can now convert the cost data developed above to RVUs as follows

Lab	Costs			RVUs		
	Sal	Nonsal	Total	Sal	Nonsal	Total
CBC	$2.00	$1.50	$3.50	1.0000	.8182	.9138
Strep	1.00	3.00	4.00	5.000	1.6364	1.0440
Urin	3.00	1.00	4.00	1.5000	.5455	1.0444
Avg. Cst	$2.00	$1.83	$3.83			

X-ray	Costs			RVUs		
	Sal	Nonsal	Total	Sal	Nonsal	Total
Chest	$5.00	$10.00	$15.00	.5883	1.1110	.8571
Head	12.00	8.00	20.00	1.4116	.8889	1.1429
Avg. Cst	$8.50	$9.00	$17.50			

Sample RVU calculation for Lab-CBC where procedure cost is divided by the average cost for all procedures studied:

Sal	Nonsal	Total
2.00/2.00 = 1.000	1.50/1.83 = .8197	3.50/3.83 = .9138

COSTING AT THE PROCEDURE/ PATIENT LEVEL

We are now ready to allocate components of costs developed using the management stepdown for each revenue-producing center to the procedure/patient level. Using our example, a comparison will be made between RCC and RVU costing for two patients. Before going further, however, I would first like to point out the following additional procedure costing methods that might be mixed and matched depending upon hospital needs, resource constraints, and applicability to certain departments and/or components of cost.

Units

Allocate a dollar value based on the number of procedure units. This might be most appropriate for the allocation of fixed capital costs. However, fixed costs allocated in this manner would not change with volume, thus creating problems of over or under applied cost as volume changes.

Multiply the number of units for each procedure by a specified ratio value (per diem cost).

Charges

Allocate a dollar value based on procedure charges. Multiply charges for each procedure by a specified ratio value (RCC). Because procedure charge information is readily available and hospitals are familiar with this type of costing for Medicare and other third parties, this method has become the method of choice by default. Obviously, after years of game playing with procedure charges, they bear little resemblance to cost. Cost may be somewhat accurate at the department level but there may be wide variations

in the accuracy of cost information derived at the procedure level using this method.

Cases

Allocate a dollar value based on the number of cases. Multiply the number of cases by a specified ratio value (per case cost).

Standard Costing

Multiply procedure volumes by the costs developed in the cost study.

EXAMPLE: RCC VS. RVU COSTING

Assumptions

1.
   Lab Total Cost = $6,500
   Total Chgs = $13,000 RCC = .500
   X-ray Total Cost = $5,500
   Total Chgs = $ 4,000 RCC = 1.375

2. Department costs by component are taken from the management stepdown. (See Steps 5–6.)

3. Total weighted departmental RVUs are calculated by multiplying procedure volumes times the individual RVU values. (See Step 2.)

Lab	Units	Sal RVU	Total Sal RVU	Nonsal RVU	Total Nonsal RVU
CBC	5	1.000	5.000	.818	4.091
Strep	2	.500	1.000	1.636	3.272
Urinalysis	3	1.500	4.500	.545	1.636
Total	10		10.500		9.000
X-ray					
Chest	3	.588	1.764	1.111	3.333
Head	1	1.412	1.412	.889	.889
Total	4		3.176		4.222

4. Total procedure costs for all procedures rendered during a specified period are determined by allocating the stepped down department costs for salary and nonsalary components based on

the Total Sal RVU and the Total Nonsal RVU above. Capital costs in this example are simply allocated to procedures based on number of units.

	Direct Fixed			*Direct Variable*	
Lab	*Sal*	*Nonsal*	*Cap*	*Sal*	*Nonsal*
CBC	$ 476.20	$ 45.26	$250.00	$1,428.00	$181.84
Strep	95.20	36.36	100.00	285.60	145.44
Urin	428.60	18.18	150.00	1,285.80	72.72
Total	$1,000.00	$100.00	$500.00	$3,000.00	$400.00

X-ray

Chest	$ 555.60	$157.90	$150.00	$1,111.20	$473.70
Head	444.40	42.10	50.00	888.80	126.30
Total	$1,000.00	$200.00	$200.00	$2,000.00	$600.00

	Indirect Fixed			*Indirect Variable*		
Lab	*Sal*	*Nonsal*	*Cap*	*Sal*	*Nonsal*	*Total*
CBC	$238.10	$113.65	$100.00	$142.86	$113.65	$3,090.36
Strep	47.60	90.90	40.00	28.56	90.90	960.56
Urin	214.30	45.45	60.00	128.58	45.45	2,449.08
Total	$500.00	$250.00	$200.00	$300.00	$250.00	$6,500.00

X-ray

Chest	$277.80	$197.37	$150.00	$166.68	$197.37	$3,437.62
Head	222.20	52.63	50.00	133.32	52.63	2,062.38
Total	$500.00	$250.00	$200.00	$300.00	$250.00	$5,500.00

Patient Costing Using RCCs

	Units	*Charges* $\times$	*RCC*	*Cost*
Patient 1				
Lab-CBC	1	$1,000 $\times$	.500	$ 500
Lab-Strep	2	5,000 $\times$	.500	2,500
Total Lab	3	$6,000		$3,000
X-ray-Chest	1	$1,200 $\times$	1.375	$1,650
Total X-ray	1	$1,200		$1,650
Patient 1 Total		$7,200		$4,650

	Units	*Charges* $\times$	*RCC*	*Cost*
Patient 2				
Lab-CBC	3	$3,000 $\times$	.500	$1,500
Urinalysis	4	$4,000 $\times$	.500	2,000
Total Lab	7	$7,000		$3,500
X-ray-Chest	2	$2,400 $\times$	1.375	$3,300
Head	1	400 $\times$	1.375	550
Total X-ray	3	$2,800		$3,850
Patient 2 Total		$9,800		$7,350

Patient Costing Using RVUs

For purposes of this example, cost will be calculated for each department's total salary, nonsalary and capital cost components only (from Step 5). In actuality, cost is calculated for each individual cost component including fixed variable and direct/indirect designations.

	Units	*Procedure RVU*	*Total Dept. RVU*	*Total Dept. Cost*	*Patient Cost*
Patient 1					
Lab-Salary					
CBC	1	$\times$ 1.000 $\div$	10.500 $\times$	$4,800 =	$457
Strep	2	$\times$ .500 $\div$	10.500 $\times$	$4,800 =	457
					$914
Lab-Nonsalary					
CBC	1	$\times$ .818 $\div$	9.000 $\times$	$1,000 =	$ 91
Strep	2	$\times$ 1.636 $\div$	9.000 $\times$	$1,000 =	364
					$455

Lab-Capital [(Units/Total Department Units) $\times$ Department Capital Cost]

CBC	(1 $\div$ 10)	$\times$ $700	$ 70
Strep	(2 $\div$ 10)	$\times$ $700	140
			$210

	Units	*Procedure RVU*	*Total Dept. RVU*	*Total Dept. Cost*	*Patient Cost*
X-ray-Salary					
Chest	1	$\times$ .588 $\div$	3.176 $\times$	$3,800 =	$704
X-ray-Nonsalary					
Chest	1	$\times$ 1.111 $\div$	4.222 $\times$	$1,300 =	$342
X-ray-Capital					
Chest		(1 $\div$ 4)	$\times$ $400	=	$100
Total Patient 1 Cost					$2,725

	Units	Proce-dure RVU	Total Dept. RVU	Total Dept. Cost	Patient Cost
Patient 2					
Lab-Salary					
CBC	4	× 1.000 ÷	10.500 ×	$4,800 =	$1,829
Urin	3	× 1.500 ÷	10.500 ×	$4,800 =	2,057
					$3,886
Lab-Nonsalary					
CBC	4	× .818 ÷	9.000 ×	$1,000 =	$364
Urin	3	× .545 :	9.000 ×	$1,000 =	182
					$546

Lab-Capital [(Units/Total Department Units) × Department Capital Cost]

CBC	(4 ÷ 10)	× $700	$280
Urin	(3 ÷ 10)	× $700	210
			$490

X-ray-Salary					
Chest	2	× .588 ÷	3.176 ×	$3,800 =	$1,407
Head	1	× 1.412 ÷	3.176 ×	$3,800 =	1,689
					$3,096

X-ray-Nonsalary					
Chest	2	× 1.111 ÷	4.222 ×	$1,300 =	$684
Head	1	× .889 ÷	4.222 ×	$1,300 =	274
					$958

X-ray-Capital				
Chest	(2 ÷ 4)	× $400	=	$200
Head	(1 ÷ 4)	× $400	=	100
				$300

Total Patient 2 Cost $9,276

SUMMARY PROFITABILITY ANALYSIS (RCC VS. RVU)

	Gross Charges	Ney Rev	RVU Cost	RCC Cost	RVU Profit	RCC Profit
Patient 1	$ 7,200	$ 4,200	$ 2,724	$ 4,650	$1,476	$ (450)
Patient 2	9,800	9,800	9,276	7,350	524	2,450
Total	$17,000	$14,000	$12,000	$12,000	$2,000	$2,000

As you might infer, the decision to use RCC vs. RVU costing will impact the accuracy of cost/profitability analysis not only at the patient level, but also by physician, specialty, payer, DRG, MDC, and product line. After years of so-called cost or charge shifting, which of the figures above would you prefer to rely upon for contractual negotiations, feasibility determinations, and other critical management decisions?

Reading 4–4

Alternative Costing Methods in Health Care

Leslie A. Davis Weintraub

Richard J. Dube

METHODOLOGY

The development of procedure level costs in a hospital can vary widely depending on the methodology used. Procedures, as referred to throughout the article, are the smallest level of detail maintained in a hospital's financial system (e.g., chest X-ray). Two common methodologies, both of which were involved in this study, are (1) ratio of cost to charges (RCC) and (2) relative value units (RVUs). All data used in this study were developed at Framingham Union Hospital in Framingham, Massachusetts, a 311-bed general medical/surgical hospital. Fiscal year 1986 data only were used. The development of RCCs involved a breakdown of costs into five separate components, thus constituting five separate RCCs for each department. These categories were as follows:

- direct labor
- direct supplies
- overhead capital
- overhead labor
- overhead supplies

This five-tiered approach is somewhat more sophisticated than the traditional single RCC

method. Two of the components of cost represent direct costs, while the other three are all indirect costs.

The RVU methodology in place at Framingham resulted from an in-depth cost accounting study performed primarily by the fiscal department staff with some outside consulting assistance. The procedural level costing study resulted in the development of 11 cost components, four of which are direct components of cost. The 11 components are

- direct variable labor
- direct fixed labor
- direct variable supplies
- direct fixed supplies
- direct capital
- support labor
- support supplies
- support capital
- overhead labor
- overhead supplies
- overhead capital

The hospital chose to distinguish between support departments and overhead departments as follows. Support departments are those such as housekeeping and dietary where a specific measurement of activity exists, allowing the department head some control over the usage of that department's services. Overhead departments include typical hospital overhead departments,

Source: Reprinted from Leslie A. Davis Weintraub and Richard J. Dube, "Alternative Costing Methods in Health Care," *Hospital Cost Accounting Advisor,* Vol. 3, No. 12, May 1988, pp. 1–5. Copyright 1988, Aspen Publishers, Inc.

such as fiscal services and depreciation, which are not usually considered within the department head's direct control.

The hospital's costing study involved determining the costs for all procedure charge codes. Once the data collection phase was complete, all data were entered into a procedure level cost management program for later integration with the hospital's mainframe cost accounting system. The hospital's cost accounting system allowed the hospital to store both departmental RCC cost values and procedural level costs as collected from the detailed study, hereafter referred to as RVU costs. The availability of these two variations of costing data allowed us to study the differences in the results of the two costing methods in much greater detail.

All data analysis was performed on the same group of patients, those treated at Framingham Union Hospital in fiscal year (FY) 1986. Preliminary analysis of the RCC/RVU cost comparison focused on an individual patient with costs detailed by department. Secondary analysis included a single diagnosis-related group (DRG) broken out by departmental costs. Comparisons at this micro level of detail proved to be unmanageable for a representative amount of data. Instead, we settled on examining all DRGs with greater than 30 cases. The number 30 was chosen as it represents a large sample size in statistical analysis. The resultant number of DRGs included in our cost comparison study was 87. These 87 DRGs represent 9,712 cases, or 74 percent of the hospital's total cases treated in FY 1986.

Statistical analysis was performed on these 87 DRGs for both sets of cost data so as to compare the statistical significance of the difference between the two methods. If the difference between the two costing methodologies was not found to be statistically significant for a particular DRG, then the two methods were considered comparable for that DRG. Conversely, if the difference was statistically significant, then the two methods were categorized as significantly different for that DRG. In order to determine statistical significance, the two-tailed t-test for paired

observations was performed on each of the 87 DRGs. Additionally, confidence intervals were calculated for all DRGs in which the difference between the two costing methods was considered statistically significant. The confidence intervals were then assessed to determine the variation in the range of the interval, indicating either a tight or loose range. All statistical tests were performed at the 99 percent significance level or .01 significance. The 99 percent significance level was selected to assure statistical significance at varying sample sizes (number of cases of a DRG), as well as to maintain a high degree of accuracy.

FINDINGS

Results of the statistical analysis are outlined below. The analysis was performed on both total cost and direct cost for each DRG. Direct costs were analyzed separately so as to eliminate the influence of indirect allocated expenses and focus solely on direct costs. Prior studies on this topic have pointed to the possible influential effect of overhead allocation on the costing methodologies. Our goal was to eliminate that effect and compare the two methods. Direct cost analysis for the RCC method thus involved only the two direct cost components: direct labor and direct supplies. The RVU methodology analysis was limited to the four direct cost components; direct variable labor, direct fixed labor, direct variable supplies, and direct fixed supplies.

When the difference between the methodologies was analyzed in terms of total cost, 29 DRGs fell into the category statistically significant, while for the other 58 DRGs the costing methodologies differential was not significant. Although these 29 DRGs represent only 33.3 percent of the total DRGs, they represent 58 percent of the total cases.

Additionally, they account for 40.3 percent of the total RVU costs and 41.2 percent of the total RCC costs. Lastly, they represent 40.7 percent of the net revenue. In comparison, a similar analysis performed with direct costs resulted in 38 DRGs in which the difference between the two costing methodologies was statistically significant. Representing 43.7 percent of the total DRGs, these DRGs constitute 65.8 percent of the total cases. The 38 DRGs account for 42.8 percent of the RVU costs and 44.2 percent of the RCC costs. These 38 DRGs also represent 43.8 percent of the net revenue of the 87 DRGs studied (see Table 4–4–1).

The analysis of direct costs resulted in a greater percentage of DRGs in which the difference between the two costing methodologies was statistically significant. One would expect this difference to occur, since direct costs do not include any overhead allocation. The allocation of overhead in the total cost methodology remains constant in both RCC and RVU costing. The equal elimination of overhead costs magnifies the difference between the methods, thus resulting in a greater number of statistically significant cases.

In order to assess the impact of the DRGs in which the difference between the two methods was deemed statistically significant, we decided to do some analysis on the basis of profitability. The hospital is able to better assess the impact of

the RVU methodology when profit/loss amounts are attached. The analysis focused on those DRGs with exceptionally high variances in total profit and profit per case between the two methods. Profit is defined as net revenue minus operating cost. The profit variance represents the difference in profit between the two costing methodologies. Another interesting observation involved DRGs that appeared to be profitable under one method, yet unprofitable under the other method. Once again the analysis was performed separately on both total costs and direct costs. Results are listed in Table 4–4–2.

Under the total cost analysis, four DRGs appeared profitable under one method and unprofitable under the other. DRG 391 (normal newborns) showed a profit of $69/case under the RCC method and a loss of $50/case under the RVU method. Although the total dollar amount of the variance is not particularly large, DRG

Table 4–4–1 Summary of Data

	Total Cost	Direct Cost
Number of DRGs where the difference between the two methods was statistically significant	29	38
Total number of DRGs in analysis	87	87
% significant DRGs of total DRGs	33.3%	43.7%
% significant cases of total cases	58.0%	65.8%
% significant DRG RVU costs of total RVU costs	40.3%	42.8%
% significant DRG RCC costs of total RCC costs	41.2%	44.2%
% significant DRG net revenue of total net revenue	40.7%	43.8%

Table 4–4–2 Total Cost Analysis

Profit per Case
DRGs with Positive versus Negative Profits

	RCCs	RVUs
DRG 24	($ 6)	$130
DRG 59	$190	($ 77)
DRG 124	($151)	$927
DRG 391	$ 69	($ 50)
DRG 374*	($190)	$ 51
DRG 379*	($ 51)	$ 86

Total Profit Variance
DRGs with > $100,000 Total Profit Variance

DRG 125	$123,346
DRG 373	($220,532)
DRG 391	$204,219

Profit per Case
DRGs with > $1,000 Profit/Case Profit Variance

DRG 1	($2,192)
DRG 124	($1,078)
DRG 125	($1,110)

*Denotes these DRGs are only statistically significant under the direct cost analysis.

391 is the highest volume DRG in the analysis, with 1,706 cases. DRG 59 (tonsil/adenoidectomy) presented a profit of $190/case under the RCC method, yet a loss of $77/case under the RVU method. Similarly, DRG 24 (seizure/headache) is unprofitable under the RCC method, with a loss of $6/case, and profitable under the RVU method, at a per case profit of $130. The fourth DRG in this category is DRG 124—circulatory disorders except AMI w/cath com dx. Here we found the largest total dollar variance, exceeding $1,000, with a loss under the RCC approach of $151/case and a profit under the RVU method of $927/case.

Continuing with the total cost analysis, three DRGs had a total profit variance of greater than $100,000. DRG 391 (normal newborns) had a positive profit variance of $204,219 and DRG 373 (vaginal delivery w/o com dxs) had a negative variance of $220,532. As mentioned earlier, newborns are the number one volume DRG at Framingham Union. The other DRG with a total profit variance of over $100,000 is DRG 125 (circulatory disorders except AMI w/cath sim dx) with a positive variance of $123,346. When profit per case was analyzed instead of total profit, three DRGs had a profit per case variance of greater than $1,000. DRG 125 was the only DRG with both a total profit variance over $100,000 and a per case profit variance of over $1,000. DRG 125 had a $1,110 profit variance per case. DRG 124 has a per case profit variance of $1,078. Lastly, DRG 1 (craniotomy) had the highest per case profit variance of $2,192. A wide variation between the RCC and RVU method is apparent in a select number of DRGs, as displayed by significant profit variances. Total profit variance for the 29 DRGs selected in the total cost analysis was a negative $329,551 for a per case variance of ($59)/case. Similarly, the total profit variance for the 38 DRGs selected in the direct cost analysis was a negative $315,401 for a per case variance of ($49)/case.

The direct cost analysis resulted in precisely similar results for those DRGs with greater than a $100,000 total profit variance, as well as those DRGs with a per case profit variance of over $1,000. The only difference was seen in the analysis of DRGs with both positive and negative profits according to the costing method selected. In addition to the four DRGs cited under the total cost analysis, two other DRGs fell into this category as well. DRG 374 (vaginal delivery w/ sterilization or D&C) appears profitable under the RVU method at $51 profit per case and unprofitable under the RCC method with a per case loss of $190. Also, DRG 379 (threatened abortion) shows a per case loss of $51 under the RCC method and a per case profit of $86 under the RVU method.

DISCUSSION

The traditional RCC approach has been accepted over the years as the standard method for cost determination. As hospitals began to shift toward strict cost containment with the advent of the prospective payment system, a more accurate method of cost determination was desired. The RVU approach, or procedural level cost determination, became the prevalent methodology for a select group of hospitals with the available resources. Procedural level cost development is a detail-oriented, time-consuming task that requires the assistance and cooperation of many individuals throughout the hospital. Subsequently, the associated cost can be very high. The results of such a study are generally accepted to be considerably more accurate than an RCC approach. The increased accuracy is attributable to the data collected in determining direct procedural costs such as labor and supplies. Actual measurements are conducted to assess the labor time involved in performing each procedure, and the associated supplies are directly assigned to the procedures as well.

Assuming that the RVU information is more accurately developed than the RCC data, we have demonstrated numerous examples where a large variance exists between the two methods. Significant differentials in profit occurred in large volume DRGs, which could have resulted in the hospital making strategic decisions on high volume DRGs on the basis of inaccurate information. The additional information garnered from the cost accounting study proved to be significantly different from the RCC data in 60 percent of the hospital's total cases. Alternatively, one could say that in 40 percent of the hospital's cases, the difference between RCCs and RVUs was insignificant and not worthy of the additional intensive data collection and analysis effort. Ultimately, the question becomes, "What level of information is necessary for the decision maker at the hospital to make critical decisions?"

Framingham Union feels they invested soundly in their cost accounting decision. As a result of the detailed RVU information, the hospital was able to realign its charge structure and conduct HMO negotiations based on accurate cost per case information. Currently, the hospital is using the data from the cost accounting study to develop a flexible budget. The future impact of the hospital's enhanced decision-making capabilities cannot be assigned a monetary value at this time; however, the hospital will continue to reap the benefits of the cost accounting data for years to come.

Even though the RCC/RVU differential was only statistically significant in 60 percent of the cases and not 99 percent, one inaccurate decision based on approximated RCC data could wreak havoc in the hospital's strategic financial plan.

Inaccurate decision-making to any degree is best avoided. A small hospital, however, may not be able to cost-justify the expense of the cost accounting study when RCC data are readily available. Although RCCs are an approximation of true cost, they are a reasonable substitute, as evidenced by our study results, for 40 percent of the cases.

Each hospital must make an individual decision whether or not to invest in a cost accounting study based on the desired uses of the resultant information in ongoing hospital managerial decisions. RCCs are an approximation and lack the validity of RVUs. However, the hospital must be willing to make a significant investment in order to pursue the development of procedural level RVU costs. A number of methods exist to reduce the investment in a cost accounting study, including the use of short-cut techniques and national RVU standards. The varying degrees of data collection involvement will determine the actual cost of the study and must be accurately assessed when considering the RCC/RVU dilemma.

ACKNOWLEDGMENTS

The authors wish to give special thanks to Mr. Harmon Jordan, Director of Biostatistics, Mediqual Systems, Inc., for his assistance and guidance with the statistical analysis, and to Mr. John Nunnelly, Regional Vice President, HBO & Co., for his consultative assistance and guidance throughout the research process.

Reading 4–5

Accounting for the Move to Ambulatory Patient Groups

Horen R. Boyagian

Randi Frank Dessingue

The imminent, and long ballyhooed, implementation of an ambulatory patient group (APG)-based prospective payment system (PPS) by Medicare and the anticipated emulation by other payers has put a premium on understanding ambulatory care costs. From the payers' perspective, the benefits are straightforward; APGs can be used to consolidate utilization and introduce cost containment incentives. For providers, however, success under such a system may require paying attention to details historically ignored. The two biggest provider considerations need to be ambulatory coding and ambulatory cost accounting. Secondary to these basic concerns, additional factors need to be considered. Are the operational processes in place to accurately bill? Will payment rates reflect? What are the costs? Will some procedures or sites of service be favored under the new PPS? While the answers to these questions will develop as implementation details are disseminated, it is clear that the introduction of APGs will result in increased demands on providers.

This article will focus on the cost accounting challenge an APG-based PPS presents to providers and the issues associated with that challenge. In particular, three topics are discussed. First,

Source: Reprinted from Horen R. Boyagian and Randi F. Dessingue, "Accounting for the Move to Ambulatory Patient Groups," *The Journal of Ambulatory Care Management,* Vol. 21, No. 3, July 1998, pp. 60–75. Copyright 1998, Aspen Publishers, Inc.

how can costs be identified? Second, what are the differences in costs associated with alternative settings? Finally, how do costs identified through a detailed resource costing methodology compare to estimates using alternative measures? Discussion will then be presented on the implications of the issues for providers and what options for response are available.

The implementation of an ambulatory PPS exposes issues previously of limited interest. For both payers and providers, the issues are both important and current. Some may be tempted to use charges as a proxy for costs as an expedient approach. This approach, however, is not without risks. The relationship between ambulatory charges and costs has been forever distorted by the introduction of PPS on the inpatient side and by the continued use of cost-based reimbursement and, in many cases, charges, on the ambulatory side. Providers responded to these obvious incentives and, accounting being a human enterprise, allocated costs to those activities that could most readily bear those costs. In fact, many consultants developed optimization models to facilitate this very behavior. While recent regulatory enforcement actions may put these practices into question, at the time, they appeared reasonable and appropriate. They did, however, undermine the relationship between charges and costs for ambulatory activities.

While payment rates for Medicare's inpatient PPS were established using hospital charges, studies (Balicki, Miller, & Nuschke, 1990) have shown that charges for outpatient services are not necessarily accurate measures of resource use. For Medicare, if payment rates are set disproportionately high for some procedures or services and disproportionately low for others, beneficiary access to services may be compromised. Some providers, with greater market share in some areas, may be advantaged to the detriment of others. To encourage appropriate provider behavior, payment rates should reflect resource use. In 1992, Health Care Financing Administration (HCFA) supported a study (Balicki et al., 1992) by the Center for Health Policy Studies (CHPS) to investigate the impact of this distortion on cost identification. The results of this HCFA study serve to highlight the need for providers to examine ambulatory costs in anticipation of APG implementation. The remainder of this article makes references to the HCFA-sponsored study performed by CHPS.

Unlike inpatient charges per case, outpatient charges per visit relate to a small number of services for which some charges are higher and some are lower than resource costs. Small numbers of charges do not provide opportunities to offset distortions in individual service charges and thus create the possibility that charges do not accurately reflect resource use. In addition, the incentives to distort cost allocations increased with the application of prospective payment to inpatient care and the continued use of charge- or cost-based payment for ambulatory services. There is, then, a need for a methodology that can accurately measure resource costs. The database developed in CHPS' study represented an important first step toward meeting this need. The study's database, however, was based on a limited sample and was intended as a research effort to provide HCFA with some data that could be used to evaluate prices for outpatient services. The focus of the study, however, was on determining the feasibility of using resource costing as a tool to measure service-specific outpatient costs.

Two aspects of the study's objectives need to be clearly understood. First, only facility costs were investigated. Although physician labor costs are an important component of outpatient costs, they are not considered in this study. Second, the study focused on the resource costs of CPT-4 (American Medical Association, Current Procedural Terminology 98) coded procedures and International Classification of Diseases, Version 9 with Clinical Modification (St. Anthony's ICD-9-CM Code Book), coded medical visits as they are categorized in the APG patient classification system. APGs were selected as the sampling framework because the system is clearly policy relevant. Each group within the system is intended to be homogeneous both clinically and in terms of resources, that is, CPT-4 and ICD-9 codes within an APG reflect the resources of other codes in the group. In addition, the system is comprehensive and includes procedures, medical visits, and ancillary services. While costs of all ambulatory activities were investigated, only ambulatory surgery results are discussed here.

Detailed data on the costs of each selected procedure/visit are available in the study's database. To demonstrate the depth of data that is available, a single resource profile is presented as Appendix 4–5–A. The profile is for CPT-4 66984, Extracapsular Cataract Removal with Insertion of Intraocular Lens Prosthesis. This procedure is the highest volume Medicare ambulatory surgery procedure.

COSTING APPROACH

Although product cost accounting has been used in many industries for decades, its principles were not applied to health care organizations until recently. Instead, health care providers focused their attention on calculating the costs of institutions, departments, and programs. Traditional health care accounting systems do not have the capability to calculate the costs of products, that is, cost per case for specific inpatient services and cost per visit for specific outpatient visits. Many providers, if they gave it any thought, relied upon special studies using management engineering and cost accounting techniques to arrive at product or product-component costs. These studies, while useful, were not consistent in either their scope or their calculation methods and, therefore, could not be used for cross-facility comparisons.

During the past 10 to 15 years, efforts have been made to introduce cost accounting systems for inpatient services. These systems allow for the calculation of product and subproduct costs and can be extended to outpatient services, but few hospitals have taken this step. At the time of the 1992 study, there were no widely used product cost accounting systems utilized by ambulatory surgery centers or physician practices, although some progress has been made since that time.

Resource costing was developed to fill the void created by the lack of health care cost accounting systems. In the simplest sense, resource costing is an approach that identifies the components of a health care activity, identifies the type and amount of resources used to complete the requirements of each component, and attaches unit costs to each resource. Unit costs multiplied by resources used yields costs of resources, and when these costs are summed, the cost of each component and the cost of the health care activity can be calculated.

Health care differs from other industries in many ways. From an accounting standpoint, the most important difference is in the number and variety of products that are produced by health care providers. In order to address the problem of measuring the cost of many diverse products, nontraditional accounting methods were introduced. The resource costing methods used identified resources for a specific service by asking clinical panels and provider staff to develop normative profiles. Unit costs incurred by each of the providers studied were then applied to the resource use profiles that each provider developed to arrive at service-specific costs. An alternative approach could rely on classical management engineering techniques to identify resources used, but such an approach would be prohibitively expensive. The large number of health care products and their diversity require the combination of normative and empirical techniques that are inherent in resource costing.

An important distinction was made between *direct* and *indirect* resource costs of outpatient services. Direct costs have been broadly defined as including any costs that can be traced to a specific procedure or visit. Direct costs include all expenses that are related to "hands-on" patient care and those that are directly assignable to a given type of surgical case or medical visit. There is no intervening basis for allocating direct costs because they can be directly traced to the delivery of specific patient services. Direct costs for outpatient procedures include direct labor time, medical supplies, special equipment, medication, anesthesia, and special ancillary testing.

Indirect costs are the other key part of the costing framework. Unlike direct costs, indirect costs are those that do not directly contribute to the production of an individual service. They cannot be measured or evaluated on a procedure-by-procedure basis. Instead, indirect costs are incurred to support all patient care activities. The cost for a surgery table at an ambulatory surgery center (ASC) is an example of an indirect cost. Although the equipment could be considered direct in the sense that it is used during the treatment of patients, its use is too broadly based to be tied to any one procedure. The purchase costs and depreciation of these and other types of nonspecialized equipment are included as part of the "indirect equipment costs" category. A more evident example of nonprocedural indirect costs is the rent or mortgage expenses for a given facility.

Measurement of indirect costs required data collectors to use different methods from those inherent in the resource profiles used to determine direct costs. First, a time period had to be selected as a basis for gathering financial information. As noted, the latest fiscal year (1991–1992) was chosen because it reflects current operations as closely as possible. Another characteristic of indirect costs, especially those that make up the largest component, which is designated overhead in this study, is that they must be allocated to each outpatient department (OPD) and ultimately to procedures. The allocation of indirect costs is a necessary step in any cost accounting system. Methods of indirect cost allocation were carefully considered, and the most significant indicators of outpatient activity or "cost drivers" known to exist in each patient care area were selected. These allocation statistics include square footage, hours of operation, volume of inpatient and outpatient procedures (if both types are offered), and average time per inpatient and outpatient procedure. Most indirect costs were allocated using procedure-specific direct contact time. Contact time is the preferred method for allocating indirect costs in cases where direct labor accounts for a significant portion of per-visit costs.

Data were collected and analyzed from a representative random sample of hospitals and ASCs. Some of the results are summarized in the subsequent sections.

FINDINGS: MEASUREMENT OF RESOURCE COSTS

The composition of resource costs for ambulatory surgery is presented in Figures 4–5–1 and 4–5–2. Based on the model and as shown in these figures, indirect costs comprise a larger portion of total costs for ASCs than for hospital OPDs. At least two factors contribute to this difference. First, indirect costs are typically spread across lower procedure volumes for ASCs because most ASCs have not attained the same volume levels for ambulatory surgery that OPDs have. Second, many hospitals consider ambulatory surgery to be a joint product that is produced simultaneously with inpatient surgery. It is possible for hospitals to gain efficiencies in indirect costs by using resources for both inpatient and outpatient services. ASCs do not have similar opportunities.

Two types of unit costs were investigated in detail because of their significance. These unit costs (i.e., costs of nursing salaries and costs of intraocular lens implants) were examined to identify their variation across providers. The weighted average mean salary for all nurses

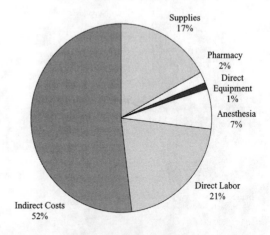

Distribution of Total Costs Ambulatory Surgery Procedures (ASCs)

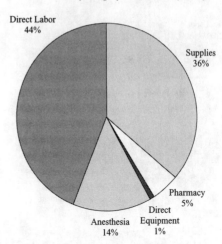

Distribution of Total Costs Ambulatory Surgery Procedures (ASCs)

Figure 4–5–1 Distribution of Total and Direct Costs of Ambulatory Surgery Procedures (ASCs). *Source:* Data from CHPS Outpatient Resource Costing Database.

working for providers included in the study was adjusted for geographic differences in wage rates. Average adjusted salary for all nurses was $36,797. There were no substantial differences in nurses' salaries across provider types and only limited differences across geographic regions for the providers included in the study. Fringe benefits per person were also found not to vary substantially for hospitals and ASCs, although

**Distribution of Total Costs
Ambulatory Surgery Procedures (Hospitals)**

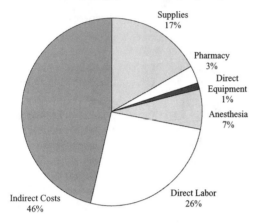

**Distribution of Total Costs
Ambulatory Surgery Procedures (Hospitals)**

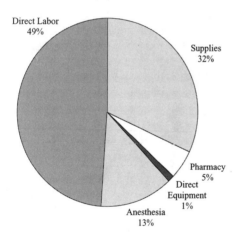

Figure 4–5–2 Distribution of Total and Direct Costs of Ambulatory Surgery Procedures (Hospitals). *Source:* Data from CHPS Outpatient Resource Costing Database.

hospitals use a greater number of full-time staff, which leads to greater aggregate fringe benefits.

Most facilities included in the study performed eye surgery, and each of these facilities performed lens replacement procedures. The costs of lenses used ranged from $80 to $722. Across all facilities, the mode for the purchase of lenses was $150.00, and the mean was $164.70. Nearly all facilities had purchased lenses at least

once during 1992 for $150.00. Differences in costs are due in part to volume of lenses used. Volume, however, did not explain many instances in which high costs were identified for lens purchases. Discussions with surgeons indicate that differences in costs of lenses are frequently associated with differences in quality. Most agree, however, that lower cost lenses are of sufficient quality to be used for most patients. It is, therefore, difficult to fully understand causes of differences in lens cost.

The analysis did not document a consistent relationship between volume and direct and indirect costs. It was expected that higher volume facilities would have lower direct and indirect costs. Direct labor costs, which depend on operating room time, were expected to be lower for facilities where higher volumes of procedures were completed. It was expected that supply, pharmaceutical, and anesthesia costs would be lower in high-volume facilities because these facilities could use volume discounts when they purchased these items.

For 2 of the top 10 procedures studied in hospitals and for 7 of the 10 procedures studied in ASCs, the lowest volume facilities have the lowest total direct costs. For some procedures, the lowest volume facilities have the lowest direct labor costs and the same pattern is found for the costs of equipment. Different patterns, however, are noted for supplies, pharmaceuticals, and anesthesia, which may imply that volume discounts have a limited effect on the costs of purchases. Supply costs are lowest in mid-volume facilities for several procedures. In the case of pharmaceuticals, high-volume and mid-volume facilities generally have the lowest costs. The lowest costs for anesthesia are distributed among different volume facilities. The pattern for all procedures studied continues to show inconsistency.

The expected relationship between volume and cost—that is, cost decreases as volume increases—was also not consistently identified for indirect costs. Failure to identify a relationship between volume and either direct or indirect cost can be due to several factors, including the vagaries of small sample size. In addition, it can be hypothesized that most providers participate in joint purchasing programs, which limits differences in prices paid across providers. Also, it appears as though low-volume providers adjust their approaches to providing services to reflect lower volumes and offset higher costs that would otherwise occur. It also cannot be assumed that all providers operate efficiently at the levels of volume that they experience.

FINDINGS: DIFFERENCES IN COSTS ACROSS SETTINGS

Using the data collected, an analysis of differences in costs across settings was completed. The analysis focused on differences in the costs of specific ambulatory surgery procedures when they are performed in OPDs and ASCs. Tables 4–5–1, 4–5–2, and 4–5–3 identify the findings from this analysis. Additional analyses included comparisons of OPDs and physician offices (POs).

The widely held assumption that ASCs are a less costly setting than OPDs was not supported by the analyses. Little difference in direct costs between ASCs and OPDs was identified. Differences in indirect costs indicated that OPDs were the less costly setting, although a statistically significant difference was measured for only one procedure. Several factors appear to contribute to the findings. First, OPDs and ASCs conduct surgery similarly; that is, the time spent by the patient from the point of arrival at the facility through recovery does not vary across settings. More importantly, operating room time does not vary nor does the use of supplies, equipment, and anesthesia during surgery. There are no systematic reasons for variation in resource use across settings. It was expected that unit costs of some resources would be less costly in OPDs that have more of an opportunity to participate in joint purchasing programs and that generally have higher volumes. As noted previously, no differences in labor costs were found across surgical settings. Although some differences in unit costs were found, they were neither significant nor consistent.

As noted, differences in indirect costs favored hospitals. Although hospitals have higher aggregate overhead, they frequently have higher volumes over which overhead can be distributed. In addition, hospitals consider ambulatory surgery to be a joint product with inpatient surgery and can distribute surgical service overhead over even greater volumes. ASCs must incur indirect costs, such as the cost of a medical director, solely for the production of ambulatory surgery services while these costs are distributed over a much larger activity in hospitals.

POs appeared to be the least costly setting for all services; the limited size of the sample of the physician practices did not provide sufficient confidence levels to support this conclusion for most procedures examined. However, some procedures were statistically less costly when provided in a PO; these were limited to certain types of medical visits. It was noted that when a surgical procedure that could be provided in a PO was conducted in an ASC or an OPD, costs were considerably greater. For example, high costs were identified for excision, including simple closure and anesthesia. These high costs resulted from patterns of care used in non-PO settings, such as the use of two nurses in operating rooms and the requirement that all patients recover from surgery using facility protocols. Indirect costs are also higher in non-PO settings.

Lower costs in POs were consistently tied to the use of fewer and frequently lower salaried staff to perform services that support physicians. For example, nurses and aides in POs are frequently cross-trained in the use of radiology and laboratory equipment. In addition, when surgery is performed in a PO, only one staff member assists the physician, whereas two are consistently used in OPDs and ASCs. Differences in direct cost between POs and other settings are significant, but differences in indirect costs are even greater. Physicians incur considerably less overhead and purchase less equipment than OPDs and ASCs. For all of these reasons, POs were found to be the least costly setting. Although this finding was consistently identified for an array of services, it must be

Table 4–5–1 Comparison of Total Direct Resource Costs, Selected High-Volume Ambulatory Surgery Procedures

| CPT Code | Procedure | Sample Size | | Mean Total Direct Costs | | Statistical Significance, 90% Confidence Level | | |
		Hospital	ASC	Hospital	ASC	Higher Hospital Mean Cost	Higher ASC Mean Cost	No Statistically Significant Difference
66984	Extracapsular cataract removal with insertion of intraocular lens	22	23	641.57	548.54	X		
45378	Colonoscopy, diagnostic	27	13	185.61	178.69			X
45385	Colonoscopy, for removal of polypoid lesion	25	15	209.65	212.40			X
49505	Repair of inguinal hernia, age 5 or over	27	20	329.46	346.53			X
43239	Upper GI endoscopy, for biopsy or collection of specimen	27	13	214.74	203.06			X
43235	Upper GI endoscopy, diagnostic	24	12	195.44	203.37			X
19120	Excision of cyst	31	23	274.84	262.57			X
52000	Cystourethroscopy (separate procedure)	26	14	261.84	256.23			X
45380	Colonoscopy, for biopsy	27	14	209.39	220.15			X
66821	Discission of secondary membranous cataract	12	12	456.59	221.24	X		

Source: Data from CHPS Outpatient Resource Costing Database.

Table 4–5–2 Comparison of Total Direct Resource Costs, Selected High-Volume Ambulatory Surgery Procedures

| CPT Code | Procedure | Sample Size | | Mean Total Direct Costs | | Statistical Significance, 90% Confidence Level | | |
		Hospital	ASC	Hospital	ASC	Higher Hospital Mean Cost	Higher ASC Mean Cost	No Statistically Significant Difference
66984	Extracapsular cataract removal with insertion of intraocular lens	22	23	305.95	387.33			X
45378	Colonoscopy, diagnostic	25	13	172.59	207.39			X
45385	Colonoscopy, for removal of polypoid lesion	23	15	186.28	282.38			X
49505	Repair of inguinal hernia, age 5 or over	27	20	242.45	420.65	X		
43239	Upper GI endoscopy, for biopsy or collection of specimen	25	13	139.11	187.83			X
43235	Upper GI endoscopy, diagnostic	22	12	115.61	188.03			X
19120	Excision of cyst	31	23	267.72	350.48			X
52000	Cystourethroscopy (separate procedure)	26	14	162.75	209.61			X
45380	Colonoscopy, for biopsy	25	14	194.93	244.23			X
66821	Discission of secondary membranous cataract	12	12	209.99	163.47			X

Source: Data from CHPS Outpatient Resource Costing Database.

Table 4–5–3 Comparison of Total Direct Resource Costs, Selected High-Volume Ambulatory Surgery Procedures

CPT Code	Procedure	Sample Size		Mean Total Direct Costs		Statistical Significance, 90% Confidence Level		
		Hospital	ASC	Hospital	ASC	Higher Hospital Mean Cost	Higher ASC Mean Cost	No Statistically Significant Difference
66984	Extracapsular cataract removal with insertion of intraocular lens	22	23	947.52	935.87			X
45378	Colonoscopy, diagnostic	27	13	345.41	386.07			X
45385	Colonoscopy, for removal of polypoid lesion	25	15	381.03	494.77			X
49505	Repair of inguinal hernia, age 5 or over	27	20	571.91	767.19		X	
43239	Upper GI endoscopy, for biopsy or collection of specimen	27	13	343.54	390.89			X
43235	Upper GI endoscopy, diagnostic	24	12	301.42	391.40			X
19120	Excision of cyst	31	23	542.56	613.05			X
52000	Cystourethroscopy (separate procedure)	26	14	424.59	465.85			X
45380	Colonoscopy, for biopsy	27	14	389.89	464.39			X
66821	Discission of secondary membranous cataract	12	12	666.58	384.71	X		

Source: Data from CHPS Outpatient Resource Costing Database.

clear that the PO sample used in this study was small and not randomly selected. These findings should be considered as suggestive of relationships but not definitive. Both procedures and medical visits are roughly half as costly when done in a PO rather than in a hospital or ASC, but laboratory and radiology procedures are about equal in cost.

FINDINGS: COMPARISONS OF RESOURCE COSTS TO OTHER MEASURES

This study included comparisons of resource costs to other relevant measures and to reported costs. Most importantly, resource costs were compared to charges and to reported costs. Charges, and the ratio of charges to charges (or cost to charges) applied to costs (charges; RCCAC) costs, are the resource measures commonly used to describe resource use in health care. Charges, however, are not necessarily accurate measures of resource use.

Medicare charges for the hospitals included in the study were compared to resource costs for the same hospitals for selected high-volume procedures. If a consistent mark-up was used for all procedures, and resource costs were an accurate reflection of resource use, the ratio between costs and charges would be consistent across all procedures. The ratio, however, was not found to he consistent for high-volume surgery procedures. Among the nine procedures studied, the ratio was found to have a range of .31 for CPT-4 49505, repair of inguinal hernia, to .66 for CPT-4 52000, cystourethroscopy. Medicare hospital charges, which range from $524 to $1,958, do not display a consistent relationship to resource costs. For low-charge procedures, the ratio is higher than for high-charge procedures. This pattern was generally found to be applicable to surgical procedures.

These findings are significant for two reasons. First, as was expected, charges, which are readily available for all services, are found not to reflect resource use as measured by resource cost. Second, and more important, it is clear that the use of charges to set relative values will result in an inequitable distribution of resources across procedures. Procedures with high charges will have relative values set too high, while lower charge services will have relative values that are too low. Economic incentives to provide high-charge services will create pressure to increase supply and utilization of these procedures. The analysis makes it clear that charges, even if reduced to relative values, have serious limitations as the basis for payment level determinations.

Procedure-specific comparisons between hospital-based resource costs and Medicare costs were completed. Medicare costs were developed by reducing hospital charges to costs using a ratio of costs to charges. As discussed, current reimbursement incentives distort the relationship between charges, cost derived from charges, and resource use. Cost reimbursement for ambulatory services or some blend thereof, combined with diagnosis-related group prices for inpatient services, creates an incentive to move costs to ambulatory cost centers or cost centers with high ambulatory utilization. The impact of specialty and payer mix on what the market will bear is an additional factor that can distort charges and RCCAC costs.

The ratio of resource cost to Medicare costs was found to range from .63 for CPT-4 49505, repair of inguinal hernia, to 1.31 for CPT-4 52000, cystourethroscopy. A clear trend was found in the data. As in the case of charges, for low Medicare cost procedures, resource costs were found to be generally higher than Medicare costs, and for high Medicare cost procedures, resource costs were found to be lower than Medicare costs. This trend has important implications for payment policy. The development of relative

values from Medicare cost data would also result in the overpayment of some procedures and the underpayment of others.

The introduction of APGs by HCFA alters many of the operational incentives currently in place. This change provides an opportunity to re-evaluate decisions made under different conditions. To meet the needs of both APGs and managed care, providers need to improve their current understanding of the underlying costs associated with ambulatory services. The results presented in the previous sections suggest that decisions made based on current measures of ambulatory cost (i.e., charge-based measures) need to be reexamined. These decisions could include which services to provide, what setting is appropriate, and where marketshare opportunities exist. In addition, managed care contracting decisions made without an accurate understanding of underlying costs can prove disastrous.

As providers prepare for success under Medicare and other payers begin to adopt APG-like methods of payment, the payback associated with accurate coding and a thorough understanding of actual costs will accumulate. The changes made on behalf of Medicare can result in benefits across payers.

REFERENCES

Balicki, B., Bialzak, M., Burnette, J., Dyckman, Z., Kellberg, E., Kelly, W., Kleinhen, B., Woodhouse, R., & Yates, T. (1992). *Measurement of outpatient facility resource costs* (Final report). Rockville, MD: Health Care Financing Administration, Office of Research and Demonstrations.

Balicki, B., Miller, H., & Nuschke, M. (1990). *Replication study of outpatient costs in 25 hospitals* (Final report). Rockville, MD: Health Care Financing Administration, Office of the Assistant Secretary of Planning and Evaluation.

Appendix 4–5–A

Resource Profile for Extracapsular Cataract Removal with Insertion of Intraocular Lens Prosthesis

Procedure: Extracapsular cataract removal with insertion of intraocular lens prosthesis
CPT: 66984
ICD: 13.41
APG: 291

Labor minutes by operating phase	Pre1	Pre2	Operating room	Pat1	Pat2	Cost/minute	Total cost
Anesthesiologist	10	15	5	1	5	0.00000	0.00
Certified registered nurse anesthetist (CRNA)	20	5	5	5	0	0.00000	0.00
Patient	55	60	50	20	30	0.00000	0.00
Physician	0	25	38	0	0	0.00000	0.00
Registered nurse (RN)	5	15	110	10	20	0.47000	90.25
Total Direct Labor:	90.25						

Disposable supplies	Quantity: unit	Unit cost	Total cost
Alcohol pad	2	0.05000	0.10
Back table drape	1	1.74000	1.74
Basin	4	0.25000	1.00
Blade–Beaver #69	1	5.71000	5.71
Blade–Beaver #75	1	3.71000	3.71
Cannula–disposable	1	2.86000	2.86
Corneal light shield	1	0.86000	0.86
Drain–Weck	1	3.43000	3.43
Drape–eye	1	9.71000	9.71
Drape–utility	1	0.86000	0.86
Electrocardiogram electrodes	3	0.23800	0.71
Eye patch	2	1.28000	2.56
Eye shield	1	1.14000	1.14
Gauze 4 × 4 sterile	1 pkg of 10	0.57000	0.57
Gloves–nonsterile	2 pair	0.34000	0.68
Gloves–surgical sterile	3 pair	0.76000	2.28
Gown–surgical sterile	3	3.11000	9.33
Head cover	7	0.10000	0.70
Inst wipe	1	1.68000	1.68
Intraocular lens (IOL)	1	238.00000	238.00
Knife–Grieshaber	1	20.86000	20.86

Disposable supplies	Quantity: unit	Unit cost	Total cost
Mask–surgical	4	0.10000	0.40
Mayo stand cover	1	1.13000	1.13
Microsponge	12	0.08900	1.07
Needle protector	1	1.14000	1.14
Needle–22 gauge Jelco	1	1.36000	1.36
Needle–27 gauge	1	0.05000	0.05
Needle–cystotome	1	2.29000	2.29
Needle	10	0.05000	0.50
Patient belongings bag	2	0.08000	0.16
Phaco setup	1	10.00000	10.00
Q-tip	10	0.02000	0.20
Shoe covers	6 pair	0.10000	0.60
Steri drape	1	4.25000	4.25
Suture–opth nylon 10-0	1	19.43000	19.43
Suture–opthalmic	1	5.00000	5.00
Suture–vicryl 9-0	1	11.43000	11.43
Syringe–10 cc	10	0.10000	1.00
Syringe–3 cc	3	0.10000	0.30
Syringe–bulb	1	2.50000	2.50
Syringe–TB	2	0.40000	0.80
Tape–1 inch paper	2 rolls	0.71000	1.42
Thermometer probe cover	2	0.02000	0.04
Tubing–BSS administration	1 roll	5.43000	5.43
Tubing–intravenous (IV)	1	5.14000	5.14
Tubing–oxygen	1	0.61000	0.61
Tubing–suction	1	2.17000	2.17
Weck Cel spear sponges	20	0.86000	17.20
Total Disposable Supplies:	404.11		

Reusable supplies	Quantity: unit	Unit cost	# Uses	Total cost
Blood pressure cuff	1	187.00000	5,000	0.04
Eye instrument set	1	3,304.00000	2,000	1.65
Forceps–cautery	2	218.90000	1,000	0.44
Goggles	1 pair	5.00000	100	0.05
Hemostats	2	3.90000	15	0.52
Phaco count	1	50.00000	100	0.50
Phaco handpiece	1	50.00000	100	0.50
Phaco tip	1	30.00000	100	0.30
Stethoscope	2	44.50000	3,000	0.03
Temperature monitor–electronic	1	400.00000	3,000	0.13
Wrist rest	1	735.00000	1,000	0.74
Total Reusable Supplies:	4.90			

Movable equipment	Quantity	Price	# of Uses	Cost/use	Total cost
Cautery machine	1	4,000	5,000	0.800000	0.80
Microscope	1	7,375	5,000	1.475000	1.48
Surgical stretcher	1	5,967	5,000	1.193400	1.19
Video system	1	20,830	3,000	6.943333	6.94
Total Movable Equipment:	10.41				

Pharmaceuticals: generic/brand names	Dosage: unit	Unit cost	Total cost
Acetazolamide/Diamox	1.00 cc	21.43000	21.43
BSS (500 cc)	500.00 cc	0.01540	7.70
H_2O irrigation solution sterile	1,500.00 mL	0.00038	0.57
Normal saline	1,000.00 mL	0.00114	1.14
Povidone iodine/Betadine swab	1.00	0.62000	0.62
Total Pharmaceuticals:	31.46		

Anesthetics: generic/brand names	Dosage: unit	Unit cost	Total cost
Bupivacaine 0.75%/Marcain 0.75%	8.00 cc	0.15000	1.20
Epinephrine/Adrenalin 1:1000	1.00 cc	1.17000	1.17
Fentanyl/Sublimaze	2.00 cc	2.29000	4.58
Hyaluronidase/Wydase	1.00 cc	4.86000	4.86
Methohexital/Brevital	7.00 cc	0.25000	1.75
Midazolam/Versed	2.00 mg	1.42200	2.84
Propofol/Diprivan	300.00 mg	0.04390	13.17
Sulfacetamide 10%/Sodium Sulamyd ointment	1.00 tube	4.50000	4.50

Total Anesthetics:	34.07		
Total Direct Cost:	575.20		
Total Indirect Cost:	259.01	[Indirect Labor Cost (19.91), Indirect Equipment Cost (38.00), & Overhead (201.10)]	
Total Cost of Procedure:	834.21		

Note: Pre, preoperative; post, postoperative; BSS, basic saline solution

Reading 4–6

Cost Allocation in the Emergency Department

Martin S. Kohn

Methods of cost allocation are intended, as part of a management control system, to help collect data needed for the planning and control of financial entities. A properly designed system helps senior management set realistic goals and measure progress toward the goals. Hospital allocation systems tend to be peculiar because of the nature of health care reimbursement procedures.

Since it is a reasonable goal for hospitals to maximize third-party reimbursement for services rendered, the administrators will tailor allocation schemes to that end. An allocation system with a reimbursement maximization aim may make institutional sense, but it may provide incentives at odds with some of the fundamental clinical goals of hospitals.

The hospital emergency department (ED) seems to have been a place that has always defied financial analysis and management. Whether this absence of financial control has resulted from the ED's traditional role of providing emergency care to all comers, irrespective of the ability to pay, or because hospitals in general have only recently grappled with cost/revenue issues, is unclear.

It had been pretty well accepted that EDs lost money directly, but compensated by generating profits on the inpatients admitted through the

Source: Reprinted from Martin S. Kohn, "Cost Allocation in the Emergency Department," *Hospital Cost Accounting Advisor,* Vol. 4, No. 9, February 1989, pp. 1–6. Copyright 1989, Aspen Publishers, Inc.

ED. The perception that EDs did not have to stand on their own financial merits probably contributed to a lackadaisical approach. No effort was made to assess material and staffing resources used by patients (or categories of patients). Frequently, a flat average fee was charged to each patient to cover overhead and staffing costs. The patients might be charged individually for specific, identifiable supplies used during treatment.

The reimbursement methodology for many states has provided no incentive for hospitals to identify cost patterns. For example, in the regulated New York environment, the hospitals are reimbursed on formulas related to average costs. In a simplified description, Blue Cross, Medicaid, and Workers Compensation each consider the average cost of treatment for a patient covered under their programs, and calculate an average visit fee. The average is calculated on data from two years earlier, and is projected forward by allowing for inflation. The hospital then receives that fee for each covered visit, irrespective of the nature of the visit. Medicare pays a fixed percentage of charges, as an interim payment for services rendered, which is supposed to approximate costs, based on data from two years earlier. A final settlement for outpatient services is completed after the year-end filing of a cost report.

The payment for each program is different, because of the nature of the patients, the kinds of services covered, and caps that may be imposed on certain expenses. An exception is the patient who is admitted to the hospital from the ED. Since admissions are reimbursed under a DRG scheme, there is no separate reimbursement for the ED component of such a visit.

An immediate peculiarity is already apparent. The patients who are usually most labor and supply-intensive in an ED are the patients who are admitted to the hospital. They may represent 10% to 30% or more of the ED patient volume. Yet, no revenue accrues to the ED for the management of its most expensive patients. To provide proper incentive and control, either appropriate revenue must be assigned to the ED for admitted patients, or appropriate costs from the ED should be allocated to the inpatient services. In the current environment, with very high hospital inpatient censuses, it has not been unusual for patients to spend several days in an ED, awaiting the availability of an inpatient bed. Under such circumstances, the absence of a reasonable allocation process can precipitate major cost/revenue discrepancies and management misdirection.

The "average" fee reimbursement system also limits the ability of hospital EDs to deal with competition. Urgent care centers (UCCs) or free-standing emergency centers (FECs) compete directly with EDs for the minor emergency patients. The UCCs attempt to provide care faster and less expensively than EDs. Part of the ability of UCCs and FECs to undercut EDs on cost is due to the typical ED cost allocation. With the standard fee being independent of service provided, patients with minor problems were clearly being overcharged. (While $75 for a severe asthma attack might be a bargain, $75 for a runny nose is clearly expensive.) The UCCs, by treating minor problems at prices more consistent with costs, are able to attract those patients from the EDs. Although one could argue that such patients should not be in the ED in the first place, the reimbursement mechanisms and cost allocations used depend on such minor emergencies for solvency. If, for example, the least seriously ill or injured 10 percent of patients leave the ED for a UCC, revenue is still down 10 percent.

In some instances, hospitals have set up charges that vary with the severity of illness or intensity of service for emergency patients. For example, in 1984, Lorain Community Hospital, in Lorain, Ohio, set up a graduated fee structure. Prior to the change, the charges were either $50 for a "minor" problem or $85 for a "major" case. With either fee, the charges for certain supplies were added on. In northeast Ohio, at that time, Blue Cross did not reimburse for emergency treatment of medical problems unless they resulted in hospitalization. The costs of most mild to moderate cases were paid out of pocket by the patients. Thus, a UCC with fees even slightly lower than the ED could be, and was, very competitive.

The fee gradation was loosely based on what was perceived as increasing utilization of nursing time. The allocation had to be approximated because of an absence of specific data. The specific charges for each level were derived by considering the estimated nursing time, and setting the requirement that total revenue had to match, or possibly exceed, revenue prior to the change. The charges also had to be within the bounds that insurance companies would accept for reimbursement. The result was a seven-level system, with charges ranging from $25 for the most minor problems (e.g., a cold) to $350 for a full cardiac arrest. In addition, a structure was instituted to allow for additional charges for each 15 minutes of intensive care nursing time above the amount allocated in the basic charge. Thus, by giving consideration to cost allocation, the ED at Lorain Community Hospital was able to restructure its charges to both compete effectively with UCCs (by advertising the reduced rates) and to receive appropriate reimbursement for its primary service objective, namely providing care for serious emergencies.

Although such a simple charge modification seems quite trivial, it is innovative enough that ED price adjustments merited front page coverage in the May 19, 1988, *Wall Street Journal.* Increased numbers of visits and increased profits were reported by hospitals that used graded charges. Such results, alone, would seem to be enough incentive to induce an administrator to refine cost allocation in the ED.

In New York, however, the "average"-cost-based method of third party reimbursement for emergency care removes most of the incentive. Also, New York Blue Cross plans, for example, pay for most of their clients' ED visits, so the attraction of a UCC's lower cost is blunted. However, the control and incentive parts of management remain. For example, would a decrease of two minor visits be offset by an increase of one visit resulting in an admission? On a strict ED revenue basis, the result would be a loss of two paying patients and a gain of one nonrevenue patient, since admissions are reimbursed as a DRG payment to the hospital. There should be an allocation method that reflects the benefit to the hospital without appearing to disadvantage the ED.

ANALYSIS OF A CURRENT ALLOCATION SYSTEM

To consider the ED allocation issue, a currently used system will be explored. The following issues will be considered:

1. Are the allocation bases rational?
2. Do the bases have any disadvantages?
3. Would a change in the allocation process provide benefit with a reasonable cost?

Fixed Overhead

Certain costs in the ED can be viewed as fixed. The largest of such costs would be depreciation for the building and capital equipment, administrative services, and supervisory nursing services. Building depreciation is assigned to the ED based on square footage as a fraction of the total hospital area. Equipment is depreciated against the actual cost of purchase. Supervisory nursing costs are assigned by actual hours of service, and administrative costs are assigned by historical patterns of the fraction of the administrators' time spent dealing with ED issues.

Currently, these costs are assigned equally to each patient, based on the year's budget for patient visits. A patient who spends 30 minutes in the ED, and utilizes 5 minutes of staff time, has the same fixed overhead allocation as a patient who spends three days.

Perhaps the overhead could be assigned by the time each patient spends in the ED. Technically, each patient's chart is supposed to have the time of arrival and the time of discharge written down. However, such notations are not always made, and when they are, the times don't always accurately reflect the useful time the patient spends in the ED. A four-hour stay could include two hours of waiting because the X-ray machine was being repaired. Thus, to be fair, the elapsed time would have to be evaluated to extract a useful "treatment time." Such a process would be cumbersome, expensive, and subjective—not desirable characteristics of a cost allocation process.

As it turns out, fixed overhead represents a small portion of the total costs of the ED, in the range of 5%. Such a ratio seems consistent with general experience. Thus, any elaborate method for fixed overhead allocation would have an undesirable cost-benefit ratio.

Variable Overhead

Like fixed overhead, variable overhead represents a small fraction of the total cost of the ED. Services such as laundry, housekeeping, power, and miscellaneous supplies account for less than 5% of total costs. They are allocated to the ED, respectively, by pounds of laundry, hours of service, floor space, and actual supply requisitions. Since the amount of money involved is relatively small, again, a complex patient allocation process is not indicated.

Variable Costs

Variable costs (salaries, pharmacy, laboratory, radiology, etc.) represent the largest fraction of ED expenses. Salaries for staff (including physicians) account for 90+% of variable costs. Salary expenses are allocated on a per visit basis, irrespective of the intensity or duration of service. A prorated allocation process makes sense when the reimbursement is independent of the actual service provided to the patient. However, it makes no sense in terms of trying to evaluate staff function.

If there were a change in patient characteristics, so that even a few more critically ill patients, requiring more personnel for more time, arrived in the ED, all that would be seen in cost data was that the average staff cost per patient increased. There would be no indication of the cause of the increase, and it could be interpreted as inefficiency on the part of the staff. Thus, even though a more sophisticated cost allocation system for salaries would not affect reimbursement for most patients, it would help interpret ED operations more effectively.

In addition, there is one group of patients whose care is reimbursed based on cost, namely, those covered by Medicare. Since the elderly patient often requires more attention and care than younger patients, a system that identifies intensity and length of care in cost allocation could result in increased reimbursement from Medicare. The much-discussed concept of ambulatory visit groups (AVGs) might reflect such differential costs.

As noted, other variable costs include laboratory and radiology. For the bulk of patients for whom reimbursement is independent of services rendered, the expenses for laboratory and radiology must be allocated to the ED. The allocation process is a prorated assignment based on total number of tests. If ED patients account for 10% of the total number of tests performed in the laboratory, then 10% of laboratory costs are allocated to the ED. The ratio is calculated on the basis of number of tests, and does not consider the cost of the test. An immunoglobulin electrophoresis has the same weight as a hematocrit determination. Since the bulk of ED patients have relatively minor problems, and the seriously ill patients have only basic diagnostic testing done in the ED, the ED utilizes the less expensive laboratory tests. Thus, allocating costs based

on the fraction of total tests inflates the cost assigned to the ED.

From the point of view of the ED, such an allocation could be unfair, because the ED absorbs some of the costs generated by other parts of the hospital. However, the process could provide an advantage to the hospital. Because of DRGs, the hospital cannot be reimbursed for individual costs for inpatients. Thus, an allocation process that assigns some inpatient costs to outpatient areas, where they will be figured into a reimbursement rate, can benefit the institution. Again, we have a conflict between institutional financial benefit and the desire to provide useful data for management and control in the ED. The ED would benefit from data about actual laboratory utilization.

Since laboratory and radiology services are ordered, and recorded, by patient, the process of assigning the associated costs would be relatively straightforward. The cost data already exist, in some fashion, since they are used to determine Medicare reimbursement.

Admitted Patients

Patients admitted to the hospital through the ED generate no revenue for the ED visit, per se. Under the DRG system, the hospital is reimbursed for the admission, with no extra consideration for the time spent in the ED. To compensate for costs that are generated in the absence of revenue, ED costs for admitted patients are allocated to the inpatient services.

The allocation process is based on the percentage of total visits that result in hospital admission. For example, if 20% of ED patients are admitted to the hospital, then 20% of total ED costs are allocated to inpatient services. As with laboratory costs, the process could be seen as inequitable for the ED.

Patients who are admitted through the ED are the sickest, most resource-intensive of the patients treated in the ED. They consume far more than a prorated share of staff and supplies, so the allocation process reassigns less cost than is actually merited. Again, however, the process may be to the hospital's advantage. If higher costs were assigned to the inpatient services, it would not result in higher revenue, because of the DRG system. Leaving the costs in the ED results in higher reimbursement since the ED is an outpatient service.

Summary of Allocation Analysis

The currently used system for allocating ED costs has these advantages:

1. It is simple.
2. It helps maximize revenue for the institution by assigning what could be considered inpatient costs to the ED.

However, it also has disadvantages:

1. It does not provide data to help control and manage ED activities.
2. A variable cost allocation could be misinterpreted with respect to staff efficiency.
3. It offers a potentially inappropriate incentive. (Minimally ill patients produce a better bottom line than sick patients requiring hospitalization.)

Because of the peculiar reimbursement mechanism, the hospital has no incentive, and in fact, great disincentive, to alter its ED cost allocation process. However, a simple process that would allow managers to understand staff utilization (which represents the bulk of ED cost) is still desirable from the point of view of control and incentive.

ALLOCATION BY INTENSITY AND DURATION

The reality is that some patients require more time and attention than others. If the patient distribution changes, and there are a greater number of seriously ill patients, staff needs increase even in the absence of an increase in the total number of patients. Therefore, an allocation process that accounts for such variation will help identify

trends, staffing needs, and operation efficiency in a way that the current system cannot.

Since staff costs represent over 80% of costs of emergency care, staff time spent with a patient seems a reasonable basis for assigning all costs. The sicker patient, requiring more staff, would also be likely to need more laboratory studies and more X-rays. Thus, staff time should also parallel other costs. For reasons already discussed, attempting to keep track of the time each patient spends in the ED is not useful. Although it would be helpful to know how much staff time is spent with each patient, such a process is too expensive and time consuming to be cost-effective.

However, grouping patients by categories would be a cost-effective and practical way of allocating starting costs. As was demonstrated at Lorain Community Hospital, referred to earlier, patients can be categorized by diagnosis and condition, in a way that reasonably predicts staff utilization. The number of categories depends on the precision you choose, and the time you have to spend. Four to seven categories seems to be common. A time-motion study can be undertaken to try to quantify the number of staff-hours consumed by patients with different diagnoses. Then the mean staff time for each diagnosis can be calculated, and the diagnoses grouped by range of staff time required (e.g., 0–5 min., 5–15 min., 15–30 min., 30–60 min., 60+ min.) in person-minutes.

Some information is available from organizations such as the Emergency Nurses Association about acuity ranking of patients. Such data can be used to verify your own conclusions, or to help get started in the process. After the categories are determined, then a weight can be assigned to each group, say in proportion to the average staff time in the category. In our example above, the mean time in each category would be (in minutes) 2.5, 10, 22.5, 45, and, say, 75. In our example, the weights would be 1, 4, 9, 18, and 30. Based on the number of patients in each category, and considering the total staff costs, the appropriate cost can be allocated to each patient.

For example, if there are 100 patients in each category, and staffing costs of $100,000, the cost per unit would be calculated as follows:

$$(1 + 4 + 9 + 18 + 30) \times 100 = 6,200$$

$$\$100,000/6,200 = \$16.13 \text{ per unit}$$

Then the cost per category would be as follows:

Category	Staff Cost
1	16.13
2	64.52
3	145.17
4	290.34
5	483.90

Then as each patient is categorized, based on diagnosis, the appropriate staff cost could be assigned. Such information would be very useful to the department director or others responsible for evaluating the ED. The result from 10 fewer sore throat patients (category 1) and 10 more cardiac arrests (category 5) would be readily apparent.

Allocation of costs for patients admitted to the hospital would then be based on the weight of the category. Most admissions would come from the higher categories, so clearly the amount of cost allocated to the inpatient services would be higher than under the simplistic prorated system.

The allocation would more accurately reflect the ED's contribution to the admitted patient's care.

Even though such information would not be useful in hospitals in some states, with respect to reimbursement at present, it is still useful for operational purposes. In addition, considering recent trends, it is unlikely that the current ED reimbursement methodology will continue. There will be more and more pressure to reduce costs, which, in itself, will require better costing information.

There is nothing in the new process that prevents the hospital from continuing to generate reimbursement figures the way it has been doing. Since the reimbursement is based on average costs, none of the needed data have been lost. The hospital can continue to use its simplistic allocation process to its financial advantage, while also developing data systems that will help it understand its ED now, and be prepared for changes in the future.

SUGGESTED READING

Asunof, L., Business Bulletin, *Wall Street Journal*, May 19, 1988 CCXI(98), p. 1.

Sabin, M.D., and P.H. Wulf in *The Hospital Emergency Department—Returning to Financial Viability.* T.A. Matson, ed., American Hospital Association, Chicago, Ill., 1986.

Janiak, B. in *The Hospital Emergency Department—Returning to Financial Viability.* T.A. Matson, ed., American Hospital Association, Chicago, Ill., 1986.

5

Costing for Nonroutine Decisions

Reading 5–1

HMO Negotiations and Hospital Costs

Steven A. Finkler

During the decade of the 1990s, it is likely that more and more hospitals will come under pressure to negotiate arrangements with HMOs and PPOs. In some cases the financial impact of such arrangements (or the failure to make such arrangements) may be critical to organizational financial viability.

Often, however, hospitals enter into such arrangements without having thought through why they are making the arrangement, and what its long-term implications are. A recent study by Kralewski et al. reported a shocking finding when they noted that "The HMO knows as much (and often more) about the target hospital's cost structure as the hospital's management."[1]

If that conclusion is in fact true, it should be disturbing information for hospital managers. Negotiations with HMOs are inherently difficult. HMOs may have information about their own mix of patients that has critical financial implications. Such information may give them an edge to begin with.

If hospitals approach negotiating sessions with less information than their adversary in the negotiation, it adds to the difficulties that already

Source: Reprinted from Steven A. Finkler, "HMO Negotiations and Hospital Costs," *Hospital Cost Management and Accounting,* Vol. 3, No. 7, October 1991, pp. 1–4. Copyright 1991, Aspen Publishers, Inc.

exist in arriving at an agreement fair to the hospital. If the HMO knows more about the hospital's own costs than the hospital knows, it removes any remaining bargaining chips the hospital may have.

WHO REALLY HAS BETTER COST INFORMATION?

Despite the claims that HMOs know more about costs than hospitals, the actual truth may be somewhat different. Perhaps HMOs just think that they know more.

For the most part HMOs get their cost information from hospital Medicare cost reports. Since these are public documents, they are easily obtained by the HMO. One can hardly assume, however, that with the hospital's cost report in hand, the HMO now knows more than the hospital. At the same time, hospital managers should realize that HMOs are likely to have some reliable sources of information.

Espionage

The Kralewski study of strategies employed by HMOs indicates that some unsophisticated industrial espionage takes place.[2] Most hospital managers would be quick to dismiss such a melodramatic possibility.

However, it would not be surprising to find that HMOs have actually obtained some inside information that would give them an edge in the negotiations. Should the Chief Financial Officer conduct monthly lie-detector tests to see which finance department staff members are leaking information? Probably the place to look for leaks is in the medical staff.

The medical staff clearly has mixed interests. On the one hand they want the hospital to thrive. On the other hand, to the extent that members of the hospital staff are also members of an HMO, there is a clear conflict of interest. The conflict becomes severe if some of the physicians who practice at the hospital share in the profits of the HMO.

This is especially true for not-for-profit hospitals. They are prevented from treating physicians as partners who share in profits. Yet the for-profit HMO is not. That means that a reduction in hospital profits and increase in HMO profits benefits those physicians directly. The implication of this problem is that hospitals must be quite judicious in sharing cost information with physicians who are also HMO members.

Even with tight security over cost information, there is the potential for physician leaks of readily available information such as the way the hospital staffs units, or the usual occupancy of various special service units in the hospital.

The Cost Report vs. Marginal Costs

If HMOs are using the hospital's Medicare cost report, this may give the HMOs more information than a hospital manager would desire them to have. Nevertheless, it should put the hospital manager in control. Knowing what is reported as costs using the appropriate cost report methodology is very different from knowing the cost implications of an HMO contract. At best, cost reports use historical average cost information. HMO contracts, however, must be considered by the hospital on the basis of marginal or incremental costs.

To calculate whether an HMO contract is beneficial, the manager must consider the hospital's financial position with the contract, and without it. In the simplest terms, what will be the total revenues and total expenses of the hospital if it has the contract, versus what will be the total revenues and total expenses of the hospital if it does not have the contract? The difference between these two calculations directly lets the manager know whether the hospital is financially better off with the contract or not.

The information needed to calculate such differences is not average costs, but rather marginal costs. The cost report may give an HMO a start in calculating marginal costs, but the hospital managers should be able to make much better estimates.

The hospital knows which units are nearly full and which are not. It knows how many more patients it can take with little or no increase in personnel costs. It knows a great deal about its fixed and variable costs. That information can be translated into approximations of marginal costs.

HMOs really cannot make good estimates of these factors. For example, based on a cost report an HMO may assume that all nursing salary costs are variable. In fact, each unit has a number of fixed personnel costs related to minimum staffing levels, head nurse salaries, and clinical specialist salaries.

If the HMOs assume that all nursing unit personnel costs are variable, it will overestimate the marginal costs of the hospital. That would lead it to believe that the hospital has less room for negotiating than it actually has. It is interesting to note that the Kralewski study, which indicates that HMOs know more about hospital costs than hospitals do, is based on a study of HMOs. Perhaps HMOs don't know as much as they think.

Careful Preparation for Negotiations

If hospitals do have less information than HMOs, the only possible explanation is one of poor preparation. The Kralewski study did note that HMOs tend to have specific strategies for dealing with hospitals, while hospitals have not seemed to have strategies for dealing with HMOs. One element of an overall strategy is the careful preparation of the financial information that forms the basis for any arrangement.

It is possible that hospitals have taken a more haphazard approach, deciding by the seat of their pants whether a contract seems financially advantageous or not. Such an approach would not seem to be in the best interests of hospitals that wish to survive in the long run.

How Low To Go

In dealing with an HMO, one question that hospitals ultimately face is how low to go. This is a difficult problem for the hospital. From a strict economic theory viewpoint, hospitals should be willing to take any additional business at any price that exceeds the marginal cost of the additional patients.

Some hospitals avoid the problem through a quick magic trick. They practice discounting through price illusion. This approach simply requires the hospital to negotiate its HMO prices as a percentage discount from charges. The benefit this has for the hospital is that once the HMO is firmly entrenched in the hospital, the hospital can raise its charges, thereby effectively recovering all or nearly all of the negotiated discount.

Given such a strategy, it would be understandable if hospital managers didn't spend much time getting too deeply involved in understanding hospital costs. However, HMOs are not likely to allow such price illusion to enter into their contracts.

The Long-Run Implications of Discounts

In trying to decide how low to go, the hospital must try to gain an understanding of why they are dealing with the HMO, and what the long-run implications are.

The most common reason to offer an HMO a discount is because there is overcapacity in the hospital industry, and the HMO promises volume. If the local hospital industry does have excess beds, and the HMO has alternatives, then hospitals are forced to negotiate.

This is not always the case. Sometimes a hospital may be the sole provider. Even if it has excess capacity, the HMO has little opportunity to steer patients to other facilities.

Sometimes there is little excess capacity. For-profit HMOs entered the New York City market with a flourish several years ago, but did not fare nearly as well as expected. New York City hospitals did not have substantial amounts of excess capacity. As a result, the HMOs did not obtain their normal discounts. They became a high-priced alternative to other types of insurance. In many markets the HMO reaction is to compete on the wide range of services they offer. However, in New York there are strong labor unions, and insurance coverage was already broad.

It is common, however, for HMOs to exist in markets that have a number of hospitals, each with excess capacity. In that case, what prices must hospitals offer, or can they afford to offer? Any price that is below charges, but above average cost, will yield a profit for the hospital.

Even if some of the volume offered represents individuals who currently would be patients of the hospital and who pay charges, the hospital should be willing to agree to a price that exceeds average cost. It is important to bear in mind that the appropriate calculation is not based on existing revenues, but on the revenues if the HMO provides the volume to the hospital, versus if the HMO takes the patients to another hospital.

What if the negotiations reach a point where the only agreeable price to the HMO is less than average cost? As long as it exceeds the marginal cost, it is beneficial in the short run. This is because the fixed costs of the hospital will be incurred in any case. If the revenue exceeds the marginal costs of the patients, the short-run profit will increase.

What about the long-run profits? If patients are paying less than average cost, the hospital may find itself in a position where it cannot afford to replace its fixed facilities as they wear out over time. If the portion of patients not paying at least average cost grows, this could become a serious problem. It is unreasonable to expect that discounting below average cost can continue for an unlimited time period for that reason.

When HMOs provide volume to one hospital, they take it away from another. In markets with excess capacity, this creates severe financial problems for some hospitals. Over the long run, this is likely to cause a reduction in the number of beds in the community. As the excess capacity problem disappears, hospitals will have less need to offer discounts to HMOs. On the other hand, the reduction in capacity should make the system more efficient. With the remaining hospitals having high occupancy levels, their cost per patient should be lower.

Your hospital must base its plan on the approach that is most likely to allow it to be one of the ultimate survivors. This might well require deep discounts, well below average cost, in order to get HMO business. What if negotiations reach a point where the price would actually be less than the marginal costs of treating the patients? In that case the hospital may well decide not to deal with the HMO. Clearly, such a contract would mean that overall profits will decline, or losses will rise.

Nevertheless the hospital must take a long-term perspective. If it accepts losses in the near term, will that result in reduced competition? There may be times when it is worth accepting losses for a period of time. On the other hand, the hospital must be careful that it does not put itself in a position of being guilty of antitrust violations. Cut-throat pricing is not legal.

CONCLUSION

The most important conclusion to be drawn from this discussion about hospital costs and their role in negotiations with HMOs is that the hospital should develop a clear strategy for its relationships with HMOs. The hospital cannot negotiate effectively until it decides whether a relationship with an HMO is seen as a necessary evil or a mutually benefiting good. It must decide if its goals concern increases in profits, or simply maintenance of existing market share. It must determine whether the HMO has control over solely its patients, or its physicians as well. And the hospital must plan with care for the financial aspects of any negotiation.

NOTES

1. J.E. Kralewski, et al., "Strategies Employed by HMOs to Achieve Hospital Discounts: A Case Study of Seven HMOs," *Health Care Management Review,* Vol. 16, No. 1, Winter 1991, p. 14.

2. Ibid., p. 12.

Reading 5–2

Capitated Hospital Contracts: The Empty Beds versus Filled Beds Controversy

Steven A. Finkler

Recently, the importance of keeping hospital beds empty under capitated arrangements has been pointed out. Although everyone would agree that there is no reason to hospitalize an individual who does not need hospital care, we would not all necessarily agree on the implications of managed care contracts.

This article contends that the financial incentives of fundamental cost accounting dictate keeping beds filled, not empty, under capitated arrangements. It argues that hospitals that equate the philosophy of keeping patients healthy and out of the hospital with the philosophy of keeping beds empty are doomed to failure.

A BASE CASE SCENARIO

To understand the financial incentives that exist under capitation, we will start with a base case situation and then examine what happens under alternative hospital payment or reimbursement approaches. Assume the following information:

Fixed costs for a hospital	$1,000,000
Original number of patients per year	1,000
Original average length of stay	10

Source: Reprinted from Steven A. Finkler, "Capitated Hospital Contracts: The Empty Beds versus Filled Beds Controversy," *Health Care Management Review,* Vol. 20, No. 3, Summer 1995, pp. 88–91. Copyright 1995, Aspen Publishers, Inc.

Hospital capacity inpatient days (i.e., hospital is full)	10,000
Variable cost per patient day	$200
Original per diem reimbursement rate	$280
Weighted average diagnostic-related group (DRG) rate	$2,800

These base data will be used throughout this article.

PER DIEM ENVIRONMENT

Historically, per diem reimbursement has been a common approach in some states. For example, until just a few years ago, care for most hospital inpatients in New York was paid for on a per diem basis. Using the base case scenario information, we can calculate the expected revenues, costs, and profits for a hospital under that form of reimbursement.

Revenue

1,000 patients × 10-day stay × $280/day	$2,800,000

Expenses

Fixed cost	$1,000,000
Variable cost, $200/day × 1,000 patients × 10 days/patient	2,000,000
Total expenses	$3,000,000
Loss	$(200,000)

Under this simple per diem approach to reimbursement, the hospital in our base case scenario will lose $200,000.

What if the hospital attempts to become more efficient by lowering average length of stay by 10 percent? How will that alter its revenues and expenses?

Revenue

1,000 patients × *9-day stay* × $280/day	$2,520,000

Expenses

Fixed cost	$1,000,000
Variable cost, $200/day × 1,000 patients × 9 days/patient	1,800,000
Total expenses	$2,800,000
Loss	$(280,000)

What impact did improved efficiency have on the hospital? The loss got greater rather than smaller. Why? Although revenue declined in direct proportion to reduced patient days, expenses did not. Variable costs declined, but fixed costs did not. This fundamental behavior of costs should indicate the desirability of increasing volume up to capacity. Revenues generally will rise faster than costs when volume increases and fall faster than costs when volume decreases. Under a per diem reimbursement approach, volume is measured in terms of patient days, and more patient days are desirable.

DRG ENVIRONMENT

Most hospitals currently have at least some of their inpatients paid on a DRG basis. What are the revenues and expenses for our base case scenario under a DRG payment system?

Revenue

1,000 patients × $2,800/discharge	$2,800,000

Expenses

Fixed cost	$1,000,000
Variable cost, $200/day × 1,000 patients × 10 days/patient	2,000,000
Total expenses	$3,000,000
Loss	$(200,000)

Note that the loss is the same as the initial per diem result in the example.

Suppose that under a DRG payment system, the hospital lowers length of stay by 10 percent? In the per diem example, we found that such an approach would increase the loss.

Revenue

1,000 patients × $2,800/day	$2,800,000

Expenses

Fixed cost	$1,000,000
Variable cost, $200/day × 1,000 patients × 9 days/patient	1,800,000
Total expenses	$2,800,000
Loss	$0

Now the loss has been completely eliminated.

There is clearly an incentive to shorten length of stay under a DRG payment system. Revenues did not change as length of stay declined, nor did fixed costs. However, variable costs were reduced as the length of stay declined. With the reduced length of stay, the hospital is no longer full. It has some empty beds. Would one conclude that we want to reduce length of stay and keep beds empty under a DRG payment arrangement? That is unlikely, as the following example demonstrates.

Suppose the hospital fills some of the newly empty beds with more patients. What if it adds 100 patients?

Revenue

1,100 patients × $2,800/discharge	$3,080,000

Expenses

Fixed cost	$1,000,000
Variable cost, $200/day × *1,100 patients* × 9 days	1,980,000
Total expenses	$2,980,000
Profit	$100,000

Now the hospital is earning a profit on those newly emptied beds. Under a DRG payment approach, there is clearly an incentive to keep the hospital full, albeit with patients that have a shorter length of stay. Note that because hospitals still want to be full, ultimately fewer hospitals will be needed. Therefore, a reduction in the number of short-term acute care hospitals is likely under a DRG payment system. In fact, during the past 10 years, there has been significant consolidation and a reduction in the number of hospitals.

MANAGED CARE AND CAPITATION

Are the same set of incentives likely to hold in a capitated environment? Suppose all patients come from HMOs and that the hospital is paid on a totally capitated basis. This is the scenario under which many have said that a hospital must learn to keep patients healthy and beds empty: The fewer inpatients the better, once all of the payments are capitated. The following examples will show the fallacy of that argument.

Suppose there are 1,100 inpatients with an average length of stay of 9 days. Suppose further:

Total population in area	1,000,000
Lives covered by arrangements with managed care providers	50,000
Per member per month (PMPM) rate	$4.50

The hospital will be paid $4.50 per covered life per month for inpatient services.

Revenue

50,000 members × $4.50 PMPM × 12 months	$2,700,000
Expenses	
Fixed cost	$1,000,000
Variable cost, $200/day × 1,100 discharges × 9 days	1,980,000
Total expenses	$2,980,000
Loss	$(280,000)

The hospital is operating relatively efficiently. It has reduced length of stay from 10 days to 9 days, and it is utilizing its facility (spreading its fixed cost) by treating 1,100 instead of 1,000 patients. However, the managed care company, perhaps an HMO, has negotiated a low price. Under the current arrangement, the hospital has a loss. This loss gives the hospital an incentive to try to achieve even greater efficiency. Suppose the average length of stay is reduced to eight days.

Revenue

50,000 members × $4.50 PMPM × 12 months	$2,700,000
Expenses	
Fixed cost	$1,000,000
Variable cost, $200/day × 1,100 discharges × 8 days	1,760,000
Total expenses	$2,760,000
Loss	$(60,000)

The reduced length of stay has helped, but the hospital is still losing money.

The HMO works to find ways to keep the members healthier, reducing the number of people needing in-patient hospitalization to 1,050:

Revenue

50,000 members × $4.50 PMPM × 12 months	$2,700,000
Expenses	
Fixed cost	$1,000,000
Variable cost, $200/day × 1,050 patients × 8 days	1,680,000
Total expenses	$2,680,000
Profit	$20,000

The hospital is now earning a profit. However, it has capacity for 10,000 patient days but is generating only 8,400 (1,050 × 8). It has 1,600 empty bed days. Does it want to keep those beds empty?

What if those beds are filled with patients who are currently part of the hospital's 50,000 covered lives? How much do costs go up per patient? For each extra patient, there will be $200 of variable cost per day for 8 days or an incremental cost of $1,600 per patient. How much does revenue go up per patient? Because payment is on a capitated basis, there is no revenue increase. This is the source of the idea that hospitals want to keep their beds empty under capitation.

However, what if the hospital *covers more lives?* Suppose it makes an additional arrangement with another HMO and covers an additional 9,000 lives. This is an 18 percent increase from the previous 50,000 lives covered. Assume that the 1,050 patients treated will increase by 18 percent to 1,239.

Revenue

59,000 members × $4.50 PMPM × 12 months	$3,186,000

Expenses

Fixed cost	$1,000,000
Variable cost, $200/day × 1,239 patients × 8 days	1,982,400
Total expenses	$2,982,400
Profit	$203,600

Profits have increased substantially. Why did the profits increase? Didn't both revenue and cost rise by 18 percent? No! Revenue rose by 18 percent and variable costs rose by 18 percent, but fixed costs did not rise at all.

Revenue-generating volume increases will generally increase profits unless all costs are variable. Volume decreases that reduce revenues will generally result in reduced profits or increased losses unless all costs are variable.

Certainly, one can argue that inpatient hospitalization should be minimized for any fixed number of covered lives. Keeping members healthy and out of the hospital may well make sense. However, that does not translate into keeping a hospital empty under capitation. Full hospitals spread fixed costs over a broad number of patients, minimizing the cost of treating each one. If capitation reduces the number of admissions, this is not likely to result in many hospitals operating at low volumes. It is more likely to result in further reduction in the number of hospitals. Managers who fail to note this key point place their hospitals at risk of closure.

EXTENDING THE CASE TO PHYSICIANS

A similar caution should be extended to physicians. At one time the economics of medical care indicated that physician supply increases were accompanied by price increases. Studies had shown that as more surgeons moved into an area, both the quantity of and price for surgery increased. This, of course, is contrary to the normal functioning of supply and demand, which dictates that as supply increases, prices fall. Quite simply, supply and demand rules did not function normally in the marketplace for physician services.

Managed care is dramatically changing that. As HMOs control utilization, especially of specialist services, the wise physician response cannot be to increase price in response to the decrease in demand. The concept of pricing physician services to attain an expected "target income" no longer holds in the new environment. Managed care will ensure that an excess of surgeons does not simply increase the number of surgeries. Nor will it allow for price increases.

In such an environment, physicians will need to keep a large number of patients to maintain an income. Just as hospitals will desire to cover more and more lives, and stay full, physicians will need to do the same. Just as some hospitals will inevitably close, some physicians will wind up leaving the profession. The last to realize this are the most at risk.

Privatization in Health Care Institutions

Yehia Dabaa
Shari Faith Fisch
Ellen Gordon

INTRODUCTION

In today's health care environment, hospitals provide services that may or may not be performed more economically by outside entities. This article concerns the relative benefits of privatizing an area of service or maintaining the status quo. A hypothetical case study of a non-routine decision is offered to help readers comprehend the benefits that may be realized and obstacles that may be faced in privatizing an area of service.

At the most basic level, privatization refers to an organization's shift from public to private ownership. Instead of being held accountable to the taxpayers, the organization is responsible to the stockholders. Advocates of privatization believe that it increases worker motivation to provide quality care. With increased health care costs, decreased government subsidies, slashed hospital budgets, and a myriad of constraints on resources, health care managers are looking to the private sector to lower costs and increase efficiency.

PRIVATIZATION: INHERENT BELIEFS AND POSSIBLE GAINS

Some health care managers believe the health care market should distance itself from public,

Source: Reprinted from Yehia Dabaa, Shari Faith Fisch, and Ellen Gordon, "Privatization in Health Care Institutions," *Hospital Cost Management and Accounting,* Vol. 4, No. 12, March 1992, pp. 1–8. Copyright 1992, Aspen Publishers, Inc.

nonprofit organizational structures and rely more on the private sector. The reliance on privatization as a cure for the health care industry's upward-spiraling costs is due to ingrained beliefs about the nature of publicly owned entities and their privately owned counterparts. Many people believe public and nonprofit organizations permit bureaucratic malaise, which in turn promotes excess capacity, inefficient uses of resources, and technical obsolescence.

Advocates base their beliefs in the primacy of privatization and the inefficiencies of public and nonprofit organizations on a basic acceptance of the economic equation by which supply and demand is influenced by market forces. The market system—which involves buyers and sellers trading their goods freely—is a function of a capitalist economic system. Other aspects of capitalism include free enterprise, private ownership of capital, and free choice.

Advocates of privatization believe that the hospital's overhead allocation of indirect costs increases the prices of goods as compared to a natural supply-and-demand environment. Through overhead allocations, hospitals subsidize cost centers with inefficiently run areas because they need to include these departments in the overall organization. In situations where costs are subsidized, resources are not utilized to their peak efficiency and prices are kept higher than they would be under competitive market conditions. These price floors are not influenced by market demand and represent an imposed inefficiency in the public sphere. Inefficiencies of this kind in the private sector may result in an organization's inability to compete, and it may eventually go out of business. In a market situation, privatization would probably ensure that the most efficient method of production is used.

Other inefficiencies also exist. Under hospital control, a department may produce a good but otherwise have little autonomy. Hospitals allocate portions of fixed and indirect costs to various departments that are not controlled by the department manager. Lack of managerial control destroys the drive for innovation in the workplace, hampers the growth of technology, and limits the development of more efficient modes of production; management makes do with an overhead allocation system that functions as a deterrent to managerial excellence.

Many people advocate a return to a purer market equation. A competitive market would increase hospital efficiency, lower costs, and increase quality. Privatization is the call to arms of those advocating less administrative, legislative, and regulatory oversight and greater reliance on market forces.

THE ROLE OF COST ACCOUNTING AND NONROUTINE DECISION MAKING

Relying on market forces for a definitive assessment of the pros and cons of privatization does not necessarily answer all the needs of today's health care manager. Managers need more information about privatizing an area of service than can be contributed by supply and demand curves. In order to do a cost benefit analysis—in which the costs associated with all viable options are compared—managers must be sufficiently versed in cost accounting applications and which costs are important for each nonroutine decision. When considering privatizing within a hospital environment, health care managers should carefully consider the nature of costs, whether they are fixed, variable, joint, sunk, direct, or indirect. For example, if one area of the hospital is privatized, hospital-incurred indirect costs and short-term fixed costs associated with the area in question will have to be reallocated to other hospital-wide departments; what may appear to be a cost savings may actually be a cost shuffling.

Within the framework of a nonroutine decision, health care managers need to identify the relevant costs (i.e., those that vary with the decision being made). Nonroutine decisions include the following.

- *Add/Drop*—adding or dropping a service. Overhead allocation of hospital indirect and joint costs should not be considered; they are not relevant to the decision to adopt a new service, because they are costs that are already incurred and they are not saved costs if management decides to drop a service.

- *Expand/Downsize*—expanding or limiting the scope of a service. All costs contingent on volume are relevant to this nonroutine decision. With this in mind, the fixed costs of providing the service are not relevant. When management decides to decrease or increase volume levels, costs of consequence are the variable costs associated with each patient and step-fixed costs associated with provision of service.

- *Make/Buy*—produce a product or service in-house or purchase it from an outside entity. If a good is produced in-house, relevant costs include capital costs and replacement costs of the fixed assets used in production, as well as all costs incurred from the production function. Managers should do a cost-benefit analysis where the measure of cost for internal production is based on the money we spend to produce the item that we would avoid spending if the item is not produced.

In most of these nonroutine decisions, joint costs (those that cannot be separated by usage) and common costs (those shared by all variables under consideration) are ignored, as are sunk costs (those associated with the original investment). Managers should attempt to avoid decisions based on irrelevant or inaccurate information. Further, irrelevant information may be misleading and lead to a wrong decision. Managers need to use critical thinking and look at all angles of a situation when doing these analyses.

THREE WAYS TO PRIVATIZE

Incorporating privatization into nonroutine hospital decision making requires an understanding of the privatization options available to health care managers. There are three ways for a publicly owned or operated organization to privatize: (1) contracting out, (2) hiring a private firm, and (3) consolidating production. Contracting out—one of the more conventional privatization methods—refers to the purchase of goods or services normally produced in-house from an outside, private company. For example, instead of manufacturing saline bags in-house, the hospital could contract with a privately owned company to provide for all its saline needs. When organizations contract out, short-run fixed costs remain, but all costs are variable in the long run; variable costs are saved in the short run but are replaced by the contract price plus ordering and carrying costs. The organization's overhead allocation costs remain the same, but department-wide indirect costs may decrease.

As with contracting for service, managers expect the costs associated with hiring a private firm to produce a desired good to be lower than those of producing it in-house. Public organizations hire private firms to manage various services or production processes. These private firms serve as consultants, lawyers, and other outside forces. For example, a private consultant may be hired to advise in-house production staff on saline production.

A third type of privatization relies on consolidating efforts among a number of public entities in a joint effort to create efficiencies of scale. Take, for example, a hospital that offers to produce saline for other hospitals in the area. The expected costs of using excess capacity to produce saline must account for a portion of fixed costs, the variable costs of production, and whatever profit margin is desirable and still within the competitive price range.

WHERE DOES PRIVATIZATION WORK BEST?

Privatization in the public/nonprofit sector works best when the area under analysis produces an actual product, as in the saline example above. The product can be compared on an equivalent level with any good in the free market. Costs relevant to the production function include production and carrying costs, and the managers must assess resources needed per volume level, and so on. The following case study illustrates the issues surrounding privatization and how cost accounting is used within the framework on a nonroutine decision.

CASE STUDY: WINTERPARK HOSPITAL

WinterPark Hospital is facing a problem experienced by many hospitals around the country. The facility was expanded in the early 1980s, when inpatient utilization was increasing and the hospital needed additional space. In an effort to remain competitive in its relatively affluent suburban service area, the hospital constructed a facility twice the size of its original plant. WinterPark's resulting elaborate structure translated into high fixed costs. In particular, management projected that volume would increase significantly; consequently, a laboratory was built to accommodate this expected volume. Management's hope was to increase the number of lab tests performed as well as the complexity (acuity) of the tests performed.

In an effort to reduce the organization's overall costs, a special task force has been established to review hospital services and find ways to reduce costs. The hospital is examining many inpatient department revenue centers as well as numerous ancillary departments. The laboratory is the first department selected for review. The task force members hope to determine if the lab contributes to the hospital's bottom line and if they should consider contracting out for all or a portion of the tests performed by the lab. Qualitative issues are always a concern when purchasing from the outside, and the task force will have to evaluate if the tests will be properly done and available on a timely basis if they choose this alternative. However, if these conditions are satisfied, they intend to make differential costing the key financial consideration (i.e., which alternative will cost less to implement).

This analysis is separated into three components or scenarios: (1) base case—all tests are performed in-house, (2) close the lab and contract out for all services, and (3) retain "Not Complex" tests and "Complex" tests but contract with an outside firm for all "Very Complex" tests (the lab performs only these three types of tests).

Base Case Scenario: Keep Full-Service Laboratory

Under this scenario, total costs and total revenues must be examined. As presented in Table 5–3–1, fixed costs for the lab are $500,000. These costs include depreciation of the building and equipment, supervisors' salaries, four technicians, the fixed-cost portion of laundry and housekeeping departments allocated to the lab,

---

Table 5–3–1 Assumptions about WinterPark Hospital's Full Service Laboratory (Base Case Scenario)

Number of tests performed annually:	10,000
Types of laboratory tests performed:	
Not Complex	A—50%
Complex	B—25%
Very Complex	C—25%
Program-specific fixed costs (includes depreciation, supervisors' salaries, two technicians, laundry, housekeeping, and other indirect costs):	A—$250,000 B— 125,000 C— 125,000 $500,000
Price/reimbursement for all three lab tests:	$ 58.00
Joint costs (these are relevant in the decision to close the laboratory, although they are not relevant when reviewing each type of test)	$100,000

and other indirect costs associated with performing laboratory services. In addition, fixed costs have been separated into program-specific fixed costs. As stated above, the lab performs three different tests, with a total of 10,000 tests annually. Test A constitutes 50 percent of all tests performed, while Test B and Test C represent 25 percent each. Joint costs are those required to perform several types of tests. It has been determined that joint costs should not be allocated when deciding whether or not to discontinue a service, primarily because these costs will exist even if Test A, for example, is discontinued. However, joint costs should be allocated when making resource allocation decisions and when calculating the cost of the entire department. Our cost objective (i.e., what we are trying to measure) is the cost of performing all three tests at the existing hospital lab.

Table 5–3–2 presents the costs of operating the lab. Total variable costs are $100,000, based on the number of tests performed and the variable cost per test. Total costs (fixed and variable) are $600,000. Total revenue for all tests is $580,000. This assumes that the hospital receives $58 per test.* Based on this calculation, the lab will lose $20,000 per year if they continue to perform all three tests in-house. More specifically, Test A produces a profit of $15,000 while Test B and Test C incur losses of $5,000 and $30,000 respectively.

As mentioned earlier, WinterPark expects to perform more Very Complex tests (Test C) than Not Complex tests (Test A). However, based on data for the past five years (which is reviewed monthly), the hospital consistently performs twice as many Not Complex tests as either Complex or Very Complex tests.

Breakeven analysis determines the volume at which a program is just financially self-sufficient. In order to calculate the breakeven for

---

Editor's note: It may be unrealistic to price all tests at the same rate. Bear in mind, however, that the objective of this case study is to focus on privatization and techniques to approach it. The specific data are of only minor significance.

Table 5-3-2 Base Case Scenario—Profits

COST OF OPERATING THE LABORATORY

Total Fixed Costs

	# Tests	% of Total	FC	VC
Test A	5,000	50%	$250,000	$ 5
Test B	2,500	25%	125,000	10
Test C	2,500	25%	125,000	20
	10,000		$500,000	

Total Variable Costs

	# Tests		VC		Total VC
Test A	5,000	×	$ 5	=	$ 25,000
Test B	2,500	×	10	=	25,000
Test C	2,500	×	20	=	50,000
					$100,000

Total Costs

	VC		FC		Total Costs	Average
Test A	$25,000	+	$250,000	=	$275,000	$55
Test B	25,000	+	125,000	=	150,000	60
Test C	50,000	+	125,000	=	175,000	70
Total cost					$600,000	

REVENUES—REIMBURSEMENT

	Price	# Tests	Total Reimbursement	Total Cost	Gain/(Loss)
Test A	$58	5,000	$290,000	$275,000	$ 15,000
Test B	58	2,500	145,000	150,000	(5,000)
Test C	58	2,500	145,000	175,000	(30,000)
Total revenue			$580,000	$600,000	$ (20,000)

Total revenue = $580,000
Total cost = $600,000
Loss incurred = $20,000

---

multiple tests, the average price and the weighted average variable cost must be calculated. WinterPark receives the same reimbursement (price) for each test; therefore, the weighted average price is $58. The variable cost per test, weighted by complexity, is $10. For the hospital to break even as a whole, it must cover all costs—including both program-specific fixed costs and hospital-wide joint costs. As shown in Table 5-3-3, in order to break even, the lab must

Table 5–3–3 Base Case Scenario—Breakeven

BREAKEVEN ANALYSIS

Weighted Average Variable Costs				Weighted Average Price			
50% ×	$ 5.00 =	$2.50		50% ×	$58 =	$29
25% ×	10.00 =	2.50		25% ×	58 =	15
25% ×	20.00 =	5.00		25% ×	58 =	15
		$10.00				$58

$$Q = \frac{\text{Fixed Costs}}{\text{Price} - \text{Variable Costs}}$$

$$= \frac{\$500,000 + \$100,000}{\$58 - \$10} = 12,500 \text{ tests}$$

BREAKEVEN FOR EACH TEST

Breakeven for Test A

$$Q = \frac{\$250,000}{\$58 - \$5} = 4,716 \text{ tests}$$

Breakeven for Test B

$$Q = \frac{\$125,000}{\$58 - \$10} = 2,604 \text{ tests}$$

Breakeven for Test C

$$Q = \frac{\$125,000}{\$58 - \$20} = 3,290 \text{ tests}$$

perform 12,500 tests annually. Of this total number, 50 percent would be Test A, 25 percent Test B, and 25 percent Test C. Although 50 percent of 12,500 is 6,250, when we consider performing Test A alone and calculate the breakeven, we determine that we need only 4,716 tests. This is because for any one service, joint costs need not be considered. The first 4,716 tests cover the direct fixed costs of the service, and each additional Test A performed contributes toward joint fixed costs in the amount equal to the difference between the price and the variable cost (contribution margin). If Test A volume will exceed 4,716,

the test would be desirable as long as the lab operates and incurs joint costs anyway.

Based on this analysis, the lab incurs a loss of $20,000. And based on the breakeven analysis performed for the entire department, additional tests must be performed if the lab is to be self-sufficient. Clearly the lab is a necessary function of the hospital, which must provide lab services in order to service its patients' needs, and the hospital may decide to absorb this loss for the overall good of the organization. Many physicians may be discouraged from admitting patients to hospitals without full labs, because of the possible inconvenience of using an outside company. In this case the overall loss would be significant, because patient volume might drop, causing a greater loss.

Another alternative might be to keep the lab and increase the volume of tests performed. Although the hospital may have difficulty attracting patients due to the competitive environment, WinterPark might consider contracting with other nearby hospitals to perform their tests. The decision to expand these services will depend on the price received for performing them. While WinterPark needs to cover its variable costs, it should also consider covering a portion of its fixed costs to contribute to the bottom line. Additional capacity constraints must also be accounted for.

Scenario 2: Contract Out for All Lab Services

This alternative requires close examination, because even though it is likely that some fixed costs—such as annual capital expenditures to replace equipment as it wears or becomes obsolete—could probably be avoided if the lab was closed, other fixed costs would remain. Under the current arrangement, some of the fixed costs cover depreciation on the building and an allocation of joint costs from the entire organization.

The lab at WinterPark Hospital generates revenues of $580,000 and costs of $600,000. If we close the lab, fixed costs of $200,000 will remain (see Table 5–3–4). Thus, by closing the lab the

Table 5–3–4 Scenario 2: Close the Existing Lab and Contract Out for All Tests

Relevant Costs and Revenues

Revenues	$0	(no tests performed)
Variable Costs:	$0	
Fixed Costs:	$200,000*	

If we close the lab entirely, the hospital will lose $200,000. This loss is $180,000 more than that of keeping the lab open.

*Includes depreciation on the building and fixed overhead allocated from other departments.

hospital would lose more money than by keeping it open. In the short run the hospital has incurred many fixed costs already and they are no longer relevant, but the overhead remains. Based on this analysis, the task force has eliminated this alternative from its options.

Scenario 3: Retain Services for Test A and Test B and Contract Out for Test C

It is important to note that the lab has additional capacity to perform more lab tests and that the equipment is relatively new. Test C is a labor-intensive test, as reflected in the higher variable cost of $20. An outside company that specializes in this type of lab test recently offered to perform all Test C lab tests for $15 per test; the contract extends for five years but will adjust in price based on volume. This is $5 less than the hospital's current variable cost. Given the special nature of the test and the large volume this outside firm services, they can perform these tests at a much lower price. The task force was excited to learn that this test can be performed at a lower variable cost, but before making a final decision they wanted to know how this would affect the entire laboratory's profitability. As presented in Table 5–3–5, fixed costs for Test C would decrease from $125,000 to $75,000—a reduction of $50,000. The remaining $75,000 would be allocated to Test A and Test B, because these costs

would still remain within the department. This will result in revised fixed costs of $300,000 and $150,000 for Test A and Test B, respectively.

Total revenues remain the same—$580,000—and total cost (including the lower variable cost associated with Test C) is reduced to $537,500. Therefore, the entire department would make a profit of $42,500. Reviewing the individual tests, however, reveals that Test A incurs a loss of $35,000 and Test B loses $30,000. These tests have more fixed costs allocated to them, so their losses rise. We have learned that careful review must be performed before services are purchased from outside the organization, because some fixed costs still remain and then must be absorbed by the entire department. In this example, the lower variable cost associated with Test C outweighs the additional overhead included in the fixed-cost component for the other tests performed.

Case Study Conclusion

The task force plans to recommend to the board of directors that the hospital accept the contract to perform Test C lab tests outside the hospital lab. However, the task force has requested that the laboratory personnel re-evaluate its fixed and variable cost components and review its cost structure to ensure that all direct costs are allocated correctly. The task force expected Test C, given its complexity, to account for greater fixed and variable costs. If these figures change, another evaluation of the cost differential is needed. The relevant costs in this example include the variable costs. The joint costs are not included, because we would not avoid these costs if Test C was not performed in the existing lab. As the lab continues to age, additional analyses will have to be completed to calculate the benefit of contracting out for the entire lab service. In addition, the hospital expects to evaluate the short run option of contracting with other hospitals to increase its existing volume and perhaps cover a greater portion of its fixed costs.

Table 5–3–5 Scenario 3: Retain Test A and Test B and Contract Out for Test C

COST OF OPERATING THE LABORATORY

Total Fixed Costs

	# Tests	% of Total	FC	VC	Revised FC
Test A	5,000	67%	$250,000	$ 5	$300,000
Test B	2,500	33%	125,000	10	150,000
Test C	0	0%	75,000	15	0
	7,500				

Test C fixed costs declined from $125,000 to $75,000 due to one less supervisor and one technician. Test C fixed costs that remain include equipment, fixed portion of allocated costs (laundry), and other fixed costs.

Total Variable Costs

	# Tests		VC		Total VC	
Test A	5,000	×	$ 5	=	$ 25,000	
Test B	2,500	×	10	=	25,000	
Test C	2,500	×	15	=	37,500	(payment to outside lab)
					$ 87,500	

Total Costs

	Revised		
	VC	FC	Total
Test A	$25,000	$300,000	$325,000
Test B	25,000	150,000	175,000
Test C	37,500	0	37,500
Total cost			$537,500

REVENUES—REIMBURSEMENT

	Price	# Tests	Total Reimbursement	Total Cost	Gain/ (Loss)
Test A	$58	5,000	$290,000	$325,000	$(35,000)
Test B	58	2,500	145,000	175,000	(30,000)
Test C	58	2,500	145,000	37,500	107,500
Total revenue			$580,000	$537,500	$ 42,500

Total revenue = $580,000
Total cost = $537,500s
Profit = $42,500

OBSTACLES FACED IN PRIVATIZATION

Like other management techniques, privatization has its supporters and opponents. Supporters believe that privatization of health care organizations could invigorate the market competition, lower costs, and improve quality and service effectiveness. Opponents, on the other hand, argue that very little is known about the effects of competition in the delivery of health care. Regardless of what the different parties believe, there are exogenous factors involved in accepting or rejecting this technique. Some of the factors impacting the privatization of health care providers include organization type and service provided, geographical location, union/employee rejection, and private providers chosen.

Organization Type and Service Provided

Successful applications of privatization principles are contingent on the type of organization and service provided. Privatization could work successfully in one market and fail in another. According to a number of sources, privatization leads to lower costs and improved cost control and service quality.[1] But the impact varies with the organization, and cost savings from the process of privatizing an area of service range from 10 percent to 60 percent.[2] As mentioned previously, production-oriented hospital services are easier to privatize than areas that are not quantifiable. Other issues that impact privatization include the organization's size, mission, and nonprofit or for-profit standing.

Geographical Location

The success or failure of privatization depends to a large extent on geographical location. One study showed that departments within a hospital increased the level of contracting out with a high level of return but another study indicated that there was a declining trend to contract out in county hospitals (some county hospitals apparently returned to public control after being privatized in the mid 1980s, due to substantial management fees charged by the private firms). Conflicting reports on the merits of privatization from broad-based studies overlook the differences in institutions located in different geographical areas, including differences in the cost of living, cost of supplies, base salaries, and qualified personnel available.

Union and Employee Rejection

Another issue of concern is the presence or absence of unions. Unions oppose privatization because they fear loss of power, and they could persuade employees and managers to oppose this technique by predicting that privatization would result in employee lay-offs and the exploitation and loss of control of managers. They might also repeat the cliché, "If it was effective, it would have been adopted long ago" and argue that better options are available. Employee resistance to privatization can damn the project before it is even implemented. Further, political infighting by the institution's Board of Directors, managers, or trustees can undermine privatization efforts; people may feel that privatizing areas of service is not consistent with the organization's mission statement.

Choice of Private Providers

In addition to the financial aspects of privatization are the issues of the relative quality of care provided by private organizations and consumer access to health care. The general consumer may fear that private firms would be interested in money alone and not in the public well-being. This is expressed as a fear of declining access to health care, and deterioration in the quality of care provided. Many believe that the budget cutting and privatization in many countries has led to serious deterioration not only of health but of education, housing, nutrition, and other social services.[3]

Choosing providers plays an important role in whether privatization is accepted or rejected. The right provider could produce satisfactory results, which would encourage further privatization. The wrong provider could cause dissatisfaction or abolishment of the technique. This highlights the importance of controlling acceptable providers. Some public organizations fall into the trap of accepting a private provider who makes the lowest bid initially but who intends to raise prices or lower quality later. They also might err by accepting high initial bid prices in their eagerness for early success and quick implementation. Public organizations should select candidates with care, weighing political, social, and economic costs against benefits. Patient satisfaction with the private provider must be a high priority, because patients who are dissatisfied with a service or good may be reluctant to pursue treatment. In a time of intense competition among providers, hospitals cannot afford to lose customers who choose not to use or to underutilize the health care facility because of privatized services.

CONCLUSION

At first glance, privatization of hospital services seems to be a panacea for the current fiscal crisis faced by health care institutions, but privatization may not always be in the organization's best interest. Advocates believe that privatization will lead to increased competition, lowered costs, and improved services. But short-term realities may not mesh with long-term needs, and hospitals must assess the full impact of privatizing any area of service. The case for or against privatization is not clear. Privatization may mean lower costs and higher profits for the area of service in question, but institution-wide costs must also be considered in the cost-benefit analysis; increased allocations to other departments may make privatization more expensive than maintaining the status quo. Privatization is not necessarily a market cure, but it can spur on an institution that may be beset with bureaucratic inertia and a lack of efficient technological changes.

NOTES

1. M.A. Walker, *Privatization: Tactics & Techniques* (Vancouver, BC: The Fraiser Institute, 1988), 218.
2. Ibid.
3. L.B. Gardner and R.M. Scheffler, Privatization in health care: Shifting the risk, *Medical Care Review* 45, no. 2 (Fall 1988):215–253.

BIBLIOGRAPHY

Burke, M. "Hospitals Seize New Opportunities in State Privatization Efforts." *Hospitals* 66, No. 7 (5 April 1992): 50–52, 54.

Clarkson, K.W. "Privatization at the State and Local level." *Privatization and State-Owned Enterprises* 3 (1989):144–207.

Cox, W. "Privatization in the Public Service: Competitive Contracting and the Public Ethic in Urban Public Transport." In *Privatization: Tactics and Techniques* by M.A. Walker, pp. 200–237. Vancouver, B.C.: The Fraiser Institute, 1988.

Crowningshield, G.R. "Cost Accounting: Principles and Managerial Applications." 2:685–692, 1969.

Finkler, S.A. *Cost Accounting for Health Care Organizations: Concepts and Applications.* Gaithersburg, MD: Aspen Publishers, 1993.

Gardner, L.B., and Scheffler, R.M. "Privatization in Health Care: Shifting the Risk." *Medical Care Review* 45, No. 2 (Fall 1988):215–253.

LeTouze, D. "The Privatization of Hospital Pharmacy Departments." *Dimensions in Health Service* 66, No. 8 (November 1989):36–38.

Lutz, S. "Officials Weigh Taking Houston Hospital District Private." *Modern Healthcare* 22, No. 19 (May 1992):6.

MacAvoy, P.W. *Privatization and State Owned Enterprise.* Boston, Mass.: Kluwer Academic Publishers, 1989.

Neumann, B.R., Suver, J.D., and Zelman, W.N. *Financial Management: Concepts and Application for Health Care Providers.* Owings Mills, MD: National Health Publishing, 1988.

Scott, L. "Hospitals Sign More Contracts for Outside Expertise." *Modern Healthcare* (24 August 1992):51–72.

Smith, S.R. "Privatization in Health and Human Services: A Critique." *Journal of Health Politics, Policy & Law* 17, No. 2 (1992):233–253.

Terris, M. "Budget Cutting and Privatization: The Threat to Health." *Journal of Public Health Policy* 13, No. 1 (Spring 1992):27–41.

Walker, M.A. *Privatization: Tactics & Techniques.* Vancouver, B.C.: The Fraiser Institute, 1988.

Reading 5–4

Considering Cost Effectiveness
in the Hospital Setting

Steven A. Finkler

The term *cost effectiveness* has been loosely applied to health care issues for many years. However, it is time to re-examine what it really implies, and try to determine how well hospitals are doing at ensuring that their actions truly are cost effective.

The word *effectiveness* focuses on whether we are accomplishing our goal. An approach is effective if it accomplishes a desired objective. However, the approach may not be cost effective if we can find a less expensive way to accomplish that same goal.

Inherent in the notion of cost effectiveness is the concept of choice. When we talk about *cost-effectiveness,* we are really presenting a comparison. Something cannot be cost effective in isolation. It is only cost effective relative to some other alternative.

Trotter indicates that there are three classes of cost-effective alternatives.[1] These are:

1. equivalent cost/superior effectiveness;
2. lower cost/equivalent effectiveness; and
3. lower cost/superior effectiveness.

Notice the essential comparative nature of these classes. Each one refers to the effectiveness of a solution in comparison to something else. Either we are concerned with being more effective or we are concerned with having a lower cost.

Be cautious to note that something is not cost effective simply because it is cheaper. A less expensive item must also be at least as effective before we can assume that it is cost effective.

COST-BENEFIT ANALYSIS

In this comparative focus, cost effectiveness differs substantially from a technique such as cost-benefit analysis. The cost-benefit approach stands in isolation. Is it worthwhile to do something? Cost-benefit is determined by dividing benefits by costs. If

$$\frac{\text{Benefits}}{\text{Costs}} > 1$$

then it pays to undertake the venture. That is, anything with a ratio of benefits to costs that is greater than 1 has benefits that exceed their cost. Therefore, such things are worth doing. However, there are a number of problems with cost-benefit analysis.

For one, the benefits are often hard to measure. Many times, the benefits relate to health outcomes, and our proxies for measuring health outcomes may be very crude. To calculate the ratio, we must not only know the change in health outcomes, but also we must be able to put a dollar value on those benefits. To measure the dollar value of those health outcomes is extremely hard to do.

Source: Reprinted from Steven A. Finkler, "Considering Cost Effectiveness in the Hospital Setting: Hospitals Benefit from Decision-Making Tool Requiring Only Limited Data Collection," *Hospital Cost Management and Accounting,* Vol. 8, No. 10, January 1997, pp. 1–4. Copyright 1997, Aspen Publishers, Inc.

Secondly, even if we can put some assessment on the benefits, this is likely to be a difficult and costly process. And if we are trying to compare alternative ways to accomplish the same objective, we will have to go through such benefit measurements a number of times. We would prefer some approach that allows for comparison of alternatives without requiring so much effort on our part.

THE COST EFFECTIVENESS CLASSES

The three cost effectiveness classes presented earlier avoid much of the problem of cost-benefit analysis. Certainly, if it is feasible and easy to measure benefits, we can do that. The first class of cost effectiveness alternatives is **equivalent cost/superior effectiveness.** If we can measure both cost and effectiveness, we will be able to assess *how much* more cost effective one approach is than another.

For example, if the effectiveness of one approach is valued at 100, and another is valued at 120, and both cost $10, then the ratio of effectiveness to cost is either:

$$\frac{100}{\$10} = 10 \quad \text{or} \quad \frac{120}{\$10} = 12$$

In this case, the more effective approach has a higher ratio, 12, and would be deemed to be more cost effective than the approach with a ratio value of 10. Note that there is not uniformity in approaching this calculation. Trotter, for example, divides cost by effectiveness,[2] which is the inverse of the above. As a result, in his approach the ideal is to achieve a ratio value as close to zero as possible. That is not intuitive. We would rather have a formulation where a larger number is more cost effective. Thus, we show effectiveness divided by cost rather than the reverse.

It is essential, however, to focus on the fact that we did not really need to measure effectiveness to determine which of the alternatives was more cost effective! All that we needed to know was which approach was more effective, not how

much more. The ratio values of 12 and 10 are helpful, but in order to determine them we had to measure the effectiveness values of 100 and 120. That measurement places an unnecessary obstacle in the process of doing cost effectiveness analysis.

Typically, the obstacle is not determining if one approach is better than another, but trying to assign a measurement value to it. We would argue that managers will be much more likely to use cost effectiveness analysis if they can bypass that measurement. And in most cases they can.

As long as we know that two different approaches cost about the same amount (the first class of cost effectiveness analysis), we need only ascertain which alternative provides a superior level of effectiveness. There is no need to determine how superior.

Although theoreticians would prefer that organizations make optimal decisions, the data generally are not available to make such decisions. There are far too many unknowns and uncertainties in the real world to be able to know the best decision with perfect insight. Therefore, managers need to spend their time making specific, clear-cut improvements rather than being frozen from any decision because they cannot find the perfect solution.

Cost effectiveness helps managers move forward. The first rule of thumb, therefore, is that we will choose the alternative that provides improved results, as long as costs don't increase.

The second class of cost effectiveness decisions relates to **lower cost and equivalent effectiveness.** This rule of cost effectiveness analysis indicates that as long as two alternatives are just as good, we will choose the one with the lower cost. Again, there is no need to put a specific measurable value on how good they are. We only need to know that neither one is superior.

This raises an interesting question related to value added. In recent years, health care managers have become very aware of only spending money on value-added items. What if one alternative is superior to another in nonvalue-added ways. In other words, we have two approaches and one does more than another. However, the extra things it does are not things that we need. They do not add true value. In that case, one method may be *superior* but it is not more *effective*. It is superior in providing things we don't need. But that doesn't move us closer to accomplishing our objectives. Therefore, the two alternatives should be viewed as having equal effectiveness. In such a case, cost effectiveness says take the less costly alternative.

The last class of cost effectiveness analysis says that we prefer choices that **cost less and provide more effective outcomes.** Many cost effectiveness studies, both by researchers and managers, rely on this principle. If we can show that one technique is more effective (it doesn't matter how much more) and is less expensive (it doesn't matter how much less), then the alternative is superior. This principle reduces the data collection burden and relieves the manager of much of the work that might otherwise be required to decide whether to make a change or not.

WHEN TO MEASURE EFFECTIVENESS

Although we can often avoid measurement, cost effectiveness analysis can sometimes be enhanced by efforts to make measurements. This occurs when it is not obvious that effectiveness is better or equal, or that cost is lower.

In some situations, we may spend more for something that is more effective. Is it cost effective to do so? In such cases, if we can measure both costs and effectiveness, we can determine whether to do the more expensive approach.

For example, suppose that one treatment costs $1,200 and another costs $1,000. The first treatment is effective and cures 90 percent of all patients. The other treatment costs only $1,000, but is less effective, curing only 70 percent of all patients. Which treatment is more cost effective?

If we divide $1,200 by 90 percent, the result is $1,333. That is the cost per patient cured. If we divide $1,000 by 70 percent, the result is $1,429. The less expensive treatment is less cost effective because it costs more per patient cured. This analysis required not only knowledge of the

costs of treatment, but also some measurement of effectiveness.

A more difficult issue arises if the numbers are slightly altered. Suppose that it costs $1,500 for a treatment that cures 90 percent of the patients, and $1,000 for a treatment that cures 70 percent. When we divide the cost by the cure rate, we find that the $1,500 treatment costs $1,667 per patient cured, while the $1,000 treatment costs $1,429 per patient. Which choice is more appropriate?

It is not clear that we would want to choose the latter treatment with the $1,429 cost per patient cured. It is less expensive, but it leaves 20 percent of the patients not cured who could have been. That is why the first three classes of cost effectiveness analysis have often been the focus. We can arrive at a clear-cut correct alternative. When more effective care costs more money, the waters become cloudy.

THINKING BROADLY

Whether we intend to make a specific measurement or simply determine if one alternative is cheaper than another, we must think broadly. By this we mean that all relevant costs must be considered. A new drug therapy may be more expensive than the old drug, but reduce length of stay by a day. The avoidable costs of that eliminated day should offset part of the higher cost of the new drug in calculating the cost impact of the new alternative.

In other words, we are interested in the total impact of each alternative on the hospital as a whole. It is not the specific cost of a new machine or drug therapy that is important. It is the overall cost to the organization that is of critical concern. Sometimes we can just replace something expensive with something cheaper that does just as well. However, sometimes you have to use a more expensive item to reduce overall costs.

A MATTER OF PERSPECTIVE

Another vital element in cost effectiveness analysis is to realize that what may be cost effective to the hospital might not be cost effective for society, and vice versa. In performing any cost effectiveness analysis, it is critical to consider whose perspective is the appropriate one for the analysis. Then cost and effectiveness must be considered from that perspective.

Suppose that a physician decides not to admit a marginal patient. The physician may be capitated and may receive a large year-end payment if admissions are kept low. The hospital may be capitated and will have to provide all care needed. The physician may have made a cost-effective decision. If the patient never needs hospital care, the year-end payment to the physician is larger than if the patient were unnecessarily admitted. And, if the patient needs hospital care after all, the physician is hurt no more than if the patient had been admitted initially. From the physician's perspective, this was a cost-effective decision.

However, what if the patient could be treated fairly simply by the hospital, at low cost, if admitted early on? If the admission comes later, the cost may be substantially higher. From the capitated hospital's perspective, it may turn out that failure to admit patients with certain symptoms is not cost effective. Employers lose the benefit of work from sick employees. Employees lose pay. Insurance companies often pay for worker's compensation costs. Each player has a different perspective. What makes sense for one may not make sense for another.

We can bemoan this fact and talk about the need for aligned incentives. When incentives become aligned, everyone will benefit by providing the most appropriate care in the least cost setting. In the meantime, each organization must closely consider its own perspective when it performs cost effectiveness analyses.

AVOIDING THE NEED TO MEASURE

As noted earlier, we don't always have to quantify in dollar terms the level of effective-ness attained. Often, we simply need to know if one approach is superior to another. If we don't measure, how will we know? The answer is that some type of rudimentary measurement is needed. However, this should not require great effort.

For example, suppose that we are discharging patients early. We might decide that if the early discharge does not result in any rehospitalizations or death, it is as good. We would need to track the number of deaths and rehospitalizations in the study group to see if it differs from current practice.

Suppose that we want to substitute a laparoscopic procedure for one currently performed by open surgery. Laparoscopic surgery takes longer and is more expensive than traditional surgery. However, the patient will be able to go back to work sooner. That is a benefit, but one that does not help the hospital. The patient may also have a shorter length of stay. That will save the hospital some money. The cost side of the equation requires determination of whether the hospital will save enough money system-wide to more than offset the higher costs in the OR. For the effectiveness side, all we really need is knowledge that the patient outcomes are at least as good. We don't have to measure the dollar value of that, but we need some assurances that all clinical results are at least as good, if not better.

Cost effectiveness is a tool with great potential value to hospitals. It can be applied to find clearly superior alternatives, and in many cases requires only limited data collection efforts.

REFERENCES

1. Jeffrey P. Trotter, *The Quest for Cost Effectiveness in Health Care,* American Hospital Publishing, American Hospital Association, 1995, p.6.

2. Trotter, op. cit.

Reading 5–5

Cost-Effectiveness Analysis in Health Care

Donald B. Chalfin

The American health care system is undergoing significant changes in the way medical care is both financed and delivered. With the failure of Congress to pass President Clinton's Health Security Act or any other health reform legislation, the major efforts have shifted to state and local governments and to the private sector, the latter evidenced by the pervasive growth and expansion of managed care. The reasons for these changes are many; however, most relate to the high cost of health care services, both in total and relative to the rest of the American economy. Health care spending has sharply and steadily increased over the past two decades and currently accounts for approximately 14 percent of the nation's gross domestic product (GDP). Many experts predict that, if left unchecked, health care will consume 15.5 to 16 percent of the GDP by the turn of the century (Ashby & Green, 1993; Lamm, 1995; Lee, Soffel, & Luft, 1992).

This sustained growth has multiple economic ramifications, especially in the face of limited resources with competing demands. From both a macroeconomic and a microeconomic perspective, resources earmarked for health care or other endeavors implicitly and explicitly imply that other worthy projects go unfunded, and

thus, needs may go unmet. To ensure equitable and desirable distribution of resources, decisions should take into account the cost-effectiveness of any program, service, or intervention. All decisions, therefore, will have to be made on the basis of clinical consequences, expected outcomes, and costs and economic consumption. As a result, as cost and purely financial considerations become increasingly clinical decisions (Udvarhelyi, Colditz, Rai, & Epstein, 1992; Weinstein & Stason, 1977), clinicians and managers will have to become more familiar with the basic approach to cost-effectiveness analysis to ensure appropriate resource allocation among competing demands. This article discusses the basic tenets of cost-effectiveness analysis and illustrates pertinent examples of cost-effectiveness analyses from the literature and practical applications to common clinical settings. Managers and clinicians alike can use the contents of this article as a foundation for the many analyses hospitals must make in the coming years.

COST-EFFECTIVENESS ANALYSIS: AN OVERVIEW

Cost-effectiveness analysis refers to the joint clinical and economic assessment of a program, service, or intervention in terms of resources expended per unit of outcome. Programs may be

Source: Reprinted from Donald B. Chalfin, "Cost-Effectiveness Analysis in Health Care," *Hospital Cost Management and Accounting,* Vol. 7, No. 4, pp. 1–8. Copyright 1995, Aspen Publishers, Inc.

expensive relative to alternatives yet may be deemed cost-effective if the incremental improvement in outcome makes up for the additional cost. Conversely, cheaper programs may be cost-ineffective if a lesser or less desirable outcome is yielded when compared with the more expensive alternative. The terms *cost-effectiveness* and *cost-effectiveness analysis* are commonly cited yet are often misused. Most commonly, cost-effectiveness is assumed to be synonymous with cost savings, even though a concurrent assessment of outcome is neglected. The basic components of cost-effectiveness analysis consist of the delineation of all costs that are incurred, the concurrent determination of all benefits or outcomes that accrue, and the calculation of a summary measure of effectiveness or cost-effectiveness ratio that relates expended resources to attained outcome. In the most commonly published cost-effectiveness analyses, those that assess the cost-effectiveness of a given medical intervention to society as whole, the cost-effectiveness ratio is commonly expressed as the cost (usually in present value dollars) per year of life gained (or added). Clearly then, an alternative with a lower ratio implies that it is the more cost-effective option, because less resources will have to be expended to obtain the same outcome.

COST-EFFECTIVENESS ANALYSIS AND RELATED ECONOMIC EVALUATIONS

Cost-effectiveness analysis is one of several analytic methods available to the clinician and administrator to assess various aspects of the economic performance of any program or intervention. The simplest method of economic analysis, cost-minimization analysis, evaluates only the costs that are expended and therefore implicitly assumes that benefits or outcomes that accrue are identical. As previously stated, monetary savings should not be confused with cost-effectiveness, because outcomes and benefits may change accordingly.

In the literature, the terms *cost-benefit* and *cost-effectiveness* are frequently interchanged, yet differences, both subtle and substantial, exist between the two methods (although both may be performed in tandem). The major difference relates to the valuation of all costs incurred and benefits gained. In cost-benefit analysis, both costs and benefits are valued in identical monetary units, a condition that does not apply to cost-effectiveness analysis. As a result, cost-benefit analysis is rarely useful in many clinical situations, because of the inherent, if not impossible, difficulty in assigning a monetary or economic value to clinical outcomes.

Cost-utility analysis is a special case of cost-effectiveness analysis in which outcomes go beyond mortality and survival estimates and incorporate morbidity and "quality-of-life" determinations into one unified measure for outcome. A common example of outcomes that are used in cost-utility analyses is *quality adjusted life-years* (QALYs), a quantitative measure that adjusts survival according to residual disability, diminished function, and perceived quality of life. Cost measurements are usually identical for both cost-effectiveness and cost-utility analysis (Detsky & Naglie, 1990; Lambrinos & Papadakos, 1987; O'Brien & Rusby, 1990; Weinstein & Stason, 1977).

COST-EFFECTIVENESS ANALYSIS: BASIC PRINCIPLES AND STEPS

Assessment of cost-effectiveness involves a comparison of two or more choices to achieve a certain clinical goal; the determination of cost-effectiveness and the calculation of a cost-effectiveness ratio implicitly and explicitly require a relative comparison among competing alternatives. From a methodologic standpoint, assessment of cost-effectiveness involves a rigorous quantitative approach that should proceed in a stepwise, sequential manner. The basic steps for cost-effectiveness analysis are described below (Detsky & Naglie, 1990; Drummond, Stoddard, & Torrance, 1987; Udvarhelyi, Colditz, Rai, & Epstein, 1992).

1. Explicit identification of all clinical choices and strategies

As previously stated, cost-effectiveness analysis requires the specification of two or more alternatives. By definition, assessment of cost-effectiveness is a relative phenomenon, and thus the calculation of a single cost-effectiveness measure (i.e., cost-effectiveness ratio) provides little, if any, quantitative insight regarding joint clinical and economic impact. To illustrate, if a hospital is considering an expansion of its intensive care facilities, it may perform a study that assesses the cost-effectiveness of two viable alternatives: the expansion of the current intensive care unit (ICU) from 10 to 15 beds or the construction of a new 10-bed intermediate care or step-down unit that will coexist in conjunction with the current 10-bed ICU.

2. Explicit identification of the study's perspective

In addition to being a relative assessment between two or more alternatives, cost-effectiveness analysis also depends on the perspective of the decision maker. Specifically, a program or intervention may be deemed to be cost-effective from the standpoint of the individual patient or from the standpoint of a specific inpatient service. However, the same program or intervention may be cost-ineffective when viewed and assessed from the overall societal point of view. This dichotomy relates to the fact that cost expenditure and benefit accrual are not uniform and show substantial variation according to different perspectives. Most published studies in the medical literature tend to evaluate cost-effectiveness from the perspective of society as a whole and thereby generally define cost-effectiveness in terms of dollars or resources spent per year of life saved (Detsky & Naglie, 1990; Drummond, Stoddard, & Torrance, 1987; Udvarhelyi, Colditz, Rai, & Epstein, 1992).

3. Determination of all costs

The precise approach to cost determination and allocation is beyond the scope to this article. However, all cost-effectiveness analyses should specify all costs that accrue for each choice, and cost assessment should include more than the direct costs alone, which usually are the easiest to assess, and attempt to capture the total incremental or marginal costs of every intervention. The total costs that accrue can be divided into the following three categories: (1) direct costs specifically linked to any health intervention, (2) cost expenditures associated with adverse events and side effects, and (3) cost savings that accrue as a result of improved health outcome (e.g., reductions in mortality and morbidity) (Weinstein & Stason, 1977). In addition, some cost-effectiveness analyses even assess indirect, or opportunity, costs. For example, indirect costs are large components of diseases that are associated with lengthy hospitalization and prolonged recovery times in terms of reduced productivity or forgone income.

4. Determination of all benefits and measures of effectiveness

The full determination of all costs and measurement of resource consumption is quite challenging and time-consuming. However, estimating benefits and objectively quantifying effectiveness is often the hardest part of a cost-effectiveness analysis because of the inherent lack of accepted objective units. Most clinical outcomes in cost-effectiveness analyses, especially those that are performed from the societal perspective, are usually reported as crude mortality and survival estimates, such as probability of survival and years of life expectancy. A growing body of literature, however, supports methods that incorporate quality-of-life measures into the more usual outcome states such as QALYs (Torrance, 1986). In addition, effectiveness may often be measured in units that more closely reflect the clinical outcomes under investigation. Examples include the number of cases identified in the case of screening tests for disease prevalence and reduction in blood pressure in the case of antihypertensive therapy.

5. Temporal relationships

Costs are rarely expended immediately and are often spent over a period time. Similarly, benefits are rarely immediately realized and often manifest at some point in the future. As a result, cost-effectiveness analyses should precisely state the time frame of the study and the period of time for which costs are expended and benefits are amassed. Long-term studies, usually defined by convention as those in which the period of time exceeds 1 year, require discounting of costs and benefits and assessment of their respective present value. This is usually not necessary for short-term studies of less than 1 year.

6. Determination of a cost-effectiveness ratio

Once costs and benefits are measured and summed, a cost-effectiveness ratio (which reflects the algebraic relation between costs and benefits) is determined. Common cost-effectiveness ratios include the cost per year of life gained and the cost per QALY; however, the ratio obviously depends on the specific units that are chosen for costs and benefits. The determination of the cost-effectiveness ratio and the expression of cost-effectiveness in terms of a sole joint clinical and economic "unit" is vital because it facilitates cross-comparisons among all alternatives under investigation. Clearly then, an alternative that yields a lower cost-effectiveness ratio is, at the baseline, the more cost-effective option because fewer resources must be spent to obtain the same, common clinical outcome. Conversely, a higher cost-effectiveness ratio implies cost-ineffectiveness because more resources must be diverted to yield a similar outcome. Inherently, then, cost-effectiveness analysis always reflects and implies a comparison; thus, an isolated determination of a cost-effectiveness ratio has little or no value.

In the same manner in which a cost-effectiveness ratio is determined, analysts also determine the marginal cost-effectiveness of a health care endeavor. *Marginal cost-effectiveness* refers to the added costs required to procure additional, or incremental, benefits and outcomes and reflects the underlying economic concept regarding diminishing returns. To illustrate, if alternative A costs *$50,000* and yields an additional life expectancy of 5 years and alternative B costs $80,000 but yields an additional life expectancy of 6 years, their respective cost-effectiveness ratios are $10,000 per year of life gained ($50,000/

5 years) and $13,333 per year of life gained ($80,000 ÷ 6 years); thus, the marginal cost-effectiveness of program B, defined as the additional costs divided by the additional benefits is $30,000 ([$80,000 − $50,000] ÷ [6 − 5]).

7. Sensitivity analysis

It is universally recommended to include rigorous sensitivity analysis to assess how changes in the baseline assumptions affect the conclusions. In real-world and real-time settings, costs that accrue may differ, and benefits may similarly vary from the model constructed by the analysis. For example, certain programs in different settings may consume more resources, and outcome data may also depend on the specific population and group to which the problem is applied. Sensitivity analysis facilitates the determination of cost-effectiveness throughout a reasonable range of values and assumptions and thus allows for more meaningful and practical comparisons among realistic alternatives.

COST-EFFECTIVENESS ANALYSIS: EXAMPLES FROM THE MEDICAL LITERATURE

Major medical and health care peer reviewed journals have begun to prominently feature more and more cost-effectiveness analyses. In fact, the *New England Journal of Medicine* recently stipulated a policy for acceptance of cost-effectiveness analyses that are submitted for potential publication (Kassirer & Angell, 1994). Most of these studies assume the perspective of society and thus usually evaluate cost-effectiveness in terms of cost per year of life saved or with related units. Several recent studies are reviewed below; topics covered include the cost-effectiveness of expensive pharmacotherapy, such as thrombolytic or mono-clonal antibody therapy, the cost-effectiveness of antitubercular masks to prevent health care workers from contracting tuberculosis from afflicted patients, and the cost-effectiveness of cardiopulmonary resuscitation for hospitalized patients.

COST-EFFECTIVENESS OF THROMBOLYTIC THERAPY

Thrombolytic agents such as streptokinase and tissue plasminogen activator (TPA) are often used to treat patients with acute myocardial infarctions. As several large multicenter trials have shown, thrombolytic agents are very effective in decreasing infarct-related morbidity and reducing mortality provided they are used under optimal clinical circumstances.

However, thrombolytic therapy raises many concerns from both a clinical and a cost-effective standpoint: Thrombolytic agents are extremely expensive (TPA, for example, has a price of more than $2,000 per dose), are associated with a small but very real risk of fatal and incapacitating events, and can be used only in certain clinical situations. In view of these factors, and because the clinical trials did not establish clinical efficacy of thrombolytic therapy in patients over the age of 75, Krumholz and colleagues (1992) used decision analysis to assess the cost-effectiveness of streptokinase in older patients. They determined that at the baseline, in which the cost of streptokinase equaled $200, a value consistent with the current acquisition cost for most hospital pharmacies, the mortality rate was reduced from 24.4 to 21.4 percent when thrombolytic therapy was given and that the cost per year of life saved for an 80-year-old patient was $21,200, a level that compares favorably with the cost per year of life saved for other less expensive therapies.

Multiple sensitivity analyses, in which the underlying estimates regarding clinical benefit, risk of adverse events, and economic cost were varied throughout a reasonable range of assumptions, were performed, and cost per year of life saved ranged from $17,000 (when the year of life gained was increased from 2.4 to 6 years) to $52,100 (when the cost of care for a stroke survivor was increased from the baseline value of $200,000 to $1,000,000). The cost per year of life increased from $21,200 to $45,900 when the acquisition cost of the drug, with all other assumptions held constant, was raised from $200 to $2,000 (Torrance, 1986).

COST-EFFECTIVENESS OF BIOTECHNOLOGY AGENTS FOR THE TREATMENT OF SEPSIS

Sepsis, the systemic response to infection, afflicts between 150,000 and 400,000 hospitalized patients each year, many of whom require admission to an ICU, and is associated with substantial morbidity and mortality. Estimated mortality rates range from 25 to 90 percent, with the highest rates occurring in those patients who develop multiorgan system dysfunction including cardiogenic shock (Bone et al., 1989). Conventional therapy for sepsis, which consists of antibiotic therapy and aggressive supportive measures including hemodialysis and mechanical ventilation, has not appreciably altered patient outcome. The sepsis syndrome and its untoward sequelae have been linked to the release of a cascade of multiple biologic mediators. As a result, researchers have developed biotechnology agents that interact with several of these mediators to halt the cascade and the resultant morbid and mortal events. Several of these agents have been studied in large ongoing clinical trials to assess their clinical efficacy. The clinical implications of these agents are vast; if they are deemed to be clinically beneficial, they may represent a major therapeutic breakthrough. However, the economic ramifications are equally onerous because, like most biotechnology products, they are extremely expensive to produce and acquire and may potentially cost several thousand dollars per dose. It has been estimated that if approved and adopted for clinical use, these agents may add $2 billion to the nation's health care bill (Wenzel, 1992).

Two studies were performed to assess the cost-effectiveness of two specific agents, both of which are monoclonal antibodies targeted against endotoxin, a substance produced by gram-negative bacteria (a class of bacteria responsible for a large percentage of sepsis cases) that triggers the deleterious septic cascade. Schulman and colleagues (1991) used decision analysis techniques to develop a model to assess the cost-effectiveness of the HA-1A monoclonal antibody. Their study was based on the data from a phase III trial that assessed the clinical efficacy of HA-1A, and cost-effectiveness was assessed for two potential strategies: (1) the empiric treatment of all patients with the agent who presented with clinical evidence of sepsis and (2) the use of a hypothetical test to screen for sepsis and to treat all patients who test positive. The empiric treatment strategy had a cost per year of life saved of $24,100, whereas the cost per year of life saved for the test strategy was reduced to $14,900. Sensitivity analysis determined a range from $5,200, when the expected years of life saved was 20, and $110,000 when the expected years of life saved was only 1 (Bone et al., 1989).

Chalfin and colleagues (1993) assessed the cost-effectiveness of monoclonal antibodies directed against gram-negative endotoxin. Like in the prior study, decision analysis techniques (including Monte Carlo simulations) were used; however, this study differed from the Schulman study in that cost-effectiveness was assessed from the perspective of the individual acute care institution and was developed from financial data derived from critically ill patients with gram-negative sepsis and two phase III trials that assessed HA-lA and ES, another investigational agent (Ziegler et al., 1991; Greenman et al., 1991). At the baseline, total expected charges for patients treated with the agent always exceeded those accrued by patients who received standard therapy alone. However, this value was significantly less than the acquisition cost of the drug because of reductions in other expenditures associated with sepsis and critical illness. The cost-effectiveness ratios for a $2,000 and $4,000 acquisition cost, in terms of cost per survivor, were $71,674 and $74,900, respectively, amounts that were less than the $80,200 for patients who did not receive the agents. Sensitivity analysis demonstrated improved cost-effectiveness when the ability to identify gram-negative sepsis rose and also demonstrated that monoclonal antibody therapy, given the underlying assumptions for clinical efficacy, was always more cost-effective than standard sepsis therapy alone, even when the acquisition cost rose above $5,000 (Wenzel, 1992).

COST-EFFECTIVENESS OF AIR FILTER RESPIRATORS TO PROTECT AGAINST TUBERCULOSIS

The studies that assess the economic impact of thrombolytic therapy and antiendotoxin agents illustrate one of the important caveats of cost-effectiveness analysis: how expensive and costly agents may in fact be cost-effective in terms of the relation between all resources that are expended relative to the clinical benefit that is realized. Yet, the converse may also be true: Inexpensive therapies and interventions may be cost-ineffective because of minimal benefit that is obtained for the resources that are expended.

A study by Adal and colleagues (1994) regarding the cost-effectiveness of air filter respirators to protect against tuberculosis highlights this point. Briefly, the increased incidence and virulence of tuberculosis has heightened the concern among hospital epidemiologists regarding the need to protect health care workers against contracting tuberculosis from afflicted patients. As a result, more vigilant protective measures have been advocated, including the use of high-efficiency particulate air-filter respirators, which are protective masks worn by health care workers. Although air filter respirators are more costly than the usual protective masks that cost between $0.06 to $0.92 each, they are nevertheless relatively cheap, averaging about $7.50 to $9.00 per mask (Ziegler et al., 1991). Yet when evaluated in terms of total resources expended to prevent a case of hospital or institutional acquired tuberculosis, air filter respirators provide minimal protection relative to the expenditures that are exhausted. Specifically, a fraction of health care workers who are exposed to patients with tuberculosis "convert" from a negative to a positive purified protein derivative (PPD) test (a screening test that demonstrates the presence of tuberculosis organisms but, in a host, usually does not mean that a clinically significant tuberculosis infection exists), and a small percentage of those who have converted eventually develop the disease.

In the study by Adal and colleagues, 0.2 percent of patients exposed had positive PPD tests, and it was assumed that 10 percent of all converters develop tuberculosis. Further extrapolations, which were based on drug sensitivity and efficacy, determined that the number of years necessary to prevent a case of occupational tuberculosis would be 41. With a cost of air filter masks between $7.51 and $9.08 and accounting for patient visits, the number of health care workers, the cost of screening and medical evaluation, and the cost of employee training, a range of $1.3 million to $18.5 million would have to be "spent" to prevent this single case (Ziegler et al., 1991). Clearly, then, inexpensive endeavors and interventions may not necessarily be cost-effective if the benefits that are attained are minimal or even minuscule relative to the additional expenditures that are allocated.

COST OF CARDIOPULMONARY RESUSCITATION

In general, many cost-effectiveness analyses only assess the cost-effectiveness of specific components of a health care process as opposed to an overall diagnostic classification or patient group. For example, the cost-effectiveness of thrombolytic therapy is but one aspect (albeit an important component) of the cost-effectiveness and economic impact of the treatment of acute myocardial infarctions. Just as accountants and managers may prefer to determine the costs associated with a certain therapeutic intervention or an entire process as opposed to a small component (e.g., the costs associated with pneumonia as opposed to the cost of a chest radiograph), health planners and clinicians may benefit from an evaluation of the cost-effectiveness of an overall process or intervention as opposed to a smaller component.

Ebell and Kruse (1994) recently studied the costs and the cost-effectiveness of in-hospital cardiopulmonary resuscitation (CPR). From a clinical standpoint, CPR is potentially lifesaving; however, the outcome depends on the primary etiology of arrest, the patient's underlying health

status and condition, patient age, and other factors. Many patients who undergo CPR have minimal chance of survival, let alone return to functional status, and evidence exists that CPR may be overused in certain circumstances (Ebell & Kruse, 1994). The actual costs and resources that are expended for each episode are relatively minimal; however, the cost-effectiveness implications are quite apparent. In view of this, Ebell and Kruse (1994) developed a decision analysis model to depict the clinical scenarios associated with CPR (i.e., immediate survival or death, expiration or survival within 24 hours of CPR, survival to discharge, and assessment of dependency at discharge). At the baseline, which assumes an average rate of survival to discharge of 12.8 percent, a direct cost of $250 per each episode of in-hospital CPR, and average costs of 1 day on the general medical ward at $1,800 and $2,600 per day in the ICU (1991 dollars), the cost per survivor was calculated to be $110,270. The amount fell to $99,055 when overall survival rate rose to 20 percent, and increased to $248,271 and $544,521 when survival fell to 1 percent and 0.2 percent, respectively. Variations in the direct cost of CPR have a negligible effect on global cost-effectiveness, whereas reductions in length of stay and increase in CPR survival and prospective prognostic assessment of patients exert a more profound influence on cost-effectiveness (Ebell & Kruse, 1994).

COST-EFFECTIVENESS: PRACTICAL POINTS AND CONCLUSIONS

These aforementioned studies, along with many others, demonstrate how cost-effectiveness can be objectively quantified, rigorously assessed, and applied to a wide variety of clinical situations. However, these studies often rely on sophisticated techniques for model building that depict clinical situations that are commonly encountered and all resultant alternatives and sequelae. Many of the studies that have been described in this article use decision analysis and associated techniques to model the appropriate scenarios, a full description of which is beyond the scope of this article and can be found in other sources (Chalfin, 1990; Weinstein et al., 1989). Although many of its techniques may not be needed in many practical situations encountered by the clinician and the manager who is faced with the task of assessing cost-effectiveness, a quantitative approach that is based on expected value decision making can provide great insight into both clinical and economic outcome and hence cost-effectiveness. Specifically, construction of a basic decision tree that depicts all possible choices and their associated sequelae, the assignment of values for probabilities of occurrence (e.g., the chance that a test result will be positive, the probability of survival to hospital discharge), the assignment of utilities for each outcome in both economic terms (i.e., cost) or clinical outcome (e.g., mortality, QALY, and so forth), the calculation of expected value on the basis of these values and assumptions, and the inclusion of multiple sensitivity analyses that vary these assumptions throughout a reasonable range will yield a significant amount of quantitative insight and information. Although many problems may need formal modeling and strict assessment, a large amount of information regarding cost-effectiveness may be obtained by framing the problem into its basic components relative to the alternative ways in which an outcome or benefit may be obtained and the depiction of all possible sequelae.

The explicit stipulation of the perspective of any cost-effectiveness investigation from the outset cannot be overemphasized. As previously stated, most cost-effectiveness studies that are published in the literature assume the perspective of cost-effectiveness to society and thus implicitly become tools for public policy. The health administrator or manager, in most cases, may be more interested in cost-effectiveness from a smaller perspective, such as the perspective of the individual institution or the perspective of a large health care network and its covered lives. From these and related vantage points, cost-effectiveness to society, while undoubtedly important in terms of overall benefit relative to

resource expenditure, needs to be balanced against other economic and noneconomic concerns, most notably affordability in the face of scarce resources and limited budgets. Thrombolytic therapy and biotechnology agents provide a vivid illustration of this conflict, for although they may be deemed cost-effective to society as a whole, individual hospitals and even health care networks have to grapple with the cost of acquiring these agents for their formularies, sometimes at several thousand dollars per dose.

Cost-effectiveness analysis, therefore, must be viewed as one of many quantitative techniques available to the health care provider and health care manager to assist in the evaluation of overall efficacy. A strategy may be deemed cost-effective relative to others; however, other equally important concerns, such as affordability, practical logistics, and underlying equity, should be factored into the decision-making process. In addition, ethical and moral concerns also should be addressed and considered. However, a formal and rigorous approach to assessment of cost-effectiveness can provide great insight into the joint clinical and economic efficiency of any program or intervention and will help to ensure that scarce and valuable resources are allocated to yield the maximal benefit and most beneficial outcome.

REFERENCES

Adal, K. A., Anglim, A. M., Palumbo, C. L., Titus, M. G., Coyner, B. J., Farr, B. M. (1994). The use of high-efficiency particulate air-filter respirators to protect hospital workers from tuberculosis. *New England Journal of Medicine, 331*, 169–173.

Ashby, J. L., & Green, T. F. (1993). Implications of a global budget for facility-based health spending. *Inquiry, 30*, 362–371.

Bone, R. C., Fisher, C. I., Clemmer, T. P., et al. (1989). Sepsis syndrome: a valid clinical entity. *Critical Care Medicine, 17*, 389–393.

Chalfin, D. B. (1990). Decision analysis and capital budgeting: application to the delivery of critical care services. *Hospital Cost Management and Accounting, 2*, 1–4.

Chalfin, D. B., Holbein, M.E.B., Fein, A. M., & Carlon, G. C. (1993). Cost-effectiveness of monoclonal antibodies to gram-negative endotoxin in the treatment of gram-negative sepsis in ICU patients. *Journal of the American Medical Association, 269,* 249–254.

Detsky, A. S., & Naglie, I.G. (1990). A clinician's guide to cost-effectiveness analysis. *Annals of Internal Medicine, 113,* 147–154.

Drummond, M. F., Stoddard, G. L., & Torrance, G. W. (1987). *Methods for the economic evaluation of health care programmes.* Oxford: Oxford University Press.

Ebell, M. H., & Kruse, J. A. (1994). A proposed model for the cost of cardiopulmonary resuscitation. *Medical Care,* 32, 640–649.

Greenman, R. L., Schein, R.M.H., Martin, M. A., et al. (1991). A controlled clinical trial of E5 murine monoclonal IgM antibody to endotoxin in the treatment of gram-negative sepsis. *Journal of the American Medical Association, 266,* 1097–1102.

Kassirer, J. P., & Angell, M. (1994). The Journal's policy on cost-effectiveness analyses. *New England Journal of Medicine, 331,* 669–70.

Krumholz, H. M., Pasternak, R. C., Weinstein, M. C., et al. (1992). Cost effectiveness of thrombolytic therapy with streptokinase in elderly patients with suspected acute myocardial infarction. *New England Journal of Medicine, 328,* 7–13.

Lambrinos, J., & Papadakos, P. J. (1987). An introduction to the analysis of risks, costs, and benefits in critical care. In: I. A. Fein & M. A. Strosberg (Eds.), *Managing the critical care unit* (pp. 358–370). Rockville, MD: Aspen Publishers.

Lamm, R. D. (1995). The ghost of health care future. *Inquiry.* 31, 365–367.

Lee, P. R., Soffel, D., & Luft, H. S. (1992). Costs and coverage pressures toward health care reform. *Western Journal of Medicine, 157,* 576–583.

O'Brien, D., & Rusby, J. (1990). Outcome assessment in cardiovascular cost-benefit studies. *American Heart Journal, 119,* 740–748.

Schulman, K. A., Glick, H. A., Rubin, H., Eisenberg, J. M. (1991). Cost-effectiveness of HA-IA monoclonal antibody for gram-negative sepsis: economic assessment of a new therapeutic agent. *Journal of the American Medical Association, 266,* 3466–3471.

Torrance, G. W. (1986). Measurement of health state utilities for economic appraisal: a review. *Journal of Health Economics, 5,* 1–30.

Udvarhelyi, I. S., Colditz, G. A., Rai, A., & Epstein, A. M. (1992). Cost-effectiveness and cost-benefit analyses in the medical literature. Are the methods being used correctly? *Annals of Internal Medicine, 116,* 238–244.

Weinstein, M. C., Fineberg, H. V., Elstein, A. S., et al. (1989). *Clinical decision analysis.* Philadelphia: W. B. Saunders.

Weinstein, M. C., & Stason, W. B. (1977). Foundations of cost-effectiveness analysis for health and medical practices. *New England Journal of Medicine, 296,* 716–721.

Wenzel, R. P. (1992). Anti-endotoxin monoclonal antibodies: a second look. *New England Journal of Medicine,* 326, 1153–1156.

Ziegler, E. J., Fischer, C. J., Sprung. C. L., et al. (1991). Treatment of gram-negative bacteremia and septic shock with HA-lA human monoclonal antibody against endotoxin. *New England Journal of Medicine,* 324, 429–436.

6

Cost-Volume-Profit Analysis

Reading 6–1

Breakeven Analysis for Capitated Arrangements

Steven A. Finkler

Breakeven analysis is a traditional cost accounting tool that is widely used in hospitals and other industries. It would be simple if we could say that every service has a price and a cost and then simply see whether the price exceeds the cost to determine whether we will make or lose money. However, the cost per unit of service is not a constant. Because generally there are fixed costs for any type of service, the greater the volume, the more these costs are shared, and therefore the lower the cost per patient. How does this play out in a capitated environment? As more hospitals start to negotiate managed care contracts that place at least some of their services on a capitated basis, this becomes an important issue.

Based on a mathematical derivation, the quantity of a service needed to break even is equal to the fixed costs divided by the price less the variable costs. This is often referred to as the breakeven formula:

$$\text{Breakeven quantity} = \frac{\text{Fixed cost}}{\text{Price} - \text{Variable cost}}$$

Source: Reprinted from Steven A. Finkler, "Breakeven Analysis for Capitated Arrangements," *Hospital Cost Management and Accounting,* Vol. 6, No. 11, pp. 1–2. Copyright February 1995, Aspen Publishers, Inc.

The price in this formula is not really the amount charged but rather the amount of money ultimately expected to be received, on average, for each additional unit of service provided.

If we want to do more than break even, we can establish a target profit and redefine the formula as the number of patients or other units of service needed to achieve that target profit:

$$\text{Target profit quantity} = \frac{\text{Target profit} + \text{Fixed costs}}{\text{Price} - \text{Variable cost}}$$

Suppose that your hospital dermatology clinic is approached by a health maintenance organization (HMO) to provide all dermatological services to its patients. The HMO proposes that your hospital provide all dermatological outpatient services for a capitated rate of \$.50 per member per month (PMPM). Is that offer acceptable? Assume that you expect to have variable costs of \$20 per patient visit and annual fixed costs of \$300,000. What other data do you need? Also assume that dealing with the HMO will cause you to incur an extra \$80,000 per year in fixed costs related to negotiations, billings, inquiries, and so on.

The basic formulas shown above still apply. We can determine how many of the new patients we need to be profitable. However, we must be judicious in the exercise of the formulas. First, what is the fixed cost? It is not \$380,000. The basic fixed cost of \$300,000 will exist in any case.

To determine whether we should take the additional patients, we would include only incremental revenues and expenses. Therefore, the fixed cost is $80,000, the extra amount incurred because of the HMO contract.

The price appears to be clearly set at $.50. However, we must be careful here as well. That $.50 is a PMPM rate, rather than revenue per patient treated. We must either convert the $20 variable cost per patient visit to an average variable cost PMPM or convert the $.50 PMPM revenue to an expected average revenue per patient treated.

In theory, either approach is identical. In practice, however, we want to be careful not to give any incentives to see extra patients. Suppose that we expect that, on average, every 20 members of the HMO will have one visit per year. Our total PMPM revenue for that visit would be $120 (i.e., $.50 PMPM $\times$ 12 months = $6 $\times$ 20 members = $120). Of course, there are likely to be some more and some less complicated patients, but, on average, the variable cost is $20 and the price is $120 in this scenario. There is a contribution of $100 per visit (i.e., price of $120 less variable cost of $20). The breakeven quantity is 800 visits:

$$\text{Breakeven quantity} = \frac{\$80,000}{\$120 - \$20} = 800 \text{ visits}$$

However, with a breakeven quantity of 800 visits, the dermatology clinic might be anxious to provide extra visits. After all, it has a contribution of $100 per visit. In reality, however, under capitation, if it has more visits, it is not likely to have any extra revenue.

On the other hand, suppose we converted the $20 variable cost per visit to an expected $.083 PMPM ($20 per visit ÷ 20 members ÷ 12 months = $.083). We would also have to convert the $80,000 fixed cost per year to $6,666.67 per month. Now the breakeven quantity is 16,000 covered lives:

$$\text{Breakeven quantity} = \frac{\$6,666.67}{\$.50 - \$.083}$$

$$= 16,000 \text{ covered lives}$$

The contribution margin of $.42 PMPM (i.e., $.50–$.083) is not likely to encourage anyone to see patients too often. In addition, stating the breakeven quantity in terms of covered lives stresses what we really want to emphasize: the effect of increasing the number of people for whom we provide care.

Breakeven analysis can be a reliable tool in a capitated environment, but it must be used appropriately and carefully.

Reading 6–2

Managed Care and Breakeven Analysis: A Clarification

Steven A. Finkler

It is becoming common in the health services accounting literature to see a new breakeven graph, designed to show how managers should act under managed care. In the graph as it is being promoted, managers should attempt to minimize services provided in order to maximize profits. This is an erroneous conclusion.

One might well want to minimize services provided per patient. However, that has been true at least as long as we have had DRGs (over 10 years).

The argument often put forth now is that overall services should be minimized. That is probably a fallacy. The following examples show why the new approach will not lead to an optimal result, by first reviewing traditional breakeven analysis, then considering the new argument being put forth recently, and finally analyzing the error in the new argument.

TRADITIONAL BREAKEVEN ANALYSIS

Breakeven analysis is based on the knowledge that some costs are fixed and some are variable. When shown in a graph with volume along the horizontal axis, and dollars on the vertical axis,

Source: Reprinted from Steven A. Finkler, "Managed Care and Breakeven Analysis: A Clarification," *Hospital Cost Management and Accounting,* Vol. 8, No. 6, pp. 1–4. Copyright September 1996, Aspen Publishers, Inc.

these two types of costs can be seen as in Figures 6–2–1 and 6–2–2.

Fixed costs are shown as a horizontal line. This is because by definition, they represent the same amount of cost as volume changes, within a relevant range. In contrast, variable costs slope up and to the right. This indicates that as volume increases, more costs are incurred. Figure 6–2–3 merely combines the fixed and variable costs of Figures 6–2–1 and 6–2–2, to arrive at total cost. The variable costs of Figure 6–2–2 are placed on top of the fixed costs of Figure 6–2–1.

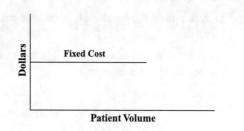

Figure 6–2–1 Fixed Costs

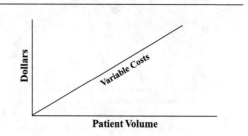

Figure 6–2–2 Variable Costs

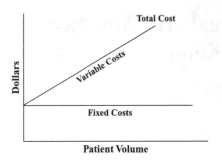

Figure 6–2–3 Total Costs

Figure 6–2–4 adds revenue into the mix. If we expect each patient to pay for his or her care (directly or through a third-party payer), then we have no revenue when we have no patients. As the number of patients increases, the revenue increases. Thus the revenue line slopes up and to the right, in a fashion similar to variable costs. The revenue line must be steeper than the variable costs line for a breakeven point to exist. That is, the extra revenue from each additional patient must exceed the variable cost of each additional patient.

Traditional breakeven analysis holds that we break even at the point on the graph where total revenue intersects total costs. If our volume is:

- greater than the breakeven point, we make profits;
- further to the right (i.e., the higher the volume), the greater the profits;

- to the left of the breakeven point, we lose money; or
- further to the left, the greater the loss.

The rationale for this argument is that at any given volume along the horizontal axis, we can go up the graph vertically to see which is higher, costs or revenues. If the total cost is higher than revenues, we are losing money. If revenue is higher than total cost, we make money.

The managerial implication of this traditional analysis is that it is important to have high volume. One must be careful to note, however, that the volume we seek is high numbers of paying patients. For any given patient we would want to keep costs as low as possible.

THE NEW ANALYSIS

The traditional analysis has come under fire as managed care has grown. In capitated situations, the HMO pays a fixed monthly premium regardless of patient resource consumption.

The graph often used to demonstrate this situation is shown in Figure 6–2–5. In this graph, revenue is shown as a horizontal line. If the revenue line is less than fixed costs, there can be no breakeven point. If, however, the revenue line is higher than the fixed costs, a breakeven volume can be found.

The main point of Figure 6–2–5 is that once a hospital is capitated, its revenue becomes fixed,

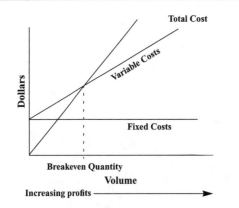

Figure 6–2–4 Breakeven Chart

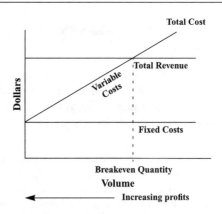

Figure 6–2–5 Fixed Revenue

similar to fixed costs. If this is true, as asserted, then the implications are that profits increase as we move to the left, and decrease as we move to the right.

This is exactly the reverse of traditional breakeven analysis. Assuming we break even at the intersection of total revenue and total cost (a logical assumption), then the distance between the total cost and total revenue lines becomes greater the further from the intersection. Since the fixed revenue line is above the cost line to the left of the intersection in Figure 6–2–5, the profits increase as volume moves closer and closer to zero.

The implication of this is that the main duty for a manager in a capitated setting is to find ways to minimize the care per member. Only by driving the variable costs per member lower and lower can profits be increased.

THE FALLACY

The problem with the new analysis is that it compares apples to oranges.

In the traditional analysis the incentive is to maximize the number of patients. The more patients, the more profit. The reason for this is that patients drive revenue. The more patients, the more revenue. Just as Activity-Based Costing (ABC) requires managers to focus on cost drivers, in breakeven analysis one must focus on revenue drivers. Note, however, that at any given volume of patients, we try to minimize the cost per patient.

In the new analysis, the argument is to minimize care provided since revenues are fixed. Thus, we not only minimize care per patient, as is true in the traditional approach. We also try to minimize total care.

This approach is similar to the new chief executive officer who decides to turn around a financially losing organization by instituting better controls over the use of paper clips. We certainly do want to avoid wasting paper clips. However, often focusing on revenue issues can be more effective.

What is not explained in the new analysis is why revenue is fixed. It is simply assumed that under capitation if you provide additional service to an individual, the monthly premium is fixed, so revenues are fixed. In a limited way this makes sense. We cannot do additional tests on a given patient and increase revenues by charging that patient more. But that hasn't been the primary focus since the introduction of DRGs.

If we can cover additional lives, then the revenue to the hospital will increase. Under capitation, we are paid per member rather than per patient. However, revenue is not fixed. As we add members we add revenue. The revenue line should continue to slope up and to the right. However, it is calibrated in terms of the number of members rather than patients. In the traditional model, how would we plot revenue if our patients were paid for under a DRG system, and we were told we had a specific fixed number of patients of each type?

Revenue would become a horizontal fixed line, the same as that shown in Figure 6–2–5. However, whether considering a fixed number of members or a fixed number of DRG patients, Figure 6–2–5 makes the unrealistic assumption that a hospital has no way to increase the population it serves. That is only true if there is no competition in the community.

The new analysis doesn't really give sound advice on how to act if payments are capitated. It adds a restriction that has not existed before, and in the real world still does not exist. The restriction is that we cannot increase revenue. In fact, revenue can be increased. Further, if any costs are fixed, it is usually a better strategy to spread those costs over as many revenue contributors as possible.

The underlying problem is that in Figure 6–2–5, the new analysis does not clearly define what is meant by "Volume" on the horizontal axis. Clearly, it should not be patients. For any fixed number of covered lives, a hospital would want to minimize the number of patients treated. But that totally ignores the revenue driver. If volume is the number of members, the revenue line is not horizontal.

An important lesson to be learned is that we must free our thinking from being overly focused on the number of patients as volume. Under a capitated setting, we should think of the revenue per member and the costs per member.

If we consider revenue as variable with the number of members, the implication is that the revenue line does slope up and to the right. In that case one would want to maximize volume, the same as in the traditional model. Adding more members will add to profits, even though they add more variable costs.

The curious thing about the analysis, is that no one has stopped to consider how HMOs react to the same set of circumstances. Their revenues are capitated. Do HMOs look at their per member per month revenue and conclude that revenue is a fixed amount, to be shown as a horizontal line?

For example, Oxford Health Plans in the Northeastern United States grew from 200,000 members in 1993 to 500,000 members in 1994 to 1,000,000 members in 1995. Nearly all of their members are capitated. Was their revenue over that three-year period a fixed amount? No—it grew at an enormous rate. Was their primary focus on minimization of services to a fixed group of members, or maximization of the number of members?

As high growth HMOs have taught us, under capitation the key to financial stability is growing volume. Move to the right on the breakeven chart, not to the left!

Reading 6–3

Using Breakeven Analysis with Step-Fixed Costs

Steven A. Finkler

In a recent issue of *Hospital Cost Management and Accounting* (Vol. 1, No. 4), a number of potential problems with the use of breakeven analysis were discussed. These included problems related to multiple products, changing prices, changing costs, and uncertainty. This article deals with one additional specific problem—step-fixed costs.

Breakeven analysis requires classification of costs into fixed and variable components. A contribution margin per unit is calculated (price minus variable cost). That amount represents how much money is available from each unit to contribute toward covering fixed costs, or toward generating a profit. The breakeven quantity is the minimal volume at which the total contribution margin from all units is sufficient to cover the fixed costs.

Thus, as long as cost behavior approximates that shown in Figure 6–3–1 or Figure 6–3–2, the model works. In Figure 6–3–1 we see that fixed costs stay constant as volume increases. For example, at a volume of B, costs would be $A. At any other volume, costs would still be $A. Variable costs increase in direct proportion with volume (Figure 6–3–2). At volume B, variable costs would be $C. At a volume lower than B, costs would be less than $C. At a volume higher than B, costs would be greater than $C.

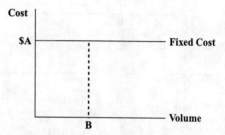

Figure 6–3–1 Graph of Fixed Costs

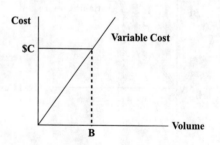

Figure 6–3–2 Graph of Variable Costs

Fixed and variable costs can be combined in one graph by adding the fixed costs at any volume (e.g., $A) to the variable costs at that volume (e.g., $C), to determine the total costs ($A + $C) (Figure 6–3–3). The traditional breakeven chart can be determined (Figure 6–3–4) by adding revenue to the graph and then comparing the total costs to total revenue. The breakeven point occurs when the total revenue and total cost line in Figure 6–3–4 intersect.

Source: Reprinted from Steven A. Finkler, "Using Breakeven Analysis with Step-Fixed Costs," *Hospital Cost Management and Accounting,* Vol. 1, No. 8, pp. 1–5. Copyright November 1989, Aspen Publishers, Inc.

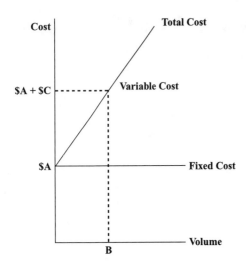

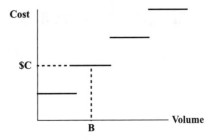

Figure 6–3–5 Graph of Step-Fixed Costs

Figure 6–3–3 Graph of the Total Costs

swings in volume, they are fixed over smaller volume changes. Therefore they are not really variable costs, nor are they really fixed costs. This article answers the question of how these costs should be treated in breakeven calculations.

A SIMPLISTIC SOLUTION

The approach often taken with respect to this problem is to ignore it. All costs are classified as either fixed or variable, and regular breakeven analysis (i.e., breakeven volume equals the fixed cost divided by the contribution margin) is applied. Implicitly or explicitly, the step costs are treated as being either fixed or variable.

In some cases this may create a reasonable approximation of reality. Suppose that we expect to have 6 hours of nursing care per 24-hour patient day. If agency nurses are hired on a daily basis, nursing labor will not be perfectly variable—it will not increase 6 hours for each extra patient day. First, agency nurses will be hired in 8-hour increments, not 6-hour increments. Second, the 6 hours needed are spread over a 24-hour day, not over a single 8-hour shift.

However, if nursing labor increases by 3 nursing shifts (i.e., 1 extra nurse per shift for 3 shifts) for each extra 4 patient days, then we can assume the cost to be variable without creating major errors in the analysis. (Note that 4 patient days @ 6 hours of nursing care per patient day implies a need for 24 hours of nursing care, or 1 more nurse per shift for that day.)

Even in this case, however, the error is somewhat greater than one might assume. If average

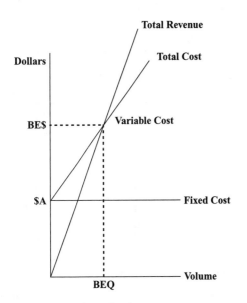

Figure 6–3–4 Breakeven Graph

Unfortunately, in most hospitals, the largest part of the hospital's costs—staffing—tends to be of a step-fixed nature, as shown in Figure 6–3–5. Hospitals do not hire an additional hour of nursing time, or housekeeping time, or dietitian time, if there is one additional patient day. While these labor costs are not fixed over wide

daily volume on a unit rises by 1 patient, that would imply 365 additional patient days over the course of a year. Suppose that we have a nursing unit with 30 beds, and this year the unit had an average census of 20. At 6 hours per patient, that would require 120 nursing hours, or 15 nurses per day. For simplicity assume that 5 nurses work each of 3 shifts.

If our census were to rise next year to 21, what would happen to staffing? We would need an additional 2 hours of nursing care per shift. Would we float in a nurse or hire an agency nurse for each of the 3 shifts (pay for 24 hours because patient needs rose by 6 hours)? Probably not.

Our staffing guide might indicate that with a census of 18–22 we staff 5 nurses on each shift. Only if census fell below 18 would we float a nurse out, or if it rose above 22 would we add staff. Therefore, within that range the staffing is a fixed cost. At a census of 18 there would be 6,570 patient days per year, while at a census of 22 there would be 8,030 patient days per year. That range represents up to 1,460 patient days. Over that range staffing cost is fixed.

It is quite possible, however, that if census was 20 patients last year, it could conceivably fall to 16 or 17 patients per day on average this year, or it might rise to 23 or 24 patients. This implies a staffing range of 12 to 18 nurses for this unit per day (4, 5, or 6 nurses per shift). In dollar terms, this range would represent a very wide possible swing for a fixed cost. But to treat the cost as variable is not very satisfactory, since there is a substantial volume range in the middle over which the cost would be fixed.

In other areas of the hospital, the step nature of costs may be even more pronounced. For example, dietitians may prepare more or fewer meals, but only a substantial volume swing would result in a change in the number of employees in that department.

A More Useful Approach

An alternative approach to this problem, although it is somewhat more complicated, will provide a substantially improved calculation.

This approach requires us to assume that we will require only the lowest staffing level possible, and to treat the step cost as a fixed cost. When the breakeven calculation is performed, the result may indicate a breakeven level at which the volume exceeds the capacity limits of the step cost item. In that case the step cost will have to be raised, and the breakeven recalculated, until a feasible solution is attained.

Example

Aspen Hospital is considering whether to open an outpatient lab. They are unsure how many tests would be processed by the lab, and would like to know the breakeven quantity. For this example we will assume that only one type of lab test is performed. That, of course, is highly unrealistic. The problem of multiple products has been widely discussed in the accounting literature (see, e.g., *Hospital Cost Accounting Advisor,* Vol. 1, No. 1, June 1985). However, in order to focus on the issue of step costs, we will not consider multiple products in the example.

Certain costs of the laboratory will clearly be variable, such as various chemicals and reagents used. Other costs will clearly be fixed costs, such as the salary of the laboratory administrator. Many other costs will be step costs, such as lab technician labor and some types of equipment.

We will assume that the variable costs per test are $.25. We will further assume that the fixed costs are $200,000 per year. In this simple example we will assume that labor has the following pattern:

Volume of Tests	Number of Techs
0– 5,000	.5
5,000–10,000	1.0
10,000–15,000	1.5
15,000–20,000	2.0
20,000–25,000	2.5
25,000–30,000	3.0
30,000–35,000	3.5

It is expected that lab tech salaries will be $25,000 including benefits.

Equipment related to this particular test has the following capacities:

Volume of Tests	Number of Sets of Equipment
0–13,000	1
13,001–26,000	2
26,001–39,000	3

The equipment for the test costs $30,000 per complete set. Aspen Hospital believes that on average they will receive $22 for each outpatient lab test performed. What is the breakeven volume?

The basic breakeven formula is as follows:

Breakeven Quantity = Fixed Cost/(Price − Variable Cost)

Therefore, if we assume that there will be only .5 technicians and 1 set of equipment, the total fixed costs would be the $200,000 basic fixed cost, plus $12,500 for one-half technician, plus $30,000 for one set of equipment, or a total fixed cost of $242,500. The price is $22, and the variable costs are $.25. Therefore,

Breakeven Quantity = $242,500/($22.00 − $.25)
= $242,500/$21.75
= 11,150 tests.

Unfortunately, when we examine our step cost items, we find that this volume is feasible with one set of equipment, but would require 1.5 technicians. Therefore, this is not a feasible breakeven solution.

The next step would be to recalculate the breakeven problem, using the staffing and equipment costs relevant at a volume of 11,150 tests. That is, we use the result from the first calculation to set the step costs for the next round of calculations. At a volume of 11,150 tests, we would need 1.5 technicians and 1 set of equipment. Therefore our new fixed costs are $200,000 plus $37,500 for 1.5 technicians plus $30,000, or a total of $267,500. Our breakeven calculation would be

Breakeven Quantity = $267,500/($22.00 − $.25)
= $267,500/$21.75
= 12,300 tests.

[Note that the result of the calculation is actually 12,299. However, some rounding is appropriate as a reminder that in real life, things seldom work out exactly according to analyses.]

The breakeven quantity of 12,300 tests is a feasible result because it requires only 1 set of equipment and 1.5 techs, which is the amount that we have built into the calculation. If the breakeven result had been above 13,000, we would have had to recalculate fixed costs to allow for additional equipment and then perform the breakeven calculation again.

Starting the breakeven analysis under the assumption that all step costs will be at their minimal values is a valuable technique, because it prevents us from failing to find the lowest possible breakeven volume. In the situation of step costs, it is quite possible for there to be more than one breakeven point.

For example, in the above situation we now know that there is a feasible breakeven point at 12,300 tests. Suppose that instead of starting at the lowest level, we had assumed that actual volume would be 13,500 tests, and then tried to find the breakeven point around that level. If we were to try the breakeven model assuming staffing and equipment costs appropriate for 13,500 tests, the cost of two sets of equipment would have to be included. In many cases this might push the breakeven point to a higher level. For instance, at 13,500 tests the fixed costs would be $200,000 plus $37,500 for 1.5 technicians, plus $60,000 for 2 sets of equipment, or a total fixed cost of $307,500. Then,

Breakeven Quantity = $307,500/($22.00 − $.25)
= $307,500/$21.75
= 14,140 tests.

We would wrongly be led to believe that there was no feasible solution unless we had over 14,000 tests, when in fact we are able to break even at a volume of 12,300 tests. This might incorrectly lead us to believe we can't achieve a breakeven without a volume higher than we can hope to attain. This creates an interesting paradox. Above 12,300 tests we are making money. However, if we exceed 13,000 tests we will start to lose money because of the $30,000 cost of the additional equipment. Should we allow our volume to exceed 13,000 tests? That depends on how much additional volume might be available. Clearly, however, the information about potential profits from 12,300 tests to 13,000 tests is more valuable than simply knowing that we are profitable above 14,150 tests. To get this information—i.e., the lowest feasible breakeven point—we must start the calculations assuming the lowest steps on our step-fixed costs. This approach to breakeven analysis might best be referred to as an iterative approach. It requires us to go around and around until we arrive at the best solution. Although it may seem to be a bit cumbersome, in an environment in which many of the costs we deal with are step costs, this method should substantially improve the accuracy and usefulness of breakeven calculation results.

Reading 6–4

Alternative Contribution Margin Measures

Steven A. Finkler

One of the most basic concepts of cost accounting is the notion of a contribution margin: the revenue received for our product less the variable costs of producing the product. However, as a management tool the specific application of contribution margin is more complicated than might at first appear.

Specifically, in maximizing a health care organization's contribution margin, we must consider constrained resources. The specific constraint will impact on the relevant approach to using contribution margin. While the organization may well desire to maximize overall contribution margin, the approach to achieve that end will not always call for trying to treat patients with the highest contribution margin per patient, nor will it always call for focusing on the highest contribution margin percent.

BASIC CONCEPTS

Before addressing the problems that arise when we apply contribution margin to management decision making, we will first discuss the basic concepts of contribution margin.

Because certain costs of operating an organization are fixed, the profitability of the organization depends largely on the volume of services it provides. Each additional patient generates revenues, and also causes us to incur additional cost. As long as the extra revenue from an additional patient exceeds the incremental cost generated by that patient, the organization will be better off.

In a definition of contribution margin, the incremental cost is often referred to as the variable cost.

Contribution Margin = Price – Variable Cost

Since fixed costs must be paid in any event, the excess of the price over the variable cost provides extra money to the organization. That money can either be used to cover fixed costs or (if all fixed costs have been covered) it provides profits.

The general rule resulting from the concept of contribution margin is that from a financial viewpoint, the organization should proceed to do anything that offers a positive contribution margin. Inherently, such output improves the overall financial well-being of the organization. The concept is important because of the great extent to which costs are allocated in health care organizations.

It is frequently the case that additional services proposed by a hospital can only be offered at a loss, if average costs are compared to revenues. However, average costs include an allocation of fixed overhead. In many cases that fixed over-

Source: Reprinted from Steven A. Finkler, "Alternative Contribution Margin Measures," *Hospital Cost Management and Accounting,* Vol. 1, No. 5, August 1989, pp. 1–4. Copyright 1989, Aspen Publishers, Inc.

head cost will be incurred whether the new service is offered or not. All that is happening is that some of that cost is being shifted from elsewhere in the organization to the new service.

Since that shifting of cost makes other areas of the organization more profitable (or reduces their loss), that benefit should be considered before deciding the new service loses money and should not be undertaken.

We can overcome that cost allocation problem by evaluating the new service based on its contribution margin. If the additional revenues generated by the new service exceed the additional costs the organization incurs, then there is a positive contribution and the service should be offered. The profits of the organization as a whole will increase, even if the specific new service shows a loss.

In applying cost-volume-profit analysis in this way, one must be aware that often additional volume causes some fixed cost items to rise as well. The usual definition of contribution margin as being price minus variable cost is not quite correct. Actually, the contribution is extra revenue less extra cost. We must subtract all costs (whether fixed, step-fixed or variable) that will be incurred only if the service or the volume expansion is undertaken.

CONTRIBUTION MARGIN PER PATIENT VS. CONTRIBUTION MARGIN PERCENT

The concept of contribution margin is extremely valuable in helping management to make correct decisions about whether or not to offer a new service, or expand volume. For example, if an HMO offers to generate an increased volume for us, at a cut-rate (less than average cost) price, we can use this notion to determine whether or not such an offer is financially attractive in the short run.

In the long run we would like to avoid it, because it fails to provide enough money to replace plant and equipment. In the short run we are already committed to depreciation and interest on our existing plant, and any positive contribution margin is better than an empty bed. Some may disagree, saying that once price cuts are started there is no stopping them. In reality, however, the only way to avoid price cuts to gain volume is to either collude (which is illegal) or reduce industry capacity. Since cut-rate pricing doesn't allow enough money to replace plant and equipment, it eventually leads to a reduction in the number of beds, and that long-run capacity decrease will allow hospitals to stop offering discounts.

In dealing with short-run decisions, we are often faced with a specific offer, such as one from an HMO, in which the appropriate contribution margin measure is straightforward. For example, if they were to guarantee 100 normal birth deliveries at a fixed price per patient, we could compare that price to the incremental costs per maternity patient to determine profitability. The volume involved is also an important consideration. One more patient might just increase variable costs, while 100 more patients might necessitate a new monitor. In either case, however, the focus is the contribution margin per patient for the maternity patients involved.

Often, however, cost-volume-profit analysis cuts across patient types. Many organizations therefore focus on the contribution margin ratio. This ratio is the contribution margin divided by the price. Thus a patient with a price of $1,000, and variable costs of $700, would have a contribution margin of $300, or a contribution margin ratio of .3 ($300/$1,000), more commonly referred to as 30%.

Now the problems for management decisions may arise. Suppose that our marketing manager has identified three different types of patients for which we might have a chance of increasing volume. The question is which type should be the first priority of our marketing efforts. Assume the following information:

	DRG X	*DRG Y*	*DRG Z*
Revenue per patient	$1,000	$3,000	$9,000
Incremental cost per patient	$ 600	$2,400	$9,100
Contribution margin per patient	$ 400	$ 600	$(100)
Contribution margin ratio	40%	20%	–1%

Which of these three types of patients would we most like to attract? Without the benefit of contribution margin analysis, the marketing director would probably pursue DRG Z. After all, without doubt our revenues rise most rapidly as we attract more of that type of patient. And, given the underlying costs, we might even find that other hospitals won't fight particularly hard to retain them.

Marketing managers tend to be oriented toward revenues. Raising revenues is a key indicator of their success. However, revenues that are accompanied by substantial cost increases are not of financial benefit to the hospital. So an immediate benefit of contribution margin analysis is to steer us away from a revenue focus and toward a profitability focus.

But should we try to attract more of DRG X or DRG Y? A conflict between the two is readily apparent. DRG Y has the higher contribution margin of $600 per patient. DRG X has the higher contribution margin percent of 40 percent of revenues. Which is the more relevant measure to use in decision making?

THE ISSUE OF CONSTRAINTS

The answer to that question depends on constrained resources within the hospital environment. Some hospital managers do generally focus on contribution margin per patient, and some do focus on contribution margin percent.

If the hospital expects its total revenues to be constrained—for example, if it is in a state that has an overall budget cap on the hospital, then the best approach is that which maximizes the contribution margin percent. In other words, for every dollar that is received, you want to keep the largest amount of that dollar as contribution margin. Thus DRG Y patients, with their high contribution margin per patient, would be less desirable, because their high price would push us to the overall budget cap quicker than DRG X patients.

On the other hand, if there is no limit on the number of patients, or the amount of revenue, DRG Y would be preferable, because for every extra patient, the contribution margin increases by the largest amount.

However, neither of these approaches is adequate. Note that in the last paragraph we said "if there is no limit on the number of patients." However, often that will not be the case. There will be some constraining factor that places a limit on the number of patients in total or of a particular type.

For example, suppose that the hospital is nearly full. Then the number of patient-days available are limited. In pursuing patients we will need to know how much of the constraining factor they consume. Suppose for example, that DRG X has an average length of stay of 4 days, while DRG Y has an average length of stay of 10 days. Then we can calculate a contribution margin per patient day:

	DRG X	DRG Y
Revenue per patient	$1,000	$3,000
Incremental cost per patient	−600	−2,400
Contribution margin per patient	$ 400	$ 600
Divided by length of stay	÷4	÷10
Contribution margin per patient day	$ 100	$ 60

As you can readily see, if the number of beds (and therefore patient days available) is limited, the desirable marginal patient switches from DRG Y, at $600 per patient vs. $400 per patient, to DRG X, at $100 of additional contribution margin per patient day as compared to $60 per day. Thus the fact that the hospital is almost full has a direct bearing on what type of patient we want to try to attract.

The specific constraint that is most pressing is likely to differ in different institutions. For example, another hospital might have a low enough occupancy that patient days were not a crucial issue. For them, $600 per patient would be better than $400, even though the patient stays much longer. But what if that hospital has limited operating room capacity, and the DRG Y patient would consume more operating room hours? In that case we would want to market ourselves in such a way as to maximize the contribution margin per operating room hour consumed.

Whenever the hospital is going to make a formal effort to increase volume in some way and to increase contribution margin in total, some resource is likely to be constrained. Even if the hospital has plenty of capacity, a simple rule of getting the patient with the highest contribution margin is unlikely to be correct. This is because different patients are not likely to be equally easy to attract.

Suppose that the marketing department can attract two DRG X patients with the same cost and effort as it would take to attract one DRG Y patient. In that case the effort to gain $600 of contribution from a Y patient would be the same as the effort to gain $800 of contribution margin from the X patients. The constraining resource in essence becomes the time and effort of the marketing department.

In most hospitals multiple constraints will exist. Beds, and operating room capacity, and marketing efforts may all be constrained. From a mathematical standpoint, all of the constraints could be built into a model that is solved using linear programming.

However, that level of sophistication is probably unnecessary. It would, as a practical point, make more sense to simply focus on one or two of the most pressing constraints, and make sure that our efforts are in accord with maximizing contribution margin to the hospital given that constraint or those constraints.

For example, suppose that both our outpatient clinic and our inpatient beds were running at 90 percent of capacity. Suppose further that the contribution margin for inpatient care is substantially higher per hour of marketing effort than for outpatient care. In that case, marketing efforts should focus on filling the inpatient beds with patients having the highest contribution margin per patient day. When the inpatient side is full, the effort can swing over to the outpatient side.

Contribution margin analysis can be an extremely valuable management tool. The key to using it effectively, however, is to move away from the limited notion of attracting patients with the highest contribution margin per patient. In many respects that approach is as naive as trying to maximize revenue per patient regardless of cost. Instead, managers should consider the constraint in the organization that is most limiting, and ensure that as we move toward the limitation imposed by that constraint, we are maximizing the contribution per unit of that constraining resource.

Part II

Cost Accounting Information for Planning and Control

A primary focus of cost accounting is on developing information that managers can use for planning and control. Once the reader is familiar with the foundations of cost accounting provided in Part I, a number of specific tools for improved planning and control can be considered. That is the role of Part II of this book.

The first chapter in this section, Chapter 7, focuses on the prediction of future costs. In order to plan for the future it is essential to be able to anticipate what costs will be in coming periods of time. Chapter 7 in the companion text, *Essentials of Cost Accounting for Health Care Organizations, Second Edition,*[1] examines a number of techniques for making such estimates. These range in sophistication from using groups of individuals to gain consensus based on opinion, to the use of regression analysis, curvilinear forecasting, and learning curves. Reading 7–1 in this book considers the problem of outliers in regression analysis. Reading 7–2 provides a discussion of the learning curve technique, and its application in the health care industry.

Chapter 8 discusses budgeting. While the companion *Essentials* text focuses on introductory and fundamental concepts of budgeting, the readings in this book provide a richness of discussion of alternative specialized budgeting approaches.

The first two readings for this chapter focus on the zero-base budgeting approach. Zero base budgeting (ZBB) is a form of evaluative budgeting. Rather than accept some prior budget level as a base, and add an annual increment to that base, ZBB requires justification of the entire budget. ZBB considers not only the justification for each and every expenditure, but also alternative ways to provide the service, alternative levels of service, and even alternative quality levels. Reading 8–1, "The Financial Evolution of Hospitals and the Zero-Base Approach," provides a thorough explanation of the technique. Reading 8–2, "Zero-Based Budgeting for a Radiology Service: A Case Study in Outsourcing," provides a specific application of the technique in a health care setting.

As health care organizations become more sophisticated, they also become more complex. In complex organizations, the development and use of a budget manual can be quite helpful. This topic is discussed in Reading 8–3.

In addition to the concern that budgeting only focuses on the annual increment, it has also been criticized at times for its focus on line-items of inputs, instead of what the organization is trying to accomplish. For example, a department knows the budgeted cost for technicians rather than the budgeted cost for a specific type of test it produces. One response to such criticism is the use of performance budgets that focus on what a department or organization is attempting to achieve. "Outcome Budgeting Shifts Focus to

---

[1]Steven A. Finkler and David M. Ward, *Essentials of Cost Accounting for Health Care Organizations, Second Edition*, Aspen Publishers, Inc., Gaithersburg, MD, 1999.

Meeting Objectives," Reading 8–4, discusses this approach in detail.

Another valuable budgeting technique is that of flexible budgeting. It is rare that an organization achieves exactly the workload it expects. Generally, either more or fewer patients will be served. It is critical to be able to anticipate the financial impact of both increases and decreases in patient volume. "Flexible Budgeting Allows for Better Management of Resources As Needs Change," Reading 8–5, provides a discussion of this technique.

Budgets are an instrumental planning tool. After actual events occur, they can become an excellent tool for control. The use of budgets for control purposes is discussed in Chapter 9. Primarily these readings are concerned with issues related to variance analysis.

The first reading, by Roger Kropf, considers a method for calculating physician cost variances. This article, "Physician Cost Variance Analysis under DRGs," Reading 9–1, looks at each physician's variance attributable to the mix of patients and to the cost of treating those patients. Many health care organizations have started to use such physician variance analyses as a cost control technique. Variance analysis is applied in a pharmacy setting in Reading 9–2, "A Contemporary Approach to Budget Variance Analysis."

Variance reports often feature current month and year-to-date information. An innovative alternative is offered in Reading 9–3, "Rolling Budgets and Variance Reports." This article proposes an alternative to the use of year-to-date information which at times provides many months worth of data, and at other times little if any additional information as compared to the current month variance.

"Statistical Cost Control: A Tool for Financial Managers," Reading 9–4 by Terrance Skantz, addresses the question of how to know when it pays to investigate a variance. Small variances caused by random fluctuations do not warrant a major investigation, taking up much of a manager's time. How small a variance can be ignored? How does a manager know when to investigate? Skantz provides a mechanism to help in making that determination.

Chapter 10 discusses management control. In addition to variance analysis, as discussed in the Chapter 9 readings, there are a number of other important aspects of control. These are addressed in the readings in Chapter 10.

The establishment of cost and revenue centers is the starting point in establishing a management control system in a health care organization. The organization must also develop a set of systems within the responsibility center structure that allow for motivation of managers through the assignment of responsibility. The development of such a management control system is discussed in Reading 10–1, "Developing a Planning and Control System for a Responsibility Unit."

Management control systems can result in organizational cost control. Reading 10–2, "Cost Control Systems," considers the three stages of cost control: planning, monitoring, and feedback. It further goes on to consider how systems can be used for cost containment, cost avoidance, and cost reduction.

One of the more difficult aspects of management control relates to the interactions among units of an organization. When one organizational unit charges another for its services, a difficult aspect is the appropriate price to charge. This is commonly referred to as transfer pricing. The general principle of management control with respect to transfer prices is to attempt to use market prices when they are available. When they are not, price setting becomes a more difficult issue. This problem is addressed in Readings 10–3 and 10–4, "Competitive Pricing Models for Intra-Hospital Services," by James Suver, and "Transfer Pricing in the Hospital-HMO Corporation," by Kyle Grazier.

7

Predicting Future Costs

Reading 7–1

Regression-Based Cost Estimation and Variance Analysis: Resolving the Impact of Outliers

Steven A. Finkler

THE OUTLIER PROBLEM

The use of regression analysis in cost estimation has been discussed in *Hospital Cost Accounting Advisor* (Vol. 1, No. 2, July 1985). One issue not discussed in that article was the impact of outliers on the results. Clearly, outliers have the potential to throw off estimates significantly. Further, when those estimates are used as the basis for budgets, the problem caused by outliers extends into the area of variance analysis. Deciding whether a variance is large enough to warrant investigation becomes less clear-cut. This article focuses on resolving a number of problems resulting from outlier and other data that can distort a regression-based analysis.

Linear regression is often used for estimating future costs of hospital departments. Many departments are able to project changes in volumes of activity. However, a 10 percent increase or decrease in activity levels does not translate into a 10 percent change in costs. Some costs in each department are fixed, and will not vary either upward or downward with a change in volume. Re-

Source: Reprinted from Steven A. Finkler, "Regression-Based Cost Estimation and Variance Analysis: Resolving the Impact of Outliers," *Hospital Cost Accounting Advisor,* Vol. 3, No. 4, September 1987, pp. 1–5. Copyright 1987, Aspen Publishers, Inc.

gression analysis uses historical information to evaluate the past changes in costs in relation to changes in volume. That information is then used to predict the likely future cost changes that would result from a given expected volume change.

When regression analysis is employed in cost estimation, the first step generally is to plot the points on a graph to allow for a visual inspection. Such an inspection has a number of benefits. First of all, the user can gain some insight as to whether a regression approach is appropriate. If the pattern detected shows seasonality, but no trend, then regression is probably a poor tool. However, if a trending effect is noted, regression analysis will generally give a superior prediction than less sophisticated estimating techniques.

Outliers are extreme data points that are sometimes caused by data collection errors or rare events. An advantage of a visual inspection of the plotted data points is that often outliers are readily apparent. For example, suppose that the data in Table 7–1–1 are being used to predict costs for the Operating Room Department for next year, when 8,550 hours of procedures are expected. These data have been plotted in Figure 7–1–1. Inspection of that figure shows that one outlier exists. The appropriate treatment of that outlier depends on what caused it.

Table 7-1-1 Operating Room Department Data

Year	Number of Surgery Hours	Cost
1980	7,300	$2,950,000
1981	7,550	3,100,000
1982	7,825	3,250,000
1983	8,200	3,610,000
1984	7,940	3,325,000
1985	8,120	3,256,000
1986	8,345	3,400,000
1987	8,450	3,458,000
1988	8,550	

If, for example, further investigation of the outlier shows that it was caused by a transposition error, then the data should simply be corrected. Perhaps the cost related to the 1984 observation was recorded as $3,610,000, but should have been $3,160,000.

On the other hand, it is possible that the outlier was not caused by any errors in calculation. Perhaps we simply had an extremely costly case-mix. Many of the patients that year had surgeries more costly than our normal average. This raises the question of whether that situation is likely to

occur again. One possibility is that a specialty hospital in town that performs only extremely costly surgeries closed their OR for six months for total renovations. Much of their normal patient load was handled by our hospital. Now that the renovation is over, such an occurrence is unlikely to be repeated for at least several decades. In that case, the outlier generates an erroneous implication about the probabilities of high-cost patients in the near future.

An alternative possibility is simply that the outlier represents a random occurrence that, given recent competition by outpatient surgery units for the less complex patients, is likely to occur from time to time. In that case, the outlier is relevant and should be retained. The key in determining whether to retain outlier data is the extent to which we believe that the data point is representative of a variation that may occasionally occur, versus the degree to which we believe that it resulted from an unusual event, and that it would be highly unlikely to occur again.

The impact of an outlier is generally to pull the estimated-line upward or downward, depending on whether it is above or below the bulk of the

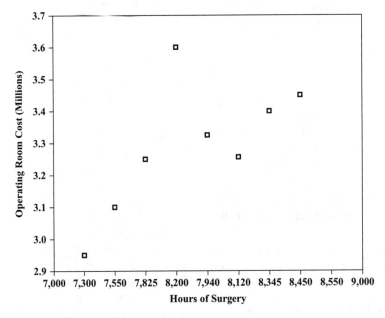

Figure 7-1-1 Operating Room Hours and Costs

observations. It is also possible for the outlier to cause the slope of the regression line to change, particularly if the outlier occurs farther away from the majority of the other data points (i.e., farther to the right or left along the X axis, as opposed to simply higher or lower along the Y axis).

A similar problem is raised by observations that are referred to as "influential points." An influential point is one that, because of its particular position among all of the data observations, happens to have a particularly strong impact on the results of the linear regression. This is more due to the nature of the regression process than to anything particularly unusual with respect to the point itself. Influential points should often be removed from the database in the same way that outliers are removed.

While outliers can often be determined by visual inspection, that is not the case with influential points. However, there are statistical techniques that can be used to check for both outliers and influential points. These techniques will not be discussed here because they are readily available in many statistical packages that would commonly be used for regression analyses, such as the Minitab software system.

Figure 7–1–2 shows the regression line based on all data points, including the outlier point. Figure 7–1–3 shows what the regression line would be if the outlier is eliminated from the data used for the analysis. Figure 7–1–4 compares the two regression lines. Note that there is a substantial difference between the lines.

This difference is particularly notable when we consider the value predicted for next year's cost based on the two regressions. When the outlier is included in the analysis, the regression analysis predicts costs to be $3,562,000 if next year's operating room activity level is 8,550 hours of surgery. In contrast, with the outlier removed, the predicted cost is $3,499,000, a difference of $63,000.

The benefits of removing an unwarranted outlier from the data are substantial. Not only is the predicted cost more accurate, but it is also subject to less random variability. In this particular example, the R-squared of the regression rose from .78 to .92 when the outlier was dropped, indicative of a better relationship between the independent and dependent variables.

Furthermore, the standard error for both the fixed cost (the Y intercept, or constant in the regression, may be interpreted as fixed cost in a cost-estimating regression analysis) and the variable cost (the X coefficient, or slope of the regression analysis, may be interpreted as the variable cost in a cost-estimating regression analysis) was halved. This implies a probability of less normal variation from the predicted cost.

Certainly, one would always prefer to have a more accurate estimate. However, in what specific way can that more accurate estimate be helpful? The remainder of this article focuses on one example, that of variance analysis.

VARIANCE INVESTIGATION

One of the most difficult decisions managers must make is whether or not to investigate a variance. Normal variations are likely to cause small favorable or unfavorable variances to occur in every budget. We have a few more patients or a few less patients. Patients are slightly more or less acutely ill than expected. Supply prices vary in some minor way from expectations. None of these variations warrants the time and effort of a thorough investigation.

Unfortunately, until the investigation takes place, one doesn't know if the variation was minor and did not really require investigation, or if the variance resulted from some major loss of control. Even if small in amount, the variance can be an early signal of a failure of management to exercise proper budgetary control, or of a marketplace shift of significant importance.

Thus, there is a desire to investigate variances, but this desire must be considered in light of the cost of the investigation. The benefits of any corrective actions that might be taken as the result of an investigation must be balanced with the costs of management time and effort to undertake the investigation.

The key question then becomes, when is a variance large enough to merit investigation? To

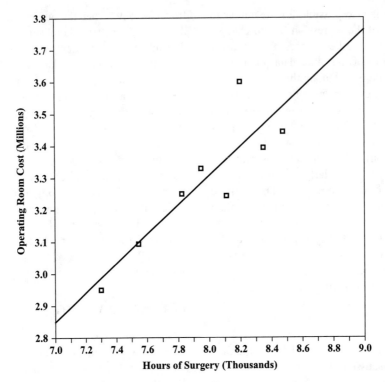

Figure 7–1–2 Operating Room Regression Results Including Outlier

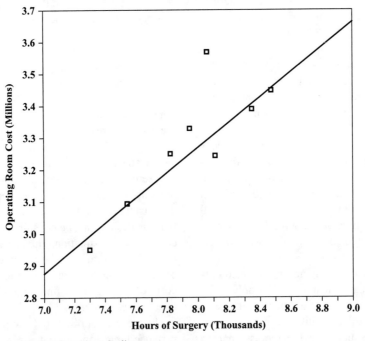

Figure 7–1–3 Regression Results without Outlier

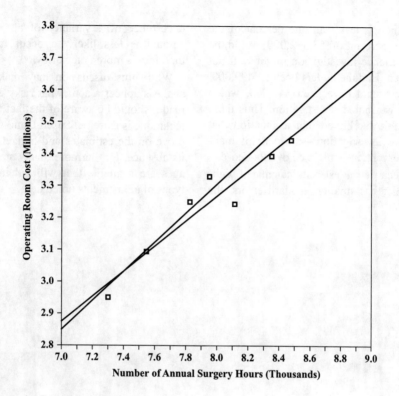

Figure 7–1–4 Regression Results Compared

some extent, managers must rely on their experience and judgment. Such judgment can always call for an investigation even if formal decision rules would not. However, formal decision rules can be a great aid.

As variances become larger, there is a greater likelihood that there are problems that management should investigate. Therefore many hospitals may set a dollar or percent limit. If a variance is below the limit, no investigation is required. If the variance exceeds the limit, then an investigation is automatically undertaken. While such approaches are better than no decision rule, they fail to take into account the degree of probability that the variance indicates an "out of control" situation, as opposed to a simple random fluctuation.

If the budget is based on costs that were developed from a regression analysis model, then the model has considered the historical dispersion of costs. If the cost for an item typically fluctuates

widely, then a somewhat large dollar amount variance might not be a particular concern. On the other hand, if historically fluctuations have been rather narrow, then a smaller variance might warrant attention.

Consider the example presented earlier in this article. Before the outlier was removed, the predicted cost for 1988 was $3,562,000. After the outlier was removed, it was determined that the predicted cost should be $3,499,000. Suppose that the department follows a rule that requires investigation of variances when they exceed the budget by more than one percent for the department as a whole. What would happen if the actual result was a cost of $3,590,000? (Note that this example looks at years in total for the sake of simplicity—actually, estimates should be made for each month, and variances investigated, when warranted, on a monthly basis.)

If the actual result is $3,590,000 and the budget was $3,562,000, the difference is only

$28,000, which is less than one percent of the budget (one percent of $3,562,000 would be $35,620). Variance investigation might well not be undertaken. Had the budget been $3,499,000, the variance would have been $41,000, which would have warranted investigation. Thus there is a reasonable likelihood that a situation that might require investigation—and perhaps management intervention—might be overlooked.

In fact, because the estimate calculated without the outlier has smaller standard errors, the occurrence of a variance of any given dollar amount is less likely to occur randomly and therefore is more noteworthy.

While this discussion may make regression analysis appear a somewhat risky approach, the reader should be aware of the fact that the basic technique is extremely useful, and will often improve on the estimates and budgets prepared in its absence. Furthermore, many statistical packages are available that will aid in making the types of adjustments noted here.

Reading 7–2

The Learning Curve and the Health Care Industry

Joann Ahrens

This article will examine the learning curve and its potential impact on the health care industry. Although the learning curve has traditionally been applied to the manufacturing industry, a labor-intensive industry like health care is a prime candidate for the benefits of the learning curve. Specifically, we will look at past research on the learning curve and discuss what effects learning might have on health care costs and outcomes in the current health care environment.

THE LEARNING CURVE

The learning curve (also called a progress function)[1] is a relationship between inputs and outputs that shows that "learning is present" by a decrease in inputs per each unit of output.[2] The curve describes the decreasing rate of savings that results from this relationship. Creating learning curves is a simple and accurate way to forecast costs and labor requirements, based on the predicted improvement as production increases. The curve can also be used as a decision-making tool and can help an organization focus on areas where organizational learning would be most cost effective.

The main concept of the learning curve is that as production volume doubles, the amount of

Source: Reprinted from Joann Ahrens, "The Learning Curve and the Health Care Industry," *Hospital Cost Management and Accounting,* Vol. 9, No. 6, pp. 1–8. Copyright September 1997, Aspen Publishers, Inc.

time and cost per unit decreases geometrically. Each time production doubles, there is a uniform percentage reduction in the amount of time it takes to produce each unit.[3] The two main effects of the learning curve are on production time (a direct effect) and cost and quality (indirect effects). The learning curve was first demonstrated in the aircraft industry, where it was shown by T.P. Wright in 1936 that when output doubled labor requirements decreased by 20 percent.[4]

It is understandable that individuals learn (and reduce the amount of time to accomplish a task) over time as a result of task repetition. The underlying concept of the learning curve, however, is that in addition to an individual learning, the organization is also learning. It is as the organization learns—through better staffing approaches, new techniques, and management approaches—that the average production time decreases.[5]

There are several important points to note regarding the learning curve:

- The learning curve does not apply solely to individuals, because it is seen in production lines that undergo changes of employees. "An organization does not lose out on its learning abilities when members leave the organization."[6]

- The learning curve can be seen in all types of industries, although its effects are most noticeable in labor-intensive industries and less noticeable in ones that rely heavily on technology.

- The learning curve has been tested most often in manufacturing industries, but can be seen in service-related industries as well.
- The learning curve is seen in both job-order and process production.[7]

HOW IT WORKS

There are several geometric versions of the learning curve. All of these rely on two basic parameters: the input resources needed for the first unit of production and the learning rate.[8] The log-linear model is the most common model and is described in the following equation as:

$$C = aV^b$$

where C is the direct labor input (or the marginal cost), V is the cumulative output, a is the cost of the first unit produced, and b is the learning elasticity.[9]

"The slope of the curve indicates the percentage cost reduction when cumulative output is doubled."[10] This means that as output is doubled, the cost per unit falls by 20 percent for an 80 percent learning curve. Initial production will see large decreases in unit costs as the output doubles often (e.g., 1 to 2 units, 2 to 4 units, 4 to 8 units). However, at higher production levels, the cost per unit will decrease the same percentage, but this decrease will occur at further and further intervals (e.g., 128 to 256 units, 256 to 512 units, 512 to 1,024 units). The graph and backup data (Figure 7–2–1 and Table 7–2–1) illustrate this effect for 75 percent, 80 percent, and 85 percent learning curves.

DEVELOPING A LEARNING CURVE

In order to develop a learning curve to predict future costs, certain data need to be collected. Models are often used to calculate costs based on a predicted volume and learning rate. One such model is displayed by NASA on the Internet. It calculates the effort for the nth unit, the cumulative average, and the cumulative total. The input data required by this model are the effort for the first unit, the number of units, and the learning percentage.[11]

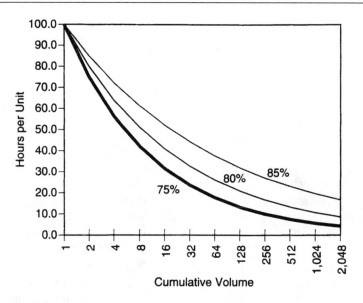

Figure 7–2–1 Learning Curves

Table 7–2–1 Backup Data for 75%, 80%, and 85% Learning Curves

Volume		Hours per Unit		
Additional	*Cumulative*	*75%*	*80%*	*85%*
—	1	100.0	100.0	100.0
1	2	75.0	80.0	85.0
2	4	56.3	64.0	72.3
4	8	42.2	51.2	61.4
8	16	31.6	41.0	52.2
16	32	23.7	32.8	44.4
32	64	17.8	26.2	37.7
64	128	13.3	21.0	32.1
128	256	10.0	16.8	27.2
256	512	7.5	13.4	23.2
512	1,024	5.6	10.7	19.7
1,024	2,048	4.2	8.6	16.7

To calculate a learning curve for a service, the volumes of the service performed over the initial period of operation need to be plotted against the cost per unit over the same period. The volume would typically be increasing as the cost per unit decreases. The curve that is plotted from these points will show the rate of learning for this service. This rate can then be applied over the next budget period to predict the cost per unit for the projected volumes of service. The per unit cost can then be multiplied by the volumes in order to determine the total cost of the service for the next budget period.[12]

APPLICATIONS

The applications of the learning curve include: estimating starting costs, determining purchasing and manpower requirements, establishing factory costs, checking the progress of individual employees, and making decisions regarding future product development.[13]

Another important use of the learning curve is for budgeting. Traditional budgeting usually allows for the same amount of money to be allotted to each department, plus additional amounts for inflation, new products, etc. The learning curve would imply, however, that the amount of money budgeted for certain products and services should be adjusted to reflect the need for less labor.[14] Studies to determine the learning curve rates of high volume or expensive services could allow managers to predict the amount of labor, and therefore the amount of budgeted cost, to allocate to each service in the next year.

A LEARNING ORGANIZATION

Because the organization itself has a large impact on the existence and rates of learning curves, some of the basics of organizational learning and how they apply to learning curves will be discussed.

A "learning organization" means learning by the system of the organization, as compared to "organizational learning," which means the learning of the individual and groups in an organization.[15] These definitions demonstrate that the learning curve is measuring both systemic and individual/group learning. A learning organization, however, would not have learning restricted to certain product lines and would be more likely to have more and higher learning curve rates.

Schein writes that an organization has to have "systemic health" in order for learning to be present. The four factors Schein includes in systemic health are: "(1) a sense of identity, purpose, or mission; (2) a capacity on the part of the system to adapt and maintain itself in the face of internal and external changes; (3) a capacity to perceive and test reality; and (4) some degree of internal integration or alignment of the sub-systems that make up the total system."[16] Specifically, the influences on a learning organization—and therefore on the learning curve—are: structure, environment, technology, knowledge acquisition, information distribution and interpretation, and organization memory.[17]

An organization's culture is the "consequence of the organization's prior experience and learning, and the basis for its continuing capacity to learn."[18] Innovative organizations have cultures where there is:

- a concern for people;
- a belief that people can learn;
- a belief that things are changeable;
- "some slack";
- a commitment to open communication;
- a commitment to "think systematically"; and
- a belief in teams.[19]

Whereas individuals may feel anxiety—in terms of both surviving in the organization and attempting to learn and fail[20]—the organization is affected on a more widespread level that can stagnate learning throughout the organization. All of these organizational factors are important because they impact the learning curve rate.

In health care, organizational learning applies because it has "become popular among organizations which are interested in increasing competitive advantage, innovativeness, and effectiveness."[21] This is exactly what many health care organizations are trying to do to survive. In addition, the ability to learn enables organizations to be more adaptable to change, which is what health care organizations have had to do in the recent past and will mostly likely have to attempt to do in the future.[22]

LIMITATIONS

A main limitation of the learning curve is the accuracy of choosing the two main parameters of the learning curve: the resources for the first unit and the learning curve rate. Failure to take all resources and associated costs of the first unit, as well as an inaccurate rate, can have deleterious effects on the predicted production volumes and costs.[23]

Another main problem is that "illusory" savings may result from errors in selecting the correct labor inputs. Savings may be attributed to learning when they are actually caused by some other factor, or when they represent cost-shifting and not actual savings. The reasons for these errors are:

- automation may decrease labor time;
- indirect labor could be increasing as direct labor time is decreasing;
- more qualified workers may be hired and change the labor mix; and
- changes in volume and not increases in learning may be producing savings.[24]

In addition to prediction and measurement limitations, there are potential problems in terms of management. (These limitations were elaborated on in the organizational learning section.) Employees may be resistant to learning because of a lack of incentives and/or bad attitudes toward the organization. Employees must believe in the idea of the learning curve, and management must ensure that the appropriate processes are in place so that the organization as a whole can learn.

Because the learning curve flattens, the amount of savings decreases significantly as volume increases. Although larger amounts of savings are seen in low-volume services, this does not mean that learning should be discounted in certain high-volume production items. For example, Finkler points out that the learning curve is applied to the area of microchips in which millions of chips are produced each year.[25]

Despite the fact that the learning curve has a limited impact in the long term, its impact in the short term is significant. In addition, each time services and production change, the learning curve slope increases to reflect the learning that is taking place in the organization once again.

A major limitation on learning in general is the reliance on technology. Although employees can learn to operate machines more efficiently, and even find new application for machines, the capability of machines is always limited.[26] Therefore, a production line's dependence on machines limits the degree of learning that can occur. Other factors, such as availability of materials and work schedules, also affect the learning curve. However, the effect of these variables depends on how much control the manager has over them and how the manager modifies these variables to reflect the learning of the organization.

THE LEARNING CURVE IN HEALTH CARE

Few attempts have been made to apply the learning curve to the health care industry. One reason is that, until recently, the major reimbursement methods did not provide any incentive for managers to control costs. Costs were also typically broken down by department and not by product. Another reason is that measuring the quality of health care is usually not as straightforward as measuring the quality of other products or services. For these reasons and others, research on learning has traditionally been done in the manufacturing sector.

Significant changes in the health care industry over the past decade (including the emphasis on cost containment and managed care and changes in reimbursement methods) warrant the investigation of the possible benefits of applying the learning curve to health services. First, the learning curve could be used as a way to predict costs and resources and to aid in creating more accurate budgets. Second, the learning curve can show which services have the potential to benefit from new processes that promote organizational learning (and the savings from these processes can be measured). Third, the curve can show improved quality in service based on outcomes measurement after an increase in the volumes of selected services.

The learning curve can be applied specifically to the impact of regionalization on hospital services. As regionalization increases the volume of services, we can determine what type of learning curve can be expected for each type of service, and exactly what effects this will have on resource consumption and quality.[27] One main obstacle in determining the effects on learning and regionalization, however, is that it is hard to measure the effects of learning vs. economies of scale.

Little research has been done to investigate these potential benefits. This research is reviewed below, but it should be noted that it is very limited and is not current. With the major developments in health care over the last decade, new research needs to be performed to see what impact learning can have on both the cost and quality of different health services.

LEARNING EXPERIMENTS IN HEALTH CARE

Most health care research on learning has focused on quality, not cost. Specifically, studies in the early 1980s showed that lower severity-adjusted mortality rates resulted from higher volumes. There is concern regarding the underlying cause of the difference in rates, most importantly that "learning from experience" was not the actual or main cause.[28] If learning is the main cause, then the regionalization of certain services would be beneficial because it should decrease the mortality rates. Smith says that if the cause was increased referrals resulting from better mortality rates, then a free market health care system would allow the best programs to dominate and mortality rates to decrease. Another reason may have been that the programs with better outcomes were more selective in choosing their patients.[29]

Smith's study, done at Temple University, looked at the effect of experience on a heart transplant program in a longitudinal study of survivors.[30] Heart transplants were chosen because they were a new service, were high cost, had a low volume, and required a team with specific skills. Smith found that whereas outcomes improved with increased volume, costs did not. Smith cited the administration as the reason that costs did not fall in line with the learning curve, identifying the absence of Belkaoui's two learning factors: faith and open-ended expectations.[31]

A 1986 study questioned whether previous results from learning and quality research were a result of individual physicians or characteristics of high-volume hospitals.[32] The study looked at the total volume of procedures, the procedures performed by the primary surgeon, board certification, and other factors concerning patient severity. The results showed the same inverse relationship between volume and patient mortality that has been seen in past studies. They also showed that board certification and medical school affiliation were related to lower mortality rates. No relationship was seen between individuals and mortality rates, "suggesting that the volume-outcome relationship reflects hospital rather than physician characteristics."[33]

Another study looked at the costs and outcomes of patients with coronary artery disease.[34] This study found that quality improved over time, with no concurrent gains in technology. Hemenway notes that such improvement "does not just happen: they require proper provider motivation."[35] Therefore, the lack of management focus on cost, under cost reimbursement, may have allowed experience to improve quality without decreasing resource use.

In a non-health care related study, a model was developed to analyze the effects of experience rates with entry barriers and market performance. The study found that experience curves could create barriers to entry and that these barriers were strongest for moderate learning rates. "Market performance increases sharply from one to two to three firms, but relatively slowly thereafter."[36] Thus, one could conclude that the learning rates of organizations can have an impact on barriers to entry into new or existing health care fields. With the increasing competitiveness and innovation within the field, organizations should analyze the impact on their current services or on services they are considering adding.

Based on the research of learning and health care, it can be concluded that there is evidence of increased quality from increased volume. This increase may be from learning, but the extent that other factors are involved has not been determined. No impact has been seen on resources or costs from increased volume. As the present health care industry has a strong focus on cost, new studies should be performed to determine what benefits learning can have in the new environment. Research on different types of services needs to be performed so that budgeting can be done accurately and so that managers can impact services through improvements in organizational learning.

A HEALTH CARE EXAMPLE

In this hypothetical example, a hospital's outpatient surgery unit recently added a radial keratotomy (RK) clinic. RK is a surgical procedure performed on the cornea to improve myopia (nearsightedness). This procedure is an appropriate one for a learning curve example, because although RK has been performed in the United States since 1978, the number of procedures performed has increased significantly over the last decade.

After its start-up year, the clinic's budgeted costs can be estimated using the learning curve instead of simply adding inflation to the current year's costs. The costs shown here are the variable costs—costs that are incurred from each procedure performed—and do not represent the total cost of the clinic's budget.

First, the learning curve rate must be calculated. By looking at a log of actual time per procedure, we can use the first entry of 80 minutes as the basis of the learning curves in the last three columns.[37] (See Figure 7–2–2.) As you can see from both the table and the graph, the actual procedure time in the clinic most closely resembles the 85 percent learning curve. More accurately, the data follow an 86 percent learning curve.

Volume		Actual Procedure Time	Learning Curves		
Added	Cumulative		90%	85%	80%
—	1	80	80.0	80.0	80.0
1	2	55	57.6	54.4	51.2
2	4	38	41.5	37.0	32.8
4	8	26	29.9	25.2	21.0
8	16	18	21.5	17.1	13.4
16	32	12	15.5	11.6	8.6

With the knowledge that the organization is learning at an 86 percent learning rate, we can perform the second step in predicting the next year's costs. The first year's total patient load was 512 patients. This means that the production level doubled nine times in the first year. Based on an 86 percent learning curve rate, the cost per procedure decreased to 26 percent of the original

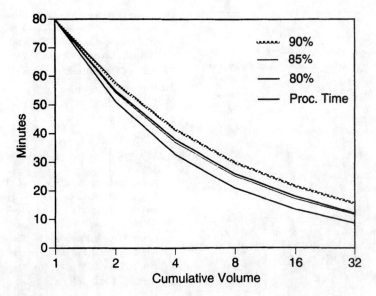

Figure 7–2–2 RK Learning Rate

cost for the last 256 patients. If the volume of patients was constant throughout the year, this means that the variable costs in the second half of the year equaled only 26 percent of the first half of the year's costs. This decrease can be seen in the following calculations.

Cost per Procedure Decrease at an 86% Rate	
Cumulative Volume	*Percent Decrease*
1	100.0
2	86.0
4	74.0
8	63.6
16	54.7
32	47.0
64	40.4
128	34.8
256	29.9
512	25.7

If we expect the clinic's procedure volume to double over the next year, we could expect the cost per procedure to drop 22 percent (25.7% × 86%) from the original cost per procedure. If the

clinic expects this volume to double twice over the next three years, the cost per procedure would decrease to 16 percent. One can see that if the volume of any procedure is growing quickly, either in the long term or during a start-up period, the savings can be significant.

CONCLUSION

As the health care industry increasingly uses elements of cost accounting to manage resources, the learning curve can play a major role in many areas of this process. The learning curve can be used in budgeting, cost control, and quality improvement, and as a measurement of organizational learning. Learning curves can also provide valuable information for total quality management and continuous quality improvement programs.[38] A focus on learning curves can lead to a competitive edge for specific services and for the organization as a whole. It can also motivate employees and be used to provide feedback on performance. The combined emphasis that the learning curve places on resource control and improved quality makes it a prime tool for health care managers at this time.

NOTES

1. NASA. *Parametric Cost Estimating Reference Curve Manual: Learning Curve Calculator* (from the Internet), p. 1.

2. Belkaoui, A. *The Learning Curve: A Management Accounting Tool.* Westport, CT: Quorum Books, 1986, p. 1.

3. Belkaoui, p. 2.

4. Ibid.

5. Finkler, S.A. *Essentials of Cost Accounting for Health Care Organizations.* Rockville, MD: Aspen Publishers, 1994, p. 134.

6. Balasubramanian, V. "Organization Learning and Information Systems." Working paper for E-Papyrus, Inc. and the Graduate School of Management at Rutgers University (from the Internet), p. 1.

7. Belkaoui, p. 2.

8. Ibid, p. 6.

9. Gruber, H. *Learning and Strategic Product Innovation.* New York: North Holland, 1994, p. 42.

10. Ibid, p. 43.

11. NASA, p. 1.

12. Finkler, p. 136.

13. Jordan, R. *How to Use the Learning Curve.* Boston: Materials Management Institute, 1965, pp. 1–15.

14. Finkler, p. 134.

15. Schein, E.H. "Organizational Learning: What Is New?" Working paper from MIT Sloan School of Management (from the Internet), May 19, 1994, p. 1.

16. Ibid, p. 2.

17. Balasubramanian, p. 4.

18. Schein, p. 2.

19. Schein. E.H. "Organization and Managerial Culture as a Facilitator or Inhibitor of Organization Learning." Working paper from MIT Sloan School of Management (from the Internet), May 19, 1994, p. 6.

20. Schein. "Organizational Learning: What Is New?" p. 2.

21. Balasubramanian, p. 1.

22. Ibid.

23. Belkaoui, p. 73.

24. Ibid, p. 80.

25. Finkler, p. 135.

26. Finkler, p. 134.

27. Flood, A., Scott, W., and Ewy, W. "Does Practice Make Perfect?: The Relation between Volume and Outcomes and Other Hospital Characteristics." *Medical Care,* Vol. 22, No. 2, 1984, p. 93.

28. Smith, D.B., and Larson, J.L. "The Impact of Learning on Cost: The Case of Heart Transplantation." *Hospital & Health Service Administration,* Vol. 34, No. 1, p. 86.

29. Smith, p. 86.

30. Smith, p. 85.

31. Ibid.

32. Kelly, J., and Hellinger, F. "Physician and Hospital Factors Associated with Mortality of Surgical Patients." *Medical Care,* Vol. 24, No. 9, 1986, p. 785.

33. Ibid.

34. Hemenway, D., Sherman, H., et al. "Benefits of Experience: Treating Coronary Heart Disease." *Medical Care,* Vol. 24, No. 2, 1986, p. 125.

35. Ibid.

36. Montgomery, D.B., and Day, G.S. "Experience Curves: Evidence, Empirical Issues, and Applications." Working paper for Marketing Science Institute—Research Program, February 1985, p. 25.

37. Finkler, p. 138.

38. Ibid, p. 370.

8

Budgeting

Reading 8–1

The Financial Evolution of Hospitals and the Zero-Base Budget Approach

Patricia S. Barry

SUMMARY

As the health care industry evolves into a highly complex and diverse sector of the economy, the need for effective budget procedures is evident in each hospital's financial management strategy. Hospitals confronting falling revenues, escalating costs, and expanding pressures to hold down prices are going out of business as a result of these demands. The zero-base budget assists managers in the effective allocation of an organization's limited resources by establishing a budget procedure that determines concurrently the answer to two questions: (1) In which areas can we most effectively spend our money? and (2) How much money should we spend?

The hypothesis behind the zero-base approach is that each manager must rationalize his/her complete budget. This approach shifts financial accountability to the departmental manager to rationalize why any money should be spent at all. The departmental manager must furnish upper management with a decision package for every activity or operation in his/her department, which includes an analysis of: expenditure, objective/
goal, varying courses of action, assessment of performance, results of not performing the activity, and benefits. Managers are also expected to devise alternative packages for a particular activity, as well as devising alternate levels of effort for performing each activity. Once the decision packages are devised, a ranking process occurs that lists each activity in order of importance. The benefit of having a ranking process is that it enables a manager to explicitly identify his priorities. In addition, the ranking process points out areas where decision packages for ongoing and new programs can be merged into one ranking. As the list of decision packages increases, the cost also increases, and top management can decide at what point on the list the added costs outweigh the benefits. Decision packages of lower priority would not be funded.

BACKGROUND

Survival is an issue threatening many hospitals throughout the United States. This issue is reflective in the closure of 342 acute-care hospitals from 1984 to 1989.[1] The organizations at risk of financial loss and even failure are those in which their health care executives fail to recognize competitive factors in management strategy formulation and implementation. In a 1990 survey conducted by Deloitte & Touche, 43 percent of 1,765 responding hospital executives believed

Source: Reprinted from Patricia S. Barry, "The Financial Evolution of Hospitals and the Zero-Base Budget Approach," *Hospital Cost Management and Accounting,* Vol. 5, No. 7, October 1993, pp. 1–7. Copyright 1993, Aspen Publishers, Inc.

that their organization could fail within a time period of five years. While the 43 percent represents a decline from 48 percent just two years previous, the primary conclusion still remains that many hospital executives, their boards, and medical staffs are legitimately concerned about corporate failure.

By formulating strategies that are linked to quality, performance and sound financial management, hospital executives can create and maintain a competitive advantage for their organizations. A recent survey that reviewed competitive strategies for successful hospital management examined financial operating data for approximately 1,000 U.S. hospitals categorized by Medicare as "large urban." The survey determined the critical relationships between business strategy and financial performance. Cost control was directly linked with quality of service and was found to be the most important factor influencing economic performance.[2]

Perhaps one of the most effective methods for controlling the skyrocketing costs of health care expenditures within a hospital is through strategic budgets. And, increasingly, budgeting procedures are becoming an activity that management must actively participate in. Hospital administrators are aware of the importance of effective management for increased growth and are pressured to become innovators and strategists with respect to cost control. Since providing quality service to patients is simply not a guarantee for success any longer, hospitals must determine their purpose and let this purpose guide the hospital in its operations. This is where budgeting is imperative to success. A strategic budget is both a planning and controlling tool and can guide a hospital around the pitfalls of financial ruin.

It is unfortunate, but many managers consider budgets to be little more than monitoring devices for cash flows. They assume that if there is enough money in the kitty to cover expenses, then the department is covering its costs. Such a flippant attitude regarding budgets clearly underutilizes a valuable resource which, if used effectively, can greatly enhance the success of an organization's financial management system. An effective, well thought out budgeting design can direct a business or hospital toward its financial goals and can augment the likelihood of a desired action taking place (i.e., controlling costs). As well as controlling costs, budgets can be used to achieve a variety of desired objectives. For example, budgets can be used to: (1) initiate new programs; (2) organize the purpose and mission of divisions within an organization; (3) examine the suitability of expense to profit budgets; and (4) assign each manager his or her responsibilities and evaluate those responsibilities. As one can see, limiting the scope of the strategic budget is indeed throwing away a valuable resource.

THE ZERO-BASE APPROACH

Background

Peter A. Pyhrr developed zero-base budgeting (ZBB) for Texas Instruments in 1970. However, it was not until President Jimmy Carter encouraged its use sometime later in the decade that Pyhrr's budgeting approach and concepts began to receive recognition. The ZBB is a practical budgetary device since its design compels departmental managers to examine and analyze *all* the expenses within their budget. In a nutshell, ZBB endeavors to analyze the following: (1) what operations are being performed within an organization; (2) why these operations are being done; (3) how tasks can be done better, as well as more effectively and efficiently; and (4) which activities are vital to the organization, as well as what they cost. This is unlike the conventional budgeting approach, which only considers the percentage increase for the next fiscal year. The conventional approach accepts the fact that all costs incurred in the preceding fiscal year were justified and new expenses that the organization will incur should be added on to the old budget. Additionally, budget negotiations would only consider the amount of the incremental increase and no further scrutiny of the preceding budget would be deemed necessary. Alternatively, the ZBB approach scrutinizes all costs, not only the incremental increase. "The concept of requiring a zero-base evaluation is attractive because it means that budgets would not be allowed to become 'fat' over time."[3]

Pyhrr defines the zero-base budget as follows:

> An operating, planning and budgeting process which requires each manager to justify his entire budget request in detail from scratch [hence zero-base] and shifts the burden of proof to each manager to justify why he should spend any money at all. This approach requires that all activities be identified in "decision packages" which will be evaluated by systematic analysis and ranked in order of importance.[4]

Pyhrr's definition is a succinct representation of how the zero-base budget operates. Beginning with management's role, the zero-base method shifts the burden of financial accountability to the respective departmental levels. Instead of top management having overall responsibility for budgets, each department's manager must accept the responsibility for the monies spent and must acquire backing for prospective expenditures and anticipated expenses. The ZBB method requires that each department manager evaluate and analyze all the programs and activities within the department, including new initiatives as well as longstanding ones. Further, managers must assess programs systematically on the significance of output or performance, as well as costs. In Cheek's viewpoint, "This method emphasizes managerial decision-making first and numbers oriented budgets second and increases analysis of designating alternatives."[5]

I. Developing Decision Packages

In addition to shifting accountability to departmental managers, it is essential that managers outline the initial steps for implementation of a zero-base approach by establishing the department's objectives. After these objectives are established, the subsequent step in the ZBB approach is to determine how these objectives will be realized. Each department defines its objectives in the form of decision packages. Often,

this results in the conceptualization of several alternative decision packages, each describing a varying level of effort. Also included within the decision packages is a description of the individuals or divisions responsible for the program or project. In addition, every decision package should include a practical evaluation of the department's program/project, which includes the projected costs and benefits of the program, as well as the potential liability, risks, and drawbacks inherent in each one. After the decision packages are defined, they can be divided into mutually exclusive packages, which identify several options for fulfilling the same function and incremental packages, which indicate the varying amounts of labor that may be expended on an individual task.

II. Ranking Decision Packages

The formulation of the different decision packages is the first step in the ZBB process and one that provides management with important information. This initial process is the essence of the ZBB approach because it is the formulation of packages that establishes which program or project to retain and which ones to eliminate. Also, it is at this juncture that the spending requests of the decision packages are challenged and must be rationalized. Programs with a less than adequate appraisal will be discontinued and resources will be directed toward efforts that will help the organization attain its objectives. The primary intention of this process is to determine not only the appropriate programs but which programs are cost-effective as well.

However, in order for the decision packages to be as effective as possible, the formulation and ranking must be carried out in cooperation with all the members of the staff who are involved in the operation. The initial process of ranking should involve all the members involved in the task or the individual responsible for the development of specific programs or projects. More individuals will become immersed in the process of ranking as the ranking procedure is steered through the levels of the organization. And, during that process, the ranking of a certain program or project may be changed. Cheek suggests that "during the ranking session, objectives should be kept in mind, managers should remain flexible, and above all, the system should be kept simple."[6] Once the ranking process is complete, management chooses the projects that produce the best results for the least amount of cost.

For example, Appendix 8–1–A is an illustration of ABC Hospital's personnel department's decision package for annual expenditures for RNs' salaries in 1993. From this illustration, ABC Hospital's personnel manager can compare four alternative decision packages, each describing a different level of staffing requirements. Each package includes a description of the number of staff required to maintain comprehensive coverage, as well as the costs and benefits of operating at each level. Before a decision package is picked, an assessment must be formulated that considers the pros and cons of operating at the varying levels. This step is crucial because it focuses attention on liability and quality assurance, instead of cost-effectiveness. After these assessments are made, a departmental manager will choose the best alternative that provides appropriate skilled nursing coverage and minimizes the hospital's costs.

STRENGTHS

As discussed previously, managers in organizations can no longer afford to adhere to budgetary methods that they have grown accustomed to and that are familiar. Instead, by implementing the ZBB technique, managers are required to delve into a department's budget and thoroughly dissect old expenses as well as new ones. This approach is simply rational since society and technology do not exist in a vacuum. Organizations evolve with technological change and it follows that these organizations will have departments with shifting financial needs.

The zero-base approach is advantageous for a variety of reasons. To begin, the zero-base approach fosters a sense of mutual understanding and commitment between upper and middle management. The ZBB approach allows upper

management to divest itself of financial responsibility for departments and relies on the departmental manager (middle management) to present decision packages that are feasible for the organization. Further, the implementation of packages and decisions regarding their ranking is jointly agreed upon. After the packages are agreed upon, upper management agrees to fund them, and the staff manager agrees to deliver the service. This approach, unlike top-down strategies, promotes a collaborative atmosphere between levels of management where middle management fully participates in key decisions and recognizes that their ideas and opinions are being given credence. Establishing this type of open-ended relationship between two levels of management facilitates a healthy working environment.

As well as establishing congruence among levels of management, the ZBB approach promotes innovation. ZBB encourages management to find inventive, efficient, and cost-effective methods to perform the identical function. Further, these objectives must formulate into a decision package and be presentable in a coherent manner. The ZBB approach initiates responsibility from individuals at all levels in the department to achieve this end. Consequently, ZBB can become a department-wide suggestion plan that stimulates ideas from individuals who have first-hand knowledge of routine tasks, i.e., housekeepers, clerks, etc.

Another apparent advantage of using the ZBB approach is that it facilitates a comprehensive control over operations. By organizing a department's operations into substantially smaller packages that are considerably smaller than a department's consolidated functional budget, it makes it much easier to understand them and to detect the excesses in each. And more importantly, by comparing these smaller packages, obvious redundancies can be readily identified and eliminated.

Another positive effect in defining decision packages is that once these packages have been accepted, they become the design of the organization's mission or planning objectives. Since the packages must be ranked in order of importance, this requires logical and consistent objectives, clearly transmitted to each department's budget manager. This approach delineates what the organization is striving to accomplish and begins to devise innovative methods whereby each department's budget can contribute to meeting some of the objectives. This produces a beneficial outcome since effective zero-base budgeting requires that communication barriers between planning and budgeting must be suspended and that the two roles must be connected.

WEAKNESSES

While the ZBB is an effective strategic tool for managing finances within departments, it is not without some shortcomings. It seems realistic to assume that implementing ZBB at departmental levels would not be an uncomplicated undertaking. Indeed, it is difficult to fathom a personnel department of a large urban medical center analyzing all expenditures annually in order to cut out the fat. This is not to say that doing so would not be better for the organization. On the contrary, it simply addresses the complexity and time involvement in implementing such a system.

One of the negative attributes of implementing *any* new operational system is the opposition it will face from administrators and staff who are comfortable with the status quo. It seems feasible that many hospitals would avoid the ZBB approach because it would encumber their smooth-running operation. Implementation of ZBB would perhaps require departments to hire additional accountants to analyze their budgets over a specified period of time. Additionally, administrators who are familiar with the old methods of budgeting for their departments would need to learn the new methods, which would necessitate extra time and effort on their part.

Another negative characteristic in the implementation of the ZBB at departmental levels is the opposition upper management might face from administrators who would not want to be involved in the scrutinization of their budgets. Realistically speaking, departmental managers

would be apprehensive about having their prior budgets being evaluated negatively and will instinctively resist the implementation of the ZBB approach. The ZBB challenges a manager's performance record by making assessments regarding the suitability of past expenses. In addition to challenging the performance of managers, ZBB requires an analysis of all expenses on an annual basis, which might seem inordinately tedious to departmental managers.

And, perhaps the most obvious criticism of the ZBB is the negative connotation of beginning from scratch. Implementation of ZBB might be damaging from a performance approach since it demands that managers defend the existence of their departments annually. The ZBB approach is *not* intended as a means for laying off workers or eliminating departments; rather it is a tool to show management how objectives can be achieved. Further, ZBB provides insight into areas where necessary cutbacks can be made with the least harm or cost to the organization. Because of the negative insinuation of beginning from a zero standpoint, many departmental managers perceive it as another stratagem of upper management to threaten if not discontinue their operations. The unwarranted focus on the zero-base aspect disregards other essential ingredients that are vital to its success. Cheek contends that the zero-base approach causes managers to become salespeople. Managers must justify their yearly expenses and scramble to elicit support for the forthcoming year's costs. Cheek believes few managers are comfortable with such a role.

As with any new theory or implementation, problems will occur, and perhaps most frequently in the first year. One of the foreseeable problems with the ZBB approach is a lack of involvement by senior management. In the same vein, a lack of support and understanding from top management can further impede the ZBB from taking hold within an organization. No budget system can realize its potential without the complete support and understanding of top management. Therefore, as well as educating middle management about the new budgeting process, top management must also undergo this educational process. In order for the implementation of ZBB to be successful within an organization, several factors must be present: reasonable expectations from upper management, comprehensive decision packages, solid communication between upper and middle management, and clear budgetary and design theories.

CONCLUSION

Considering the zero-base budgeting approach from an economic standpoint, an assertion can be made that zero-base budgeting's objective is simply to compare the alternative uses of scarce resources. Clearly, this is the objective of any perceptive businessman/woman when considering whether a new factory should be constructed or whether the older facilities should or can be used to more capacity. Realistically speaking, the principal role of a business person is to assess the various resources their company pos-

sesses in order to decide how best to employ them. After these assessments are formulated, decisions can be made regarding the implementation of plans or projects. The zero-base theory can be utilized to require such assessments on a regular basis.

NOTES

1. Deloitte & Touche, "U.S. Hospitals and the Future of Health Care," June 1990.
2. Buzzell, R. and B. Gayle, "Profit Impact on Market Strategy: Linking Strategy to Performance." New York: Free Press, 1987.
3. Finkler, Steven A., *Budgeting Concepts for Nurse Managers*, 2d Edition, W.B. Saunders, 1992, p. 143.
4. Pyhrr, Peter A., *Zero-Base Budgeting, A Practical Management Tool for Evaluating Expenses*, New York: John Wiley & Sons, 1973.
5. Cheek, J.M., *Zero-Base Budgeting Comes of Age*, 1977, AMACOM, p. 12.
6. Ibid.

Appendix 8–1–A

DECISION PACKAGE LEVEL 1
ABC HOSPITAL

RN Salary Expenditures 1993
Personnel Department

(1) **Package Name**
RN Salary Expenditures

(2) **Organization**
Personnel Dept.

(3) **Purpose; Expected Benefits (Describe)**
Provide patients with the maximum amount of comprehensive coverage with two nurses per shift for a total of 20 stations.

(4) **How Will This Be Accomplished? (Describe)**
The personnel department must hire at least 120 RNs in order to provide coverage for vacation, illness, and personal days.

(5) **Consequences of Not Approving This Package**
This package provides complete, comprehensive care with the assumptions that *all* beds will be filled for each attending station. If ABC Hospital fails to provide adequate nursing coverage, possible adverse consequences could take place such as liability and negligence suits.

(6) **Resources Required**

	Cost
Wages/Salaries	$3,600,000
Benefits	150,000
Total	$3,750,000
Employees	120

DECISION PACKAGE LEVEL 2
ABC HOSPITAL

RN Salary Expenditures 1993
Personnel Department

(1) *Package Name*   (2) *Organization*
RN Salary Expenditures   Personnel Dept.

(3) *Purpose; Expected Benefits (Describe)*
Provide patients with comprehensive coverage with two nurses for first and second shifts and one nurse per third shift.

(4) *How Will This Be Accomplished? (Describe)*
The personnel department must hire at least 100 RNs in order to provide coverage for vacation, illness, and personal days.

(5) *Consequences of Not Approving This Package*
This package provides complete, comprehensive care with the assumptions that *most* beds will be filled for each attending station. If ABC Hospital fails to provide adequate nursing coverage, possible adverse consequences could take place such as liability and negligence suits.

(6) *Resources Required*   *Cost*

Wages/Salaries $3,000,000
Benefits   150,000
Total $3,150,000

Employees   100

DECISION PACKAGE LEVEL 3
ABC HOSPITAL

RN Salary Expenditures 1993
Personnel Department

(1) *Package Name*   (2) *Organization*
RN Salary Expenditures   Personnel Dept.

(3) *Purpose; Expected Benefits (Describe)*
Provide patients with adequate RN coverage with two nurses for first shift and one nurse for second and third shift.

(4) *How Will This Be Accomplished? (Describe)*
The personnel department must hire at least 80 RNs in order to provide coverage for vacation, illness, and personal days.

(5) *Consequences of Not Approving This Package*
This package provides complete, comprehensive care with the assumptions that *half* of the beds will be filled for each attending station. If ABC Hospital fails to provide adequate nursing coverage, possible adverse consequences could take place such as liability and negligence suits.

(6) *Resources Required*   *Cost*

Wages/Salaries $2,400,000
Benefits   70,000
Total $2,470,000

Employees   80

DECISION PACKAGE LEVEL 4 ABC HOSPITAL
RN Salary Expenditures 1993 Personnel Department

(1) **Package Name**
RN Salary Expenditures

(2) **Organization**
Personnel Dept.

(3) **Purpose; Expected Benefits (Describe)**
Provide patients with the minimum level of required RN coverage with one nurse assigned for each shift.

(4) **How Will This Be Accomplished? (Describe)**
The personnel department must hire at least 60 RNs in order to provide coverage for vacation, illness, and personal days.

(5) **Consequences of Not Approving This Package**
This package provides complete, comprehensive care with the assumptions that *less than half* of the beds will be filled for each attending station. If ABC Hospital fails to provide adequate nursing coverage, possible adverse consequences could take place such as liability and negligence suits.

(6) **Resources Required** — **Cost**

Resources Required	Cost
Wages/Salaries	$1,800,000
Benefits	50,000
Total	$1,850,000
Employees	60

DECISION PACKAGE SUMMARY ABC HOSPITAL
RN Salary Expenditures 1993 Personnel Department

Level	Service Implications	Employees	Annual Cost
1.	Provide patients with complete, comprehensive coverage with two nurses per shift for a total of 20 stations with the assumption that all hospital beds will be filled.	120	$3,750,000
2.	Provide patients with comprehensive coverage with two nurses for first and second shifts and one nurse per third shift with the assumption that most hospital beds will be filled.	100	$3,150,000
3.	Provide patients with adequate RN coverage with two nurses for first shift and one nurse for second and third shift with the assumption that half of the hospital beds will be filled.	80	$2,470,000
4.	Provide the minimum level of required RN coverage with one nurse assigned for each shift with the assumption that less than half of the hospital beds will be filled.	60	$1,850,000

RECOMMENDATIONS:

ABC might consider picking level 2 or 3, which is probably the level at which hospital beds will be utilized.

Reading 8–2

Zero-Based Budgeting for a Radiology Service:
A Case Study in Outsourcing

Tara A. Cortes

In this era of cost control and quality care, all health care organizations are being scrutinized to see where and how more can be done with less. This attitude has given significance and credibility to the concept of reengineering or restructuring that is currently common in all organizations. Reengineering eliminates the traditional boundaries of organizations and allows for visionaries to discover new ways to perform business processes and thereby reduce operating costs (McManis 1993). Tangential to this is the total quality management approach, which continuously examines the processes of an organization to improve its function (Walton 1986).

Contracting for services is one practice that is becoming increasingly prevalent in health care, because it allows hospitals and other agencies to use the resources and expertise that may be available in other organizations and find services at lower cost from systems with greater volumes. Many of these services are those that the organization previously performed itself (Heinbuch 1993). Contracting allows for the provision of efficient services if decisions are made carefully in planning and negotiating the provisions of the contract. Smaller hospitals with more limited resources or specialized interests can gain much

Source: Reprinted from Tara A. Cortes, "Zero-Based Budgeting for a Radiology Service: A Case Study in Outsourcing," *Hospital Cost Management and Accounting,* Vol. 8, No. 2, pp. 1–6. Copyright May 1996, Aspen Publishers, Inc.

from contracting services. This is the case of Nightingale Hospital.

Nightingale Hospital is a 40-bed university-affiliated hospital, fully approved and accredited by the Joint Commission on Accreditation of Healthcare Organizations and the state department of health. The present management of the hospital has begun to contract for services in an effort to capitalize on the cost savings related to high volume as the hospital "piggybacks" on to purchase orders and services that are at a lower price. Some examples of this are in the following areas of service.

PREVIOUS OUTSOURCING EFFORTS

Nightingale Hospital had its own laundry servicing the hospital and the university. The cost per item of laundry varied but ranged from two to three times the amount charged by any other hospital laundry contacted, including City Hospital. A contract was negotiated with City Hospital's laundry that reduced Nightingale Hospital's total laundry cost per year by nearly two-thirds. The university is now negotiating with City Hospital for services to cover the laundry needs of its custodial personnel, and the laundry that has existed at the university is closing. This outsourcing will eliminate five positions, approximately $350,000 in energy consumption, and 1,500 square feet of occupied space.

The next service to be reengineered was pharmacology. The hospital had employed two full-time pharmacists to provide service for 8 hours a day, 5 days a week at a salary plus a benefits package of approximately $150,000. Outside of normal operating hours, nurses would enter the pharmacy to procure those items they had not anticipated needing. In addition, a review of the functions of the pharmacists showed that 80 percent of their time was being spent on purchasing drugs and filling prescriptions at cost for university employees and extended families while 20 percent of the time was being spent on the research and patient care mission of the hospital.

To cut costs and improve the quality of work devoted to research and patient care, management decided to refocus the pharmacy activities to the hospital mission and to eliminate both pharmacist positions. A contract was negotiated with City Hospital to supply Nightingale Hospital with a pharmacist for 40 hours a week. This person would remain part of the City Hospital staff in order to maintain a relationship with an academic-based pharmacy department and would be covered by another pharmacist from that department during vacation, holidays, or sick days.

In addition, the hospital would have 24-hour coverage from City Hospital to provide any drugs needed when the pharmacy at Nightingale Hospital was closed. Furthermore, the administration has eliminated the sale of drugs for employee prescriptions and personal needs and arranged for Nightingale Hospital employees to use the pharmacy at City Hospital for their personal needs.

This contract has provided Nightingale Hospital with a research-oriented pharmacist who benefits from the continuing education and collegial rapport of an academic medical center; the hospital gains 24-hour coverage at a total cost of $113,000, thereby reducing the cost of the service by 25 percent. In addition, drugs are now ordered through the same supplier as City Hospital at 1 percent above cost instead of the 6 percent Nightingale Hospital was paying to its supplier.

Another area of service negotiated and contracted for was central supply. The hospital had been doing its own purchasing, storing, and stocking. Because purchases were at low volume, prices were high. In some cases, the hospital ordered 1,000 items because it was impossible to purchase at a lower volume. This bulk purchasing resulted in surplus stock that needed to be stored. It was calculated that the cost of personnel to manage this process was $60,000 per year. The volume of inventory stock was $45,000, and the cost of storage was $20,000 per year based on space rental. The contract negotiated with City Hospital included a $7,000 service fee for one time per week delivery to the hospital, at which time City Hospital personnel would stock the supplies. This contract has enabled Nightingale Hospital to reduce its stock substantially and free up all but one storage area (it is planned that after 1 year there will be no storage of supplies), free up staff to do research and patient care activities instead of inventory and purchasing, and set a realistic level of supplies geared to the needs at any particular time.

The next area that is being targeted for change is the radiology department. It appears that the radiology department may not be cost-effective and is not providing the best quality of service for cost. A zero-based budget decision package has been developed to decide how to best deliver the service.

RADIOLOGY RESTRUCTURING DECISION PACKAGE

The purpose of the radiology department at Nightingale Hospital is to provide cost-effective radiological services to clinicians as needed to carry out patient care research efficiently and effectively.

Radiological studies performed at the hospital are primarily done in the clinic, which is used for screening potential subjects for participation in research studies. The purpose of the study may be to rule out a disease that would eliminate a potential subject from participation or to confirm a disease process that is being studied. Diagnostic radiology studies are also done on inpatients, and the volume depends on the protocols approved by the Institutional Review Board at any given time.

At this time, a study involving patients with pulmonary disease requires radiological studies before each bronchoscopy done and again on the following day. These radiological studies are predictable because they are driven by the protocol and are consistently performed on specific days of the planned protocol.

Another study on patients with acquired immune deficiency syndrome (AIDS) always requires a preadmission film and sometimes requires stat radiographs if and when the patient develops pulmonary symptoms. Although almost all radiographs done by the department are chest radiographs, there are rare occasions when a radiograph might be done on a university employee or on a patient who may need a radiograph of an extremity. Any needed specialized procedures such as magnetic resonance imaging are done by City Hospital.

Table 8–2–1 shows an upward trend in the number of films and the number of readings per year for the past 5 years.

In a research hospital, the number of films taken and read is driven by the research protocols. The sharp increase in 1993 was related to new protocols that study tuberculosis and AIDS. The next increase in 1994 was related to a new protocol studying the effects of therapy in pulmonary diseases. It is predicted the ratio would

go up the same for 1995 because of several protocols studying patients with human immunodeficiency virus and AIDS.

Based on the trend, one would anticipate doing about 775 films and 350 readings during 1995. The discrepancy between the number of films taken and the number read is because many films done are read by the physicians on a particular service for the purpose of research findings and do not need a radiologist's diagnostic report on the chart.

The existing program and the costs per year for personnel service in this department are as follows:

	Salary	Benefits	Total
Radiological technician 20 hours per week	$30,000	+ $10,500	= $40,500
Coverage for nonproductive time	$ 4,500		= $ 4,500
Radiologist to read radiographs (salary paid to City Hospital)	$25,000		= $25,000
On-call films when radiological technician is not "in house"	$150 per film		= $ 7,500
		Total	= **$77,500**

There are many disadvantages to this program. One is that this technician is being paid a salary of $30,000 per year for 20 hours per week while a salary for a full-time technician is $32,000 on the market. This technician's hours are fixed to 5 hours Monday through Thursday, and he or she is not available on Friday.

This technician carries a beeper and responds to calls when not at work; these films cost an additional $150 per procedure. There seem to be more stat films on Friday than during the "after hour" periods.

When the technician is on vacation or ill, he or she arranges for someone to cover his or her hours. This substitute is often a person who is unfamiliar with the system and needs orientation.

In addition, the radiologist is contracted through City Hospital at a fixed salary regardless

---

Table 8–2–1 Number of Films and Readings Performed during the Past 5 Years

	No. of Films (Excluding Autoradiographs)	No. of Readings
Calendar year 1991	425	197
Calendar year 1992	181	203
Calendar year 1993	490	250
Calendar year 1994	674	300
Calendar year 1995	775*	350*

*Projected figures

of volume. This salary is increased by 3 percent per year regardless of use. Films are read once a week and a note is dictated to a tape; the tape is returned to Nightingale Hospital where it is transcribed.

Negotiation had taken place with various community sources to provide resources to fulfill the above services. Assuming the need for services will continue to grow at the same level it has for the past 2 years, there are alternative approaches to provide radiological services to Nightingale Hospital.

The options for service are as follows:

Option A

Radiological technician	Hire full-time (37.5 hours per week) technician. The salary ($32,000) + benefits ($11,200) total $43,200. Coverage for vacation and sick time for this person is estimated for 6 weeks. The cost of this time is estimated to be (6 × $32,000 ÷ 52) = $3,692. **Cost of service for technician = $48,892**
On-call films	Contract with City Hospital for hours of 5 PM through 9 AM Monday through Friday and for weekend/holiday coverage. Estimated to be approximately 20 per year at $100 per procedure. **Cost $2,000**
Radiologist	Contract with private radiologist to do readings. Estimate 350 readings per year at $40 per read. **Cost $14,000** Off-hour stat wet readings would need to be done at City Hospital at a set cost per year regardless of volume. **Cost $ 1,000** **Total cost for Option A $65,892**

The advantages of this package are that there would be a full-time technician in the hospital from 9 AM to 5 PM Monday through Friday. This arrangement allows the physicians flexibility in their scheduling because they are ensured that a film can be done anytime during these hours. By having a person at the hospital 37.5 hours per week, the number of stat films needed to be done through an outside contract is decreased.

The disadvantages are that with an estimated 750 radiographs per year, a full-time technician is not fully occupied, with an average of three films per day of work. It would be necessary to have this person job share with another department to fully utilize the position. In addition, when this person is on vacation or sick, an agency would have to provide temporary coverage. This person would not be familiar with the hospital.

The advantage of the radiologist contract in this option is that the total fee is generated by volume, so if only 100 films were done, the cost would be $4,000, but if 1,000 readings were done, the cost would be $40,000. Furthermore, a written report will be faxed to Nightingale each day for every radiograph read, thus eliminating the need for transcription.

Option B (Contract entire radiology personnel service with City Hospital)

Radiological technician	Contracted with City Hospital at 15 hours per week (.43 full-time equivalent) at a salary of $15,000 + benefits ($5,000). To provide coverage for 52 weeks would involve an additional 20 percent of .43 full-time equivalent or .08 full-time equivalent. This would cost an additional $3,800. **Cost for technician = $23,800**
On-call films	Contracted with City Hospital at 15 percent discount of institutional rate of $100 per chest film. It is estimated that outside of hours covered at Nightingale Hospital there would be approximately 60 films per year. **Cost is .85(100) × 60 = $5,100**
Radiologist	Contracted with City Hospital to include: (A) 350 general films (estimated) per year at $40 fee less discount of 15 percent = **$11,900** (B) 12 hours of administrative services per year for in-service education and Joint Commission and agency inspection at $150 per hour = **$1,800** (C) After hours wet readings (provided by radiology house staff) = **$1,000** **Cost = $14,700** **Total cost for Option B = $43,600**

The disadvantage of this system is that the technician would be on site 3 hours per day. However, the time could be arranged to provide 2 hours in the morning such as between 9:30 and 11:30 AM and 1 hour in the afternoon such as between 3:00 and 4:00 PM. This should cover the prime times of patient visits in the clinic or admissions to the inpatient units. In addition, ambulatory patients could walk to City Hospital, if necessary, and have a radiograph done there at any time. The 3 hours per day could vary if the hospital's needs were in the afternoons on some days of the week or in the mornings on other days.

Advantages are that the technician will be part of a larger radiology department at City Hospital and will receive in-service training and updates on the regulatory issues and mandates. In addition, when the technician is on vacation another technician from that department will be trained to provide coverage that will ensure consistent quality.

Another advantage is that on-call films can be set up in advance if the hospital knows a patient is being admitted at 10:00 PM and needs a radiograph with personnel who are familiar to the Nightingale Hospital staff. Even stat radiographs can be set up with people who know the system at Nightingale Hospital.

The radiologist fee is based on volume so the cost could increase or decrease if the hospital's needs change. The reports will be faxed to Nightingale Hospital daily, so there is no need for a transcriber. In addition to this, administrative services are built into the cost. This is a service the hospital does not presently have and it will assist it in meeting regulatory mandates.

Table 8–2–2 shows an analysis of the quality issues related to cost-benefit issues of the above options for delivery of services for the radiology department.

The analysis shows clearly that the system that is least cost-effective and least efficient for the hospital is the existing system. The most cost-effective and quality efficient system is Option B, which is to contract for the entire service with City Hospital. Negotiation is ongoing with this

Table 8–2–2 Quality/Cost-Benefit Analysis of Options

Options	Radiological Technician	Radiologist	On-Call Radiographs
Existing program	Moderate/ minimum	Moderate/ minimum	Minimum/ minimum
Option A	Moderate/ best	Moderate/ best	Moderate/ moderate
Option B— City Hospital	Best/best	Best/best	Best/best

contract, and it is expected that there will still be an overhead added to the amount for the technical services, which usually ranges from 10 to 20 percent in the other contracts negotiated with City Hospital. Even with this overhead, the cost is still less than the other two options and the consistency of quality and service cannot be underestimated.

With the knowledge that the ability to do radiographs is an essential service for this hospital, a question that must be dealt with in this decision package is the level of output. How many productive hours need to be allocated to meet investigators' needs? Because almost no radiograph films are done on an emergency basis, they can almost all be preplanned and scheduled during the 3 specified hours each day.

The system still needs to provide for the few outliers or films that need to be taken outside of scheduled hours. As the system evolves, continuous evaluation needs to be done to consider the ongoing cost-effectiveness and quality of the program.

If the 3 hours per day are not sufficient, costs will increase because of more "on-call" radiographs, and investigators will be dissatisfied because they will not be able to meet the requirements of their research protocols in an effective and timely manner. If 3 hours per day are more than what is needed, there will be a loss of productive time by the technician, thus decreasing cost-effectiveness. For these reasons, flexibility needs to be built into the contract so if evaluation shows a need for change in hours of technician availability, the contract can be changed accordingly.

REFERENCES

Heinbuch S. E. (1993). Walk the talk: Applying TQ principles to an element of management development-contracting. *Journal of Management Development 12*(7), 60–70.

McMannis, G. L. (1993, October 5). Reinstating the system: The reengineering process will launch a new era of health care delivery. *Hospital Health Network,* 42–48.

Walton, M. (1986). *The Deming Management Method.* New York: Perigee Books.

Reading 8–3

Developing and Using a Budget Manual

Steven A. Finkler

Today's hospitals have complex budgeting procedures that are generally performed by managers throughout the organization, who complete a series of forms. Budgeting is a fairly recent addition to the hospital management process. Prior to the introduction of Medicare, just a quarter-century ago, most hospitals did not have formal budgeting procedures. Over the last 25 years the hospital budgeting process has been constantly changing and developing.

Today, the budgeting performed in most hospitals is stable enough to allow them to develop manuals to guide the process. The complexity of the budget process necessitates the use of manuals—yet many hospitals have not yet documented their budget process in manual form. The reason for this lapse may be that the managers who could prepare the manual aren't aware of the need for it.

However, the budget process in most hospitals has become increasingly decentralized. The basic elements of the budget are prepared by individuals who are not necessarily comfortable working with financial information and who could benefit greatly from a manual. This is especially true with new managers of clinical departments, who often have no background in the budget process.

Source: Reprinted from Steven A. Finkler, "Developing and Using a Budget Manual," *Hospital Cost Management and Accounting,* Vol. 4, No. 7, October 1992, pp. 1–4. Copyright 1992, Aspen Publishers, Inc.

WHAT IS A BUDGET MANUAL?

Willson defines a budget manual as "an orderly presentation of directives, instructions, or facts concerning a given activity or repeated procedure."[1] Most hospitals have, at least, a set of written directions for filling out various forms. Without a formal manual, however, a manager may not be able to acquire an adequate understanding of the budget process.

A budget manual should provide a comprehensive portrait of the budget process. It should not be limited only to the information a manager needs to complete a specific form. Managers' dissatisfaction with budgeting may be attributed largely to their lack of information about the entire process. Factors that seem unfair when taken out of context may seem reasonable when viewed as part of a larger picture.

Therefore, the most important element of a budget manual is not the specific instructions it contains but the overview it provides to every manager about the organization's whole budget process.

Budgeting has acquired a mysterious aura in many hospitals—a mystique that tends to be destructive. Instead of focusing on a common effort to best serve the hospital's patients, managers vie for maximum resources. The best way to create a cooperative effort is to share information openly.

Managers at all levels of the organization should understand that the hospital has a long-range plan and that it has established priorities to help it move in that direction. They should also understand that the hospital reviews its environment to ensure that the approved budget reacts adequately to the threats and opportunities the organization faces.

A budget manual can convey the complexity of the budget process while also simplifying it. Managers who find themselves buried in forms that must be completed for their unit's or department's operating budgets may feel that the process is unduly complicated. If they are given a wider perspective on the process, however, they are more likely to understand how their particular pieces fit into the larger picture. The interrelationships between the operating, capital, and cash budgets can be explained to help line managers understand the rationale for what they are doing and why a process of negotiation is often necessary.

Willson asserts that preparing a specific manual of budget procedures offers the following advantages:

- it clearly defines authority and responsibility in budget matters
- it promotes standardization and simplification because, presumably, the best procedures for developing the budget or plan are stipulated and a uniform or standard format for presenting the plan is identified
- it encourages coordinated effort by identifying what procedures should be followed and by whom
- it provides a convenient reference guide when questions of procedures, format, or responsibility arise
- it permits better supervision, because supervisors do not have to spend time explaining procedures that are covered in the manual
- it assists in the training of new employees and in transfer of duties because many phases of the job have been described in writing
- it assists in "selling" the budget by explaining the advantages of the procedure[2]

As noted above, however, an additional important advantage of a budget manual is that it communicates the entire budget process, providing each manager with an understanding of the overall budget framework.

WHAT GOES INTO A BUDGET MANUAL?

In describing the budget process, budget manuals should start with a clear statement of the objectives of the hospital's budget process. Although budgets are required by federal regulation in order for the hospital to be eligible for Medicare payments, the other expected benefits of the budget process should be noted as well. These might include such issues as Board mandates for balanced budgets, requirements imposed by bond covenants, or the need to reach certain profit levels to provide for future expansion.

Next, the lines of responsibility for the budget should be clearly stated. The Board's role in approving the budget should be explained, as well as the roles of the CEO, CFO, and other hospital managers. The authority of various managers and their responsibility for budget preparation should be explained, including specification for which managers are responsible for preparing what parts of the budget and who has the final authority over the amounts that will appear in the approved budget.

The manual should include descriptions of specific procedures to be performed by all managers with budget responsibility throughout the organization. All necessary budgeting forms should be contained in the manual, along with instructions for completing them so that managers do not have to figure out how to fill them out or try to learn it from the previous occupant of a position. Furthermore, procedures in such areas as budget review and revision should be explicitly described.

The manual should include a time schedule for budget preparation that establishes when various tasks must be undertaken and completed. It will be especially useful for managers to observe the overall schedule rather than to know only their own deadlines. They are more likely to recognize that their deadlines are reasonable if they are aware of the critical timing involved in bringing the various pieces of the budget together.

A discussion of departmental interrelationships is a critical aspect of the budget manual. Budgets should not be considered secret documents. Sharing information between cost centers will result in a more accurate budget than if each manager keeps within his or her own domain. For example, if the operating room is considering a new procedure that will shorten the length of stay of a specific type of patient, the med/surg units should be informed so that they can reduce their expected number of patient days.

Hospital budgeting is a dynamic process; over the last several decades it has been subject to continuous modification and improvement. Therefore the budget manual should be prepared in a loose-leaf format, which allows specific revisions to be made without redoing the entire manual. Further, managers will pay closer attention to new procedures as they review each change before entering it into their budget manuals.

WHO DOES WHAT?

One of the major potential benefits of the budget manual is its capacity to convey to each manager what his or her specific budgeting responsibilities are. For each element of the budget, there should be a section specifying who is responsible for what activities, how they are to be carried out, and when they must be done.

Conveying this information can, of course, be somewhat complex. One approach is to simply specify who does what as the manual progresses and various procedures are described. While this does provide the necessary information, it means that managers must frequently review the entire manual to locate their required activities. A more workable approach is to create a set of *responsibility charts*. Each chart shows all of the budget responsibilities for one specific job title. An alternative is a chart for each type of budget that lists the functions allotted to each job title.

DEVELOPING A BUDGET MANUAL

The development of the budget manual is a major undertaking, and hospital financial managers should not attempt to carry the full burden. It will be easier to develop the manual—and the results will be enhanced—if the tasks are divided among a larger number of people.

While financial managers may need to coordinate the process, widespread participation makes sense. Managers are more likely to want to use the manual, and more likely to accept its usefulness, if they have contributed to its development.

The hospital's budget committee should assume the role of making budget goals and objectives explicit. The financial managers should develop explanations of the various elements of the hospital's master budget and how they interrelate. Each cost center, however, should have the primary responsibility for drafting the parts of the manual concerned with budget preparation in its own area.

As the parts of the manual are prepared, drafts should be widely circulated to generate as much feedback as possible. During this process, suggestions will probably be made that will impact not only the manual but the budget process itself. The preparation of a budget manual invariably results in managers' taking an in-depth look at how the budget is currently prepared in each cost center. Things that have previously been accepted as fact are likely to be questioned, resulting in improvements to the budget process.

Further, managers will gain insights about the entire budget process as the manual takes shape. They will learn how their pieces fit, which will also lead to suggestions that could improve the process. Thus manual development is not simply a codification of existing budget policies and procedures but also provides for refinement of the process.

Once drafts have been reviewed and revisions to the budget process made, the final manual must be reviewed and approved by the top management team. Then a list of the individuals (and their positions) who should receive a manual can be made and copies produced and distributed.

UPDATING THE MANUAL

Revision of the budget process should not be limited to the period when the manual is being prepared. As the hospital changes over time, or as regulations and reimbursement policies change, it will be necessary to revise budget procedures. The manual should occasionally be reviewed to ensure that it is up to date. We have already noted that a looseleaf format allows for easy insertion of changes. One department should be responsible for making sure the manual is properly maintained.

Willson suggests that

- all revisions should be handled on a systematic, scheduled basis
- any changes should be coordinated with all affected units
- typically, users will forward suggestions for change; *all* the procedures should be periodically reviewed for currency and applicability
- preferably, the revision should indicate the date it was made and the issue it supersedes
- it may be helpful to indicate (by, for instance, an asterisk) a segment that has been modified
- the procedure-issuing organization should maintain in its files the background of the change (i.e., the reasons, who suggested it)
- most important, manual changes do cost money, so the necessity of each change should be considered carefully.[3]

NOTES

1. J.D. Willson, *Budgeting and Profit Planning Manual,* Second Edition. Boston: Warren, Gorham & Lamont, 1989, p. 46–1.
2. Ibid, p. 46–2.
3. Ibid., p. 46–11.

Reading 8–4

Outcome Budgeting Shifts Focus to Meeting Objectives

Steven A. Finkler

The health care industry has had a growing awareness in recent years of the need for improved outcome measurement. As managed care continues to expand and, in many areas, dominate the industry, there are growing concerns about quality of care. Newspapers around the country carry frequent anecdotal evidence of patients receiving too little care. Improved outcome measurement has become a hot topic for researchers, as we try to get a better handle on how we can measure improved health. It may take some time before a system is developed that really helps us to better measure the impact of our efforts on patient health status.

However, while researchers are attempting to solve that problem, we do not have to sit idly by. Hospitals already have enough knowledge about their goals and objectives to start to improve results by budgeting for outcomes. Essentially, we can convert our existing budgets into budgets that consider, plan for, assess, and measure our immediate goals and how good a job we are doing of attaining them. That will be the focus of this article.

Source: Reprinted from Steven A. Finkler, "Outcome Budgeting Shifts Focus to Meeting Objectives," *Hospital Cost Management and Accounting,* Vol. 8, No. 5, pp. 1–8. Copyright August 1996, Aspen Publishers, Inc.

FAILURE OF CURRENT FOCUS ON INPUTS

In preparing budgets, we generally do use at least one outcome proxy as the starting point. Nursing may use the number of patient days. The operating room may use the number of hours of surgery. Housekeeping may use either the number of square feet or the expected hours of service. Sometimes more than one measure is used. Nursing may consider not only the number of patient days, but also their acuity level. That is, how sick the patients are expected to be.

Once we have accepted the one or two outcome measures, we then proceed to focus entirely on inputs. How much labor will be needed? Who will provide that labor? How much will we pay them per hour? What supplies will be used? How much of those supplies? What price will we pay for those supplies? All of these questions, which are answered during the budget process, determine the required resources to achieve one volume measure such as 5,000 hours of surgery.

The problems related to a focus on resources without full consideration of outcomes can be seen every time a hospital has a financial crisis and implements an across-the-board budget cut. Suppose that an operating room expects to provide 5,000 hours of surgery during the year and has a

$1 million budget. In an emergency situation, hospital management might implement a 10 percent budget cut on the expense side, while hoping to keep patient volume and revenue constant.

What are the implications of a 10 percent cut in spending, while keeping surgery hours at 5,000? It would seem that we will produce the same outputs with fewer resources. Therefore, we are providing just as much care, at a lower cost. However, it is unlikely that will be the case. Some activities currently undertaken will no longer be done. Will that impact directly on the patients' health outcome? It may or may not. Whether it does or not depends largely on what activities are changed within the operating room. However, the budget provides no information on that. The budget merely says that we expect to provide 5,000 hours of surgery.

The reality is that every department has many goals and objectives. The work in each department consists of a set of activities designed to achieve each of those various goals and objectives. When more resources become available, if we use them efficiently, we can attain either more of those goals and objectives, or do a better job of achieving them. When resources are cut, unless there was substantial fat in the original budget, we will scale back either the amount or quality of accomplishment of some of those goals and objectives.

Unfortunately, traditional budgeting does not make those goals and objectives explicit. We list neither the goals, nor the budgeted level of accomplishment for those goals. Since we have no budget for them, we cannot explicitly assess how good a job we are doing of accomplishing them. When cutbacks are made, we have no way of assessing the potential negative impact of those cutbacks.

BENEFITS OF OUTCOME BUDGETING

American industry is often accused of being extremely shortsighted. We tend to focus on the organization's bottom line today, without considering the long-term implications of our actions. That is probably due, at least in part, to our failure to explicitly assess what we are doing, why we are doing it, and what the implications are of not doing it. That is where outcome budgeting comes in.

Budgeting for outcomes is an advancement on management by objectives. The technique of management by objectives asserts that managers should be evaluated not only on their current financial performance (achieving profit goals, or staying within expense budgets), but also on their accomplishment of a variety of objectives set up for their responsibility center.

The outcome budgeting discussed in this article goes beyond that. We intend to budget for the amount of each objective to be accomplished, and the amount of resources to be consumed in the process of achieving those objectives. When the budget period ends, the manager should know not only the total amount spent and the total volume of service produced by the department, but also how well the department did in each of its major objectives areas. The approach used to budget for outcomes in this article is sometimes referred to as "performance budgeting."

THE TECHNIQUE

The technique for budgeting for outcomes consists of the six steps described below.

1. Define objectives.

The first step is for the department or unit to explicitly identify its major objectives. Every department of every hospital has many things that it is trying to achieve. Clearly, the specific service of the department, such as hours of surgery, must be delivered. Further this specific service must be delivered at a certain desired quality level; efficiently; and in a way that keeps the department's customers happy. Customers may be patients but may also be a variety of other individuals within the hospital. The department must keep its staff satisfied. It should keep its equipment properly maintained and functioning.

Selecting the outcome area is a difficult part of this process. Most managers could list many different things that they are trying to achieve. As this technique is first adopted, it is probably worthwhile to limit the number of outcome areas to only those that are most important. That will keep the approach manageable. Once a manager has used the approach for a while, additional performance areas can be added to further refine the model and its benefits.

Thus, the department must assess what its most important goals and objectives are. This process is a very introspective one. It has the potential of forcing the manager to reconsider the different things the department does, and why it does them. This assessment will help the manager with the important activity of determining how much of the department's scarce resources should in fact be devoted to each of the department's objectives.

2. Identify operating budget.

The second step is straightforward. Since hospitals all currently prepare operating budgets, rather than start from scratch, we will make use of the operating budget normally prepared for each department. That way, individuals can learn how to improve their budgeting, starting from a known base of information.

3. Determine percentage of resources to devote to each objective.

Upon examining the operating budget, the manager and department staff must make an assessment of the portion of each resource to be devoted to accomplishing each objective. One may approach this in several ways. One approach is to try to assess how much of each resource is currently devoted to each objective or outcome area. That is reasonable for a first pass. However, keep in mind that we are developing a budget, and therefore want to allocate resources based on what we believe is an appropriate allocation. One must ask, "How should the manager and staff spend their time?" That is, "What are the priorities of the department?" One of the main benefits of the process should be to reorient resources from where they are going to where they should be going.

4. Assign operating budget costs to objectives.

The next step, assignment of the operating budget to the various outcome areas, is fairly mechanical. This process will be demonstrated in the example discussed later in this article.

5. Define measure of performance for each objective.

One of the aspects of the process that managers are likely to have the most difficulty with is defining measures of performance for each area. One aspect of this process is to determine how the performance of the department can be better evaluated. How can we understand what the department really does, and how can we measure how much it does, and how well it does it?

6. Prepare outcome budget.

The last step is to take all of the information that has been gathered and combine it into the form of a budget. The budget should contain information on what each outcome or objective area is, how it is to be measured, the amount of that objective which is budgeted, and the total and average cost of accomplishing that objective.

AN OUTCOME BUDGET EXAMPLE

In order to better understand the process of budgeting for outcomes, a numerical example is provided below. In this example, we will consider a materials management department in a hospital. The numbers are all hypothetical. The approach used can be modified and adapted to almost any hospital department.

1. Define objectives.

As noted earlier, a department could undoubtedly prepare an extensive listing of objectives. The outcome budgeting approach moves away from the simplistic notion that a department simply treats patients, or cleans pounds of laundry. On the other hand, the list of objectives must be manageable.

For a materials management department, we might consider the key objectives to be as follows:

- Process purchase orders.
- Improve client satisfaction.
- Reduce invoice discrepancies.
- Improve staff productivity.
- Control supply cost per patient day.

Processing purchase orders is probably similar to the output measure currently used as the basis for the department's operating budget. Ultimately patients are the customers of the department. However, managers and staff in other departments throughout the hospital are the materials management department's customers or clients as well. As hospitals try to work more as unified teams, rather than departmentalized advocacy groups, customer satisfaction takes on a growing importance.

In many hospitals, numerous invoice discrepancies arise. These take substantial amounts of time on the part of both the materials management department and the accounts payable department. At times they can result in lost discounts, higher prices from alternate suppliers, and in some cases stockouts on certain items. Materials management often considers a major objective of their department to process purchase orders (POs) in such a way as to minimize the number and size of invoice discrepancies.

As with most areas of the hospital, this department is likely to be seeking ways to improve staff productivity. By making it a key objective, we can budget for the amount of productivity increase, assess the cost of altering processes to attain the productivity improvement, and then measure to see what actually occurs.

Finally, a major concern of the hospital is controlling supply costs. But the major buyer of supplies, materials management, ultimately is not charged for those supplies. The cost is passed on to the departments that consume them. A clear example of the need for improved budgeting is that we have no idea how much materials management spends on explicit efforts to control supply costs; nor do we have any sense of the return on investment for those efforts. By incorporating this objective into the outcome budget, it

becomes explicit, measurable, and something that can be evaluated after the fact.

2. Identify operating budget.

We will assume for this example that the budget for the department for one year is as follows:

Materials Manager	$ 80,000
Staff Salaries	500,000
Education	20,000
Internal Supplies	10,000
External Overhead	50,000
Total	$ 660,000

3. Determine percentage of resources to devote to each objective.

As discussed above, we can either use historical information or make judgments as to what resource allocation among objectives is desirable. If we choose to use historical information, we may have to collect some data. It is unlikely that any department currently tracks the kind of information we need.

One approach to gathering the historical data is simply to ask each staff member to keep a log for a week or two to gather the information. Alternatively, individuals can be asked to give their best estimate of how their time and other resources are currently used in the department. Assuming that individuals have provided their best estimates of how resources are currently consumed, we could complete the following resource allocations.

Allocation of manager's time to key objective areas

	Percent
Process Purchase Orders	10
Improve Client Satisfaction	10
Reduce Invoice Discrepancies	20
Improve Staff Productivity	20
Control Supply Cost/Patient Day	40
Total	100

We can see from this allocation that the manager spends relatively little time directly processing POs. In fact, the manager spends just as much time working on direct efforts to improve client satisfaction. This might take the form of communications with clients, or it might take the form of developing new procedures that will result in happier clients. Clearly, some of these objectives could be subdivided into several distinct activity areas.

The areas that receive more of the manager's attention are reduction of invoice discrepancies, improving staff productivity, and controlling the supply cost per patient day. Whether this is an appropriate or inappropriate use of the manager's time can only be assessed by the manager and the individual to whom the manager reports.

The staff are likely to use their time in a substantially different way than the manager. Staff are likely to be more highly preoccupied with completing POs. However, they also do things that are related to the other performance or objective areas. Their allocation is:

Allocation of staff time to key objective areas

	Percent
Process Purchase Orders	70
Improve Client Satisfaction	5
Reduce Invoice Discrepancies	10
Improve Staff Productivity	5
Control Supply Cost/Patient Day	10
Total	100

Note that nearly a third of staff time is going toward efforts to accomplish objectives of the department that are not measured in the simplistic volume measure of POs. As activity-based costing is incorporated into hospital management, we are learning to look to activities that are cost drivers when allocating costs. Product costing can be made substantially more accurate when costs are allocated based on the activities that cause them to be incurred, rather than on simple volume measures. It turns out that budgeting can similarly be improved when we focus on how the resources are consumed, rather than simplistically making budgets as if all costs are either

fixed, or vary with volume of one measure, such as patient days or POs.

The department in our example has an education budget for staff development. Many hospitals would link that budget to full-time equivalent (FTE) employees. So, if the volume of POs increases, the number of FTEs may increase, and therefore, the education budget will increase as well. What are we doing with that money? What are we getting for it? In many cases we do get good value. However, because we have not been able to explicitly incorporate the benefit into the budget and actual results, it is often transparent. Decisions to cut budgets may result in cutting education costs. Such cuts may have a negative financial impact. The budget for education for this example might be allocated as follows:

Allocation of education resources to key objective areas

	Percent
Process Purchase Orders	0
Improve Client Satisfaction	0
Reduce Invoice Discrepancies	0
Improve Staff Productivity	10
Control Supply Cost/Patient Day	90
Total	100

Most of the education here is going toward teaching our staff how to reduce the supply cost per patient day. If we eliminate the education, we can still process the same number of POs. When we view education simply as consumption of resources, with no linkage to outcomes, it seems safe to eliminate the cost. As soon as we start to link the resource more directly with departmental objectives, a warning signal comes on. What will happen to supply costs if we cut this item? We will return to this question at the end of this article.

The materials management department consumes some supplies, and the manager of the department, together with staff, have estimated that the supplies are used as follows:

Allocation of supplies to key objective areas

	Percent
Process Purchase Orders	80
Improve Client Satisfaction	0
Reduce Invoice Discrepancies	10
Improve Staff Productivity	5
Control Supply Cost/Patient Day	5
Total	100

As you can see, the bulk of supplies are used for the day-in-and-day-out processing of POs.

Overhead is a particularly difficult area to assess. A satisfactory allocation would require a detailed study of the underlying causes of overhead. This is more advanced than we need to go into at this time. Rather, the example will simply assign all costs allocated from other departments as being for the purpose of processing POs. Once hospitals have adopted and become used to the overall outcome budget method, managers can determine whether a more accurate allocation of overhead costs would be worth the additional effort required.

Allocation of overhead to key performance areas

	Percent
Process Purchase Orders	100
Improve Client Satisfaction	0
Reduce Invoice Discrepancies	0
Improve Staff Productivity	0
Control Supply Cost/Patient Day	0
Total	100

4. Assign operating budget costs to objectives.

The next step in the process is to recreate the operating budget, incorporating the resource allocation information we have just established. Table 8–4–1 summarizes the above allocation information. Table 8–4–2 applies the percentages in Table 8–4–1 to the operating budget information. For example, in Table 8–4–1, we note that the manager spends 10 percent of his or her time processing POs. In Table 8–4–2 we see that the manager's cost to process POs is budgeted at $8,000. That is the amount we see in the "Process POs" column in Table 8–4–2, in the row for the manager. In a similar fashion, each value in Table 8–4–2 is calculated.

Table 8–4–2 does not represent an outcome budget. It provides no measures of how much of each objective we expect to be able to accomplish or attain during the coming year. However, it does provide some useful insight into how the department is spending its money. Of the $660,000 budget, only $416,000 is spent on the direct process of processing POs. The department devotes $33,000, or 5 percent of its budget, to improving customer satisfaction. More than twice that amount is spent on reducing invoice discrepancies. Over $100,000 is spent on efforts to control the supply cost per patient day.

Without a more fully developed budget for each outcome area, it is difficult to draw any conclusions about the resource allocation at this time. However, a manager can look at this and get some sense as to whether money is going

---

Table 8–4–1 Summary of Percent of Resources Devoted to Each Objective

Cost Item	Total	Process POs	Improve Client Satisfaction	Reduce Invoice Discrepancies	Improve Staff Productivity	Supply Cost/ Patient Day
Manager	100%	10%	10%	20%	20%	40%
Staff	100	70	5	10	5	10
Education	100	0	0	0	10	90
Supplies	100	80	0	10	5	5
Overhead	100	100	0	0	0	0

where the manager thinks it ought to go. A sense of priorities can be developed by looking at the totals for each column. Note how little information we get from the "Total" column in Table 8–4–2, which simply tells how much we are spending on inputs, compared to the "Total" row in that table, which specifically shows how much we have budgeted to spend in each of our key objective areas.

5. Define measure of performance for each objective.

In order to actually develop an outcome budget based on the information in Table 8–4–2, we need to also have specific measures of performance for each objective area. This may be the most difficult aspect of the process. Researchers are working hard at developing better outcome measures for health care. However, we do not have to wait for that research to be completed before we can make substantial progress. While we may have trouble measuring health improvement, we have a number of proxies available that can aid us in the outcome budget process.

Determining the proxy for processing POs is not a problem. We can either use the number of POs, or the number of lines on POs. This represents an evolution. At one time hospitals measured the dollars purchased. However, that simple volume measure does not take into account the effort required. A PO that is quick and easy-to-process but is for a large dollar amount may not take as much resources as a much smaller, but more complicated order.

Hospitals that allocate purchasing costs based on the number POs or PO lines have moved in the direction of activity-based costing. Ultimately, we need to improve on the volume measures of the number of POs or lines, and move even closer toward the activities that drive costs. However, we can use current measures such as volume of POs or lines on POs and still get improved information from the outcome budget. For this example, we will assume that there are 20,000 POs budgeted.

Improving client satisfaction is a worthy goal, but how can it ever be measured? In fact, there *are* a number of ways that satisfaction can be measured. For example, a survey could be done annually to determine satisfaction with the services of the department. That might provide a rich data set of information.

However, it is also time consuming for everyone involved. An alternative, perhaps less accurate but also less costly, is to count the number of complaints. Complaints may represent only the tip of the iceberg. There may be only 20 complaints a year, but these might represent 200 occasions on which individuals were dissatisfied. Not all dissatisfied customers complain. Complaints, however, are readily measurable. Furthermore, if we reduce the number of complaints by 20 percent, it is likely that we have improved the overall satisfaction level. Therefore, it is a low cost, useful proxy for client satisfaction. We will assume that there were 48 complaints, and

Table 8–4–2 Allocation of Operating Budget to Objectives

		Objective Area				
Cost Item	Total	Process POs	Improve Client Satisfaction	Reduce Invoice Discrepancies	Improve Staff Productivity	Supply Cost/ Patient Day
Manager	$ 80,000	$ 8,000	$ 8,000	$16,000	$16,000	$32,000
Staff	500,000	350,000	25,000	50,000	25,000	50,000
Education	20,000	0	0	0	2,000	18,000
Supplies	10,000	8,000	0	1,000	500	500
Overhead	50,000	50,000	0	0	0	0
Total	$660,000	$416,000	$33,000	$67,000	$43,500	$100,500

the budget for the coming year is to reduce that number to 36.

Reduction of invoice discrepancies is more straightforward. We will simply measure the reduction in the number of invoices that have discrepancies when compared to POs. A more advanced application of this technique might categorize discrepancies by the percent or dollar amount of the discrepancy. In this example, however, we will use singular measures for each outcome area, to keep the example relatively uncomplicated. We will assume a budgeted reduction in discrepancies from 3,000 currently to 2,000 for the budget period.

Improving staff productivity is an objective that can be approached subjectively or objectively. For our needs, rather than simply assess whether we subjectively feel that productivity is improving, we will look for some more objective measure. Specifically, we will use the number of POs processed per FTE. The budget will be to increase the number of POs per FTE from 2,000 to 2,100.

Controlling the supply cost per patient day is both challenging and important for hospitals today. With lengths of stay falling, and patient severity rising for the remaining days of stay, it becomes harder and harder to avoid increases. Our measure of performance will be the percent increase in per patient supply costs. Specifically,

we will assume that the budget is for a 4 percent increase, in an environment where costs would otherwise be expected to rise by 6 percent.

These proxies are not meant to be the only "correct" ones any more than the outcomes being addressed here are the only appropriate objective areas for a department. They merely represent examples of how this approach could be used as a helpful tool for managers. Specific details of applications must depend on the judgment and experience of each manager throughout the hospital.

6. Prepare outcome budget.

Table 8–4–3 shows the completed outcome budget for our example. The first column shows each outcome area. The second column explains the activities that must be undertaken to accomplish our goals for that outcome area. The third column explains the proxy we will use to measure the amount of each outcome that we achieve. The fourth column tells how much we have budgeted for each outcome. The fifth column explains how much of our budget we expect to devote to achieving the outcomes for this objective area. (These total costs come from the data in Table 8–4–2.) Finally, the last column divides the total cost by the budgeted output to get a cost per unit for each of our outcome areas.

The resulting information tells us that we expect it to cost $20.80 for each PO processed,

Table 8–4–3 Outcome Budget

	Type of Activity	Output Measure	Budgeted Output	Total Cost	Average Cost
Process POs	Normal processing	Number of POs processed	20,000	$416,000	$20.80/PO
Improve Client Satisfaction	Accommodate special requests	Number of complaints	Reduce number of complaints from 48 to 36	$ 33,000	$2,750 per complaint eliminated
Reduce Invoice Discrepancies	Improve price verification procedures	Number of invoice discrepancies	Reduce number of discrepancies from 3,000 to 2,000	$ 67,000	$67/eliminated discrepancy
Improve Staff Productivity	Redesign work to allow more POs/FTE	POs processed per FTE	Increase POs processed/FTE from 2,000 to 2,100, i.e., 5% increase	$ 43,500	$8,700 per percent increase in productivity
Control Supply Supply Cost/ Patient Day	Work on vendor contracts, work with clinical staff to buy only needed supplies	Supply dollars per patient day	Constrain increase to 4% versus expected industry 6% increase	$100,500	$50,250 per percent below industry expectations

$2,750 per complaint eliminated, $67 per discrepancy eliminated, $8,500 per percent increase in productivity, and $45,750 per percent that we hold per patient day supply costs below the expected industry average. Are these amounts reasonable? Each manager must decide whether or not we are allocating our resources in the best manner.

In trying to interpret these numbers, one must bear in mind that while $2,750 may seem like a high cost to eliminate each complaint, the goal is to improve customer satisfaction. The number of complaints is simply a proxy. We believe that there are many unstated complaints. Therefore, the cost per satisfied customer may be much less. On the other hand, we may still feel that the approach we are taking is too costly for the level of improvement in satisfaction.

If the budget of this department were cut, the manager now has a quantifiable way of assessing the impact. Where should less time and effort be used? In each outcome area we can see the financial savings from reductions, as well as the likely effect of those reductions on our output in that outcome area.

One way to help assess the appropriateness of our spending is to perform a cost-benefit analysis. For example, should we spend $50,250 to save just 1 percent in supply costs? Suppose that there are two different hospitals. One hospital orders $4 million of supplies annually, while the other orders $40 million of supplies. The savings for each 1 percent reduction in supply cost would then be as follows:

	Hospital A	*Hospital B*
Supply Cost	$4,000,000	$40,000,000
Percent Saved	× 1%	× 1%
Dollar Savings	$ 40,000	$ 400,000

Now compare that savings to the cost:

Savings	$40,000	$400,000
Cost	$50,250	$ 50,250
Savings/dollar	$ .80 savings	$7.96 savings

What we learn from this is that for a small hospital to pay $50,250 to reduce supply cost increases by 1 percent would not be worthwhile.

For every dollar spent on this activity, the supply cost savings is only $.80. On the other hand, for a larger hospital, this would be worthwhile. In the example above Hospital B saves $7.96 for every dollar it invests in this activity.

Consider the implications of this information. If we worked with a standard budget, instead of an outcome budget, we would not have quantified measures, and expectations about the various outcomes of this department. If a budget cut is proposed, the POs would still have to be processed. Should the cut come from our efforts to reduce supply costs? That will have a negative impact on the hospital. While the materials management department will he able to survive without a major problem if it eliminates its supply cost control efforts, the supply costs charged to departments throughout the hospital will increase substantially more than the savings from cutting the department's budget.

Earlier, we raised the issue of looking at education simply as consumption of resources, with no linkage to outcomes. Many departments might cut costs in the education area. That is because budgets are normally viewed as a list of inputs, unrelated to outputs. In our example, however, the education costs were 90 percent directed at reducing the supply cost per patient day. When we go to cut costs, we can use Table 8–4–2 as a guide. Rather than focusing on which row should be cut (education costs, staff, etc.), we can focus on what column can best sustain cuts. That focus must be done with consideration of the information in the last column of Table 8–4–3, and any cost-benefit analysis that we are able to do.

Hospitals are becoming more and more dependent on having good information. To survive and thrive, hospitals must make cost-effective decisions. Those decisions often depend on the information available when we make them. Budgeting for outcomes moves the manager from a focus on resources consumed, to a focus on the various objectives of the department, and the level of outcomes obtained. This cannot help but provide the manager with a substantially improved ability to make sensible decisions.

Reading 8–5

Flexible Budgeting Allows for Better Management of Resources As Needs Change

Steven A. Finkler

Budgeting for hospitals is a field that is still evolving. Prior to the advent of Medicare, hospital budgeting was very unsophisticated. Medicare and Medicaid created a necessity for having a formalized budgeting process.

In the years since then, the budget process has grown more and more complex. Recent trends in health care have created a situation in which the budget process needs to be flexible enough to adjust to significant changes that occur within a budget year, rather than simply from year to year. Flexible budgeting is a tool to improve hospital managers' ability to cope with the rapidly changing health care landscape.

For the last several decades, hospitals have gone through a complex annual process that results in the development of "the budget." After the fact, variance analysis is employed to examine the variations from budget, which are expected to be relatively minor for the most part. However, given the major changes that are occurring in the health care industry, a more flexible budgeting approach is needed.

Flexible budgeting provides managers with the ability to keep their budget current by anticipating in advance the impact that changes will have on the budget. The initial development of

Source: Reprinted from Steven A. Finkler, "Flexible Budgeting Allows for Better Management of Resources As Needs Change," *Hospital Cost Management and Accounting,* Vol. 8, No. 3, pp. 1–5. Copyright June 1996, Aspen Publishers, Inc.

the budget creates not one unique budget, but rather a range of budgets based on volume achieved. As the organization succeeds (or fails) with its attempts to increase volume, the budget adjusts automatically and provides a guiding tool for the organizational responses that are needed.

THE STARTING POINT

For many years, hospital financial managers have realized that knowledge of fixed and variable costs were critical for optimal management. However, all data come at a cost. In many hospitals, the cost of developing and implementing a sophisticated cost accounting system that provides detailed information on fixed and variable costs has been deemed a desirable but unaffordable luxury. In recent years, the cost of such systems has fallen as technology has advanced. At the same time, the need for such systems has increased. We may have reached the point at which hospitals in a competitive environment *must* have a handle on their fixed and variable costs. Such information is vital to the effort of developing a flexible budget.

The essence of flexible budgeting is to be able to respond to changes in volume or activities. The impact of such changes is to alter the spending on variable costs. By developing a sophisticated flexible budgeting model, a hospital is in a position to rush resources to different areas as needs change. The hospital is also in a position to more closely monitor resource consumption in areas where the spending is not justified by the activities being carried out.

Under a flexible budget approach, a range of possible budget outcomes is approved rather than a single, fixed, static budget. While this does create a somewhat more complex budget process, an advantage is that there is planning for what will be done if things do not go according to specific expectations. Reactions to change become swift and decisive, since change doesn't throw everyone for a loop, but rather has been anticipated and a response developed in advance.

DEVELOPING A FLEXIBLE BUDGET

The starting point in developing flexible budget is recognition that volume changes cause variable cost elements to change in turn. Therefore, the goal is to develop a budget that indicates anticipated spending at a variety of volume levels. In order to do so, one needs to identify fixed costs, develop a relationship for the impact of volume changes on variable costs, and then apply this relationship to actual utilization (Kerschner and Rooney, p. 59).

In rudimentary flexible budgets, three to five specific volumes are projected, and a budget is prepared for each volume level. This provides stark information for management, making the impact of volume on success immediately apparent. For example, suppose that the following budget existed for a hospital that was not using a flexible budget approach:

Table 8–5–1 Operating Budget

ABC Hospital Operating Budget for the Coming Year

Net Patient Revenue	$100.000
Less Operating Expenses	
Salaries	50,000
Benefits	10,000
Supplies and Other Expenses	30,000
Depreciation	4,000
Interest	1,000
Total Expenses	$ 95,000
Excess of Revenues over Expenses	$ 5,000

The projected profit margin for this hospital is a reasonable 5 percent ($5,000 profit per $100,000 revenue). Since the hospital is making a profit on its patients, no manager wants patient volume to fall. A 10 percent drop in patient volume will cut profits and, given what is known about fixed costs, will likely cut profits by more than 10 percent. With volume levels 10 percent lower, the final result will likely be a profit of less than $4,500 (90 percent of the current $5,000 excess of revenues over expenses). How much lower? That depends on the degree of fixed costs in the mix. Clearly the depreciation and interest are fixed costs. They will not drop by 10 percent. However, in a normal budget, we do not know the extent to which salaries, benefits, and supplies are fixed costs. Hence the need for a flexible budget.

A three-alternative flexible budget might appear as shown in Table 8–5–2.

Table 8–5–2 Flexible Operating Budget

ABC Hospital Flexible Operating Budget for the Coming Year

	Volume		
	Low	**Medium**	**High**
Net Patient Revenue	$90,000	$100,000	$110,000
Less Operating Expenses			
Salaries	$47,000	$ 50,000	$ 53,000
Benefits	9,400	10,000	10,600
Supplies and Other Exp.	28,000	30,000	32,000
Depreciation	4,000	4,000	4,000
Interest	1,000	1,000	1,000
Total Expenses	$98,400	$ 95,000	$100,600
Excess of Revenues over Expenses	$ 600	$ 5,000	$ 9,400

In this example, it is assumed that $20,000 of salaries are fixed. That simply means that they are salaries that are unlikely to be affected by relatively small volume changes. Salaries dropped and rose by $3,000 in the lower and higher volume scenarios. That represents a direct proportional change for the portion of the salary costs that are variable. Similarly, only $20,000 of the supplies and other expenses were assumed to be variable. Benefits changed in proportion to the changes in salaries.

This example provides a lesson about the leveraging effects of fixed costs. If volume falls by just 10 percent, profits will fall by 88 percent (from $5,000 to $600). In contrast, just a 10 percent increase in volume results in a near doubling of profits (from $5,000 to $9,400). The greater the proportion of fixed costs, the greater the magnitude of the gyrations in profitability caused by volume swings.

In fact, the results can be even worse. Whether by use of a flexible budget or some other device, hospitals must plan what they will do in response to a drop in volume. Unless there is a contingency plan, it is likely that volume drops will not be accompanied by staff decreases. Some costs that are variable, if anticipated, may not decline as volume drops. Thus, the salary and benefits savings may not be achieved, and the drop in volume in the above example could easily throw the hospital into a deficit position. In ratchet-like fashion, unexpected volume increases are more likely to result in increased staffing costs than unexpected decreases are to result in reduced staffing costs.

However, armed with a flexible budget, managers are immediately aware of the specific financial implications of a volume decline. They are therefore more likely to aggressively adjust variable costs downward as volume declines.

In the flexible budget above, the revenue has decreased and increased in proportion to volume changes. The real world is more complex. Depending on the source of the patients, revenues might rise and fall slower or faster. For example, HMO patients may generate less revenue per patient. For this reason, it is beneficial to develop the flexible budget as a computer model that allows all numbers to be modified as necessary. The model need not be overly sophisti-

cated. A spreadsheet program such as Excel™ or LOTUS™ can easily handle the budget adjustments resulting from the modification of any number.

However, while we need to consider the revenue and be able to adroitly adjust for changing levels of revenue per patient, the essence of flexible budgeting rests on a good knowledge of fixed and variable costs (Suver, Neumann and Boles, p. 175). Each hospital must continue to decide the amount of effort to put into the determination of these costs. Clearly, the need for improved determination of variable costing is increasing.

Many consulting firms are selling costing systems that can quickly assess the cost impacts of volume changes, based on detailed breakdowns of variable costs. These programs can be very useful, but are also very costly. Less formalized systems can also help. For example, one can ask managers to prepare many different budgets at different projected volumes. However, doing so is likely to be extremely time consuming.

Alternatively, we can ask managers to specify which costs are fixed and which costs are variable. That approach sounds good, but is not necessarily workable. Managers often have trouble objectively identifying any staff as being variable, even though in practice they do adjust the number of staff hours consumed as volume changes.

A somewhat simpler and potentially more accurate approach is to ask managers to prepare two budgets rather than one, based on two different volumes. While this increases their work somewhat, it is not likely to require an unbearable amount of time. Given two budgets at two different volume levels, it becomes a relatively simple matter to assess fixed and variable costs.

For example, consider the high and low volume flexible budgets presented earlier. In that example, the salary cost was $47,000 for the low volume and $53,000 for the high volume. Let's assume that the low volume is 90 patient days, while the high volume is 110 patient days. The change in volume is 20 (110 high volume less 90 low volume 20 change in volume). The change in the salary cost was $6,000 ($53,000 at the high volume less $47,000 at the low volume = $6,000). If we divide the change in cost by the change in volume, we determine the change in salary cost for each extra patient day. That is, we will have found the variable cost per unit. Dividing $6,000 by 20 generates a variable cost of $300 per patient day for salary cost.

We can also estimate the fixed costs using the same information. If 90 patient days have a variable cost of $27,000 (90 patient days times $300 variable cost per patient day), and a total salary cost of $47,000 (from the flexible budget presented earlier), the difference of $20,000 must be the fixed cost ($47,000 total salary cost less the variable cost of $27,000 = $20,000 fixed cost). We could also calculate this using the 110 patient days that have a variable cost of $33,000 (110 times $300) and a total cost of $53,000. The difference between the $53,000 and the $33,000 is the fixed cost of $20,000. Note that this is the same as the fixed cost calculated at the lower volume. By definition, the fixed cost does not change as volume changes.

We could employ this method to estimate the fixed and variable costs for all departments and for all line items within each department. The results can be used to provide a *continuous* flexible budget. By continuous we mean that we could create a budget that shows the costs at any volume within a reasonable range (over which fixed costs are unlikely to change). This means that each month, managers can evaluate everything against the flexible budget for the specific volume attained in their department. This holds managers much more accountable for adjusting spending as volume is changing, as opposed to several months later.

Textbooks often object to determination of variable and fixed costs by comparison of just two data points as was done above. However, the objections to the so-called "high-low" method are voiced when historical data are used. A textbook approach to estimating costs is to use historical data, or data from a number of years in the past; regression analysis can then be used to project costs into the future. However, the high-

low method simplifies the historical approach by simply selecting the highest and lowest volume points and employing the approach described above, eliminating the need for using regression. The problem with high-low is that it is likely to select outliers. Why is one year the highest or lowest? Often because something unusual happened. We don't want to base our predictions of the future on the occurrence of something that is not likely to occur.

The approach described here is *prospective* rather than retrospective. We are not selecting two points that are likely to be wild outliers, but rather two very reasonable points, each representing volumes that might well occur for the coming year and be handled in the routine course of events. The trade-off of the likely quality of the data, versus its cost, must be considered as in all cases.

An alternative approach, as mentioned above, would be to use historical data and regression analysis to get a reasonable estimate of fixed and variable costs. The data can then be used to develop a flexible budget, showing the expected results of departments and the organization at a wide variety of different volumes. Although regression analysis is a complicated statistical technique, many software programs, such as SmartForecasts for Windows®, make the process quite feasible for the average manager with little statistical background.

ORGANIZATIONAL BUY-IN

As the rate of financial distress in the health care industry continues to increase, it becomes more and more important for boards of hospitals to have an understanding of what is happening. Overall, the number of inpatient days continues to decline. The flexible budget, rather than being too complex for the board to understand, may be the one tool that can best convey to the board the difficulties faced by hospital management. Many of the members of the board are likely to have come from organizations that benefit from continuous growth. A presentation of profit levels at different volumes can show the board what is happening in the health care industry. Therefore, it would not be unreasonable to ask the board to vote on a flexible budget rather than the traditional static budget.

NEGOTIATION

Flexible budgets are also advantageous in that they generate information helpful in the process of negotiating new arrangements. The importance of volume to profitability is driven home by the flexible budget. The immediate impact of a discount arrangement can be seen by considering both the change to the total revenue line, as well as the various cost responses to the implied change in volume.

NEW SERVICES

As an organization becomes comfortable with flexible budgeting, the next step is to broaden its usefulness by expanding it to cover the addition of new services. Hospitals of the future will tend to be more integrated providers of care. If for no other reason, it just doesn't make much sense to keep wings of the building closed down and nonproductive. The information generated by a flexible, volume-related approach can be used to more readily determine the impact of adding (or removing) services.

For more information on SmartForecasts III, call Smart Software at 800/SMART-99.

REFERENCES

Kerschner, Morley I. and Jeffrey M. Rooney. "Utilizing Cost Accounting Information for Budgeting," *Topics in Health Care Financing,* Summer 1987, pp. 56–66.

Suver, James D., Bruce Neumann, and Keith E. Boles. *Management Accounting for Healthcare Organizations,* 4th Edition, Chicago, Precept Press and HFMA, 1995.

9

Flexible Budgeting and Variance Analysis

Reading 9–1

Physician Cost Variance Analysis under DRGs

Roger Kropf

Cost variance analysis can be used to improve management's understanding of how the cost of treating patients admitted by individual physicians is changing over time. It is an alternative to two other common methods of assessing physician behavior with respect to patients of varying case-mix.

The first of these common methods is examination of the costs incurred by the individual patients of each physician. This approach is time consuming and doesn't focus the manager's attention on those physicians whose costs are changing. The second is to start by examining high-cost and/or low-profit DRGs and study only physicians whose patients fall into those DRGs. Because patients in only a few DRGs are examined, the manager may not see the overall direction of the physician's costs, either upwards or downwards.

The cost variance analysis method presented in this article provides information on trends (as well as absolute variance amounts) that is not provided by the other two approaches.

Table 9–1–1 shows the number of cases admitted and the average cost per patient for a physician during January–June and July–December of

1985. In order to study the effect of case-mix, the data are presented by DRG. For this example, only four DRGs are shown. The method can easily be extended to all DRGs.

The total operating costs incurred in the treatment of patients admitted by this physician dropped by $10,243.99 or approximately 5.5 percent, while the total number of patients treated dropped by 11 percent.

These two percentages do not adequately describe what has occurred, however. The effect of a drop in admissions on costs will depend on whether admissions are reduced in high- or in low-cost DRGs. While total costs are going down, an increase in the use of resources for low-cost DRGs could be masked by decreases in the admission of patients in high-cost DRGs.

The question that needs to be raised is the extent to which the variance in cost between these two periods was due to changes in case-mix (the number of patients in each DRG) and the extent to which it was due to changes in the cost of treating the average patient in each DRG. Other possible causes for the variance will be discussed later in this article.

PHYSICIAN COST VARIANCE

The physician cost variance is the difference in the cost of treating the patients admitted by a

Source: Reprinted from Roger Kropf, "Physician Cost Variance Analysis under DRGs," *Hospital Cost Accounting Advisor,* Vol. 1, No. 12, May 1986, pp. 1, 3–5. Copyright 1986, Aspen Publishers, Inc.

Table 9–1–1 Number of Cases and Operating Cost per Case, R. Smith, MD, 1985

		PRIOR PERIOD January–June				CURRENT PERIOD July–December		
	Cases		Operating Cost Per Case	Total Cost	Cases		Operating Cost Per Case	Total Cost
DRG 1	24	×	4,365.88	= 104,781.12	16	×	4,815.88	= 77,054.08
DRG 2	9	×	4,863.75	= 43,773.75	10	×	5,073.75	= 50,737.50
DRG 3	7	×	2,645.47	= 18,518.29	8	×	2,962.93	= 23,703.44
DRG 4	4	×	4,638.40	= 18,533.60	5	×	4,777.55	= 23,887.75
	44			$185,626.76	39			$175,382.77

	Total Operating Cost
January–June	$185,626.76
July–December	$175,382.77
Increase/(decrease)	($10,243.99)

physician between the current and a prior period. The variance can be expressed in total dollars or as a percent of prior period costs. The physician cost variance in this example is a negative $10,243.99 or 5.5 percent.

In order to interpret the meaning of the variance, it must be broken down into a number of other variances, as shown in Table 9–1–2.

CASE-MIX VARIANCE

This variance summarizes the effect of changes in the number of patients in each DRG. The effect of changes in cost per DRG is removed by using the current cost in both parts of the equation (see equation 1 in Table 9–1–2, as well as Table 9–1–3). The case-mix variance is

Table 9–1–2 Physician Cost Variance Analysis, R. Smith, MD, 1985

Physician cost variance = case-mix variance + cost variance
($10,243.99) = ($25,712.81) + $15,468.82

Where
(1) Case-mix variance =

Σ(Current volume per DRG × current cost per DRG)
Minus
Σ(Prior volume per DRG × current cost per DRG)

Case-mix variance = $175,382.88 – $201,095.58
= ($ 25,712.81)

(2) Cost variance =

Σ(Prior volume per DRG × current cost per DRG)
Minus
Σ(Prior volume per DRG × prior cost per DRG)

Cost variance = $201,095.58 – $185,626.76
= $ 15,468.82

Table 9–1–3 Calculation of the Case-Mix and Cost Variances

(1) Case-Mix Variance

	Current Volume		Current Cost		Total Cost
DRG 1	16	×	4,815.88	=	77,054.08
DRG 2	10	×	5,073.75	=	50,737.50
DRG 3	8	×	2,962.93	=	23,703.44
DRG 4	5	×	4,777.55	=	23,887.75
	Σ(Current Volume	×	Current Cost)	=	$175,382.77

	Prior Volume		Current Cost		Total Cost
DRG 1	24	×	4,815.88	=	115,581.12
DRG 2	9	×	5,073.75	=	45,663.75
DRG 3	7	×	2,962.93	=	20,740.51
DRG 4	4	×	4,777.55	=	19,110.20
	Σ(Prior Volume	×	Current Cost)	=	$201,095.58

Case-Mix Variance = $175,382.77 − $201,095.58
= ($25,712.81)

(2) Cost Variance

	Prior Volume		Current Cost		Total Cost
DRG 1	24	×	4,815.88	=	115,581.12
DRG 2	9	×	5,073.75	=	45,663.75
DRG 3	7	×	2,962.93	=	20,740.51
DRG 4	4	×	4,777.55	=	19,110.20
	Σ(Prior Volume	×	Current Cost)	=	$201,095.58

	Prior Volume		Prior Cost		Total Cost
DRG 1	24	×	4,365.88	=	104,781.12
DRG 2	9	×	4,863.75	=	43,773.75
DRG 3	7	×	2,645.47	=	18,518.29
DRG 4	4	×	4,638.40	=	18,553.60
	Σ(Prior Volume	×	Prior Cost)	=	$185,626.76

Cost Variance = $201,095.58 − $185,626.76
= $ 15,468.82

a negative $25,712.81, which is two and one-half times the physician cost variance and 14 percent of the total operating costs in the prior period.

COST VARIANCE

This variance summarizes the effect of changes in the costs incurred by patients in each DRG. The effect of changes in the volume of patients in each DRG is removed by using the prior volume of patients in both parts of the equation (see equation 2 in Table 9–1–2, as well as Table 9–1–3). The cost variance is a positive $15,468.82, which is one and one-half times the physician cost variance and 8 percent of the total operating costs in the prior period.

INTERPRETATION

Table 9–1–4 shows a number of cost ratios that are useful in interpreting the meaning of the cost variances.

The analysis shows that the change in case-mix was more important than the change in the

Table 9–1–4 Physician Cost Variance Analysis Cost Ratios

	Ratio
Case-mix variance/prior period operating costs	(14%)
Cost variance/prior period operating costs	8%
Case-mix variance/cost variance	(166%)
Cost variance/case-mix variance	(60%)
Case-mix variance/physician cost variance	251%
Cost variance/physician cost variance	(151%)

cost per DRG in determining the magnitude of the drop in total operating costs. The case-mix variance was 166 percent of the cost variance and 251 percent of the physician cost variance.

On the other hand, the cost variance is positive, showing that the costs incurred by the patients admitted by this physician are increasing. If the number of patients admitted by this physician increases in the next period, management may see an increase in total costs.

Admissions may, however, continue to drop, resulting in even lower total costs while the costs incurred in treating the remaining patients continue to rise.

FURTHER ANALYSES

Since managers have a very limited amount of time to examine the reason for variances, establishing priorities is important. This physician's situation might be examined further if it is part of a continuing trend of both higher costs and lower admissions or if an examination of the net revenues received from the physician's patients shows a significant and negative effect on the hospital's profits.

In addition to looking at the revenues received from this physician's patients, one could analyze the effect of changes in input costs and the volume of inputs consumed on changes in cost per case. The cost variance described in this article includes the effect of changes in both the cost of inputs and the volume of inputs consumed. For example, the same number of nursing hours may have been used to treat patients, while nursing wages increased substantially between the two periods. The action required by management obviously differs substantially depending on whether input costs are rising or whether the physician is increasing the quantity of inputs used for a given type of patient.

We have also assumed that the severity of illness of the patients treated has remained constant and had no effect on the resources consumed. The physician may have been treating fewer patients in a DRG, for example, while those patients were sicker and required additional resources. If data are available on severity of illness as well as on the volume of inputs and

the cost of inputs consumed by patients in each severity category, this issue can be pursued.[1]

LIMITATIONS

The method described in this article attributes all of the costs incurred by a patient to the physician who admitted the patient to the hospital. A number of other physicians may be responsible for treating the patient during a hospital stay, and the responsibility for ordering services may shift to another physician as the condition of the patient changes. The method is likely to be most useful, therefore, in describing the effect of physician referrals to the hospital, rather than in accurately estimating the effect of physician treatment patterns.

In hospitals where the vast majority of care is ordered by the admitting physician, the physician cost variance analysis suggested will indicate the effect of ordering and practice patterns on hospital costs.

Managers need to examine the changes in costs incurred by physicians. Looking at data on the costs of treating the individual patient is too time consuming. Data aggregated by DRG do not reveal how the behavior of individual physicians is affecting costs.

By carrying out a physician cost variance analysis, managers can gain some understanding of how changes in the costs attributed to specific physicians are related to changes in case-mix and the cost per patient.

NOTE

1. For a discussion of the use of patient acuity or severity in cost variance analysis, see Steven A. Finkler, "Flexible Budget Variance Analysis Extended to Patient Acuity and DRGs," *Health Care Management Review* (Fall, 1985), pp. 21–34.

Reading 9–2

A Contemporary Approach to Budget Variance Analysis: A Pharmacy Application

Sharon Minogue Holswade

David P. Vogel

In most hospitals, the pharmacy department manager routinely evaluates monthly expenses as they compare to budgeted expenses and explains significant variances. This exercise can be either fruitful or frustrating, depending on a number of variables. These variables include the manner in which the budget was created, the availability of substantial detail in support of expense lines, and the knowledge of the pharmacy manager concerning the factors that can cause fluctuations in expense, particularly drug cost.

A number of articles have been written in an attempt to assist pharmacy managers with budget variance analysis. Excellent analyses of factors affecting budget variance have been written by O'Byrne[1] and Buchanan[2] in *Topics in Hospital Pharmacy Management.* Other articles provide helpful insights to the manager relative to the other two variables. Buchanan,[3] Miller,[4] and Williams[5] have suggested thoroughgoing approaches to projecting realistic budgets. Hunt,[6] Nold,[7,8,9] and Mehl[10] have suggested approaches to data collection that help to support and explain variations in expenses during the year. The present authors will make some recommendation regarding these variables in the discussion that follows; however, the reader is encouraged to review the articles just cited to supplement our comments and to enhance his or her understanding of budgeting and budget variance analysis.

THE PROBLEM WITH THE TRADITIONAL APPROACH TO VARIANCE ANALYSIS

Until January 1987, monthly budget variance analysis at the Robert Wood Johnson University Hospital (RWJUH), as at many others, resulted in a report comparing actual expenses to budgeted expenses when an individual variance was greater than 5 percent and more than $1,000 over budget or under budget. The report listed the relevant line items, the amount of the variance, and a brief explanation of the variance.

Explanations were relatively straightforward. For example, some annual or quarterly payments were budgeted monthly, creating wide variances in both directions. Expenses for newly approved positions or market adjustments in salary were not added to the budget, resulting in salary variances. Seasonal availability of pharmacy students as *per diem* employees created wide variances in full-time-equivalent positions (FTEs) and salaries in certain months. An unexpectedly high turnover of pharmacists created variances in the form of advertising expenses.

The most significant pharmacy expense variances, however, were the most difficult to explain. These expenses were drug and IV costs. For variances in these expenses the explanation frequently included some reference to change in

Source: Reprinted from Sharon Minogue Holswade and David P. Vogel, "A Contemporary Approach to Budget Variance Analysis: A Pharmacy Application," *Topics in Hospital Pharmacy Management,* Vol. 9, No. 2, August 1989, pp. 1–10. Copyright 1989, Aspen Publishers, Inc.

volume or activity as a justification. It was very difficult, however, to quantify the change in activity. The use of percentage changes in admissions or patient days as an indicator of volume or activity never seemed to be sufficient to explain the percentage increase in expense. This was true because it is not possible to correlate an admission with the type of pharmacy resources consumed. For example, a 20 percent increase in admissions relating to maternity might affect the pharmacy budget very little, while a 5 percent increase in oncology admissions may have a significant budget impact.

This problem with pharmacy variance analysis was common to many departments with significant direct patient care responsibilities. In the traditional approach to hospital budgeting and budget analysis at RWJUH, many departmental activity levels were not integrated in such a way as to correspond to monthly expense levels. Activity reports typically relied on traditional measures such as visits, procedures, and admissions, but this type of measure is not always indicative of the activity experienced by the department. For example, a first visit to a physician may consume one hour of time, while a revisit may consume 15 minutes. To count these simply as two visits does not reflect the resources consumed to provide these services. Similarly, there is a substantial difference in resource consumption between the preparation and dispensing of one dose of IV chemotherapy versus the preparation and dispensing of a 24-hour supply of oral propranolol.

A CONCEPTUAL CHANGE

In late 1986 it was determined that a new method of variance reporting should be established that would address the explanatory deficiency of the traditional system. The new system would incorporate department-specific workload data that would be weighted to reflect resource consumption and departmental expenses more appropriately. The weighted workload data would be totaled and divided into departmental expenses that vary with activity to establish a unit cost for producing one unit of activity. In theory this number should remain constant, regardless of changes in volume or activity at the departmental level.

The goals of the new system would be to: (1) relate variances in departmental expenses more closely to actual changes in activity; and (2) produce reports that were easy to prepare in a minimum of time and that could be easily read and interpreted by a wide range of individuals, including senior administrators, finance officers, and board members.

The outcome of implementing this concept was a new report entitled the relative unit cost (RUC) report, which would be completed each month by departmental managers and submitted in lieu of the traditional budget variance report. The administration felt that implementation of this report could be made with minimal impact on management time, since the necessary data were already available and the education of staff would not be a restrictive variable.

A different approach to this problem was described by Coarse[11] in 1985. He thoroughly described the concept of flexible budgeting but did not make any reference to its implementation or use in his own institution. He did acknowledge that "its use [in hospitals] is not widespread. This is partly due to its complexity and partly due to lack of understanding of its basic elements by hospital managers, including pharmacy managers."[12] In contrast, the approach implemented at RWJUH is markedly less complex, an attribute that has substantially affected its success and acceptance.

THE RELATIVE UNIT COST REPORT

The RUC report is a one-page cumulative summary of cost and activity data for an entire year. It must be completed and submitted with two supporting documents: a workload statistics report and a RUC variance report. The RUC report (Table 9–2–1) contains two fixed columns with comparative data. One column has the previous year's monthly averages; the other column

Table 9–2–1 Relative Unit Cost Report for November 1988

Department	1987 Average	1988 Budget	Adjusted Unit Cost	Jan	Feb	Mar	Apr	May	June	July	Aug	Sept	Oct	Nov	Dec	YTD
PHARMACY																
No. of orders	78,993			84,446	80,672	84,600	78,036	83,372	81,596	85,713	90,141	80,064	85,838	83,301		83,434
Total weighted units	249,209	255,938		273,395	256,108	269,465	246,846	265,770	256,786	277,204	288,233	262,303	281,562	271,664		268,121
Ratio of activity to budget	1.09	1.03		1.07	1.00	1.05	0.96	1.04	1.00	1.08	1.13	1.02	1.10	1.06		1.05
Salary																
Cost per activity unit ($)	0.32	0.33	0.39	0.34	0.34	0.35	0.36	0.35	0.38	0.40	0.37	0.39	0.37	0.42		0.37
Nonsalary																
Cost per activity unit ($)	1.21	1.21		1.19	1.22	1.53	1.26	1.34	1.39	1.12	1.39	1.31	1.11	1.24		1.28

contains budget data for the current year. A third column for use in variance analysis contains adjusted budget data. The remainder of the columns on the form contain data for each month, as well as a year-to-date (YTD) column.

For the pharmacy department there are only five reportable lines of data in each column: total numbers of orders, total weighted activity units, the ratio of actual activity units to budgeted activity units, the salary cost per activity unit, and the nonsalary cost per activity unit. These five pieces of data can be calculated from two sources: departmental workload statistics and the monthly budget report from the finance department. The RUC report is customized for each department and may contain other relevant lines of data for other departments.

The preparation of the November 1988 RUC report of the pharmacy department will be explained in detail to illustrate how the report is used.

Workload Activity

The first step in the preparation of the monthly RUC report is to collect and total relevant workload statistics. The November 1988 Pharmacy Statistics Report is shown as Table 9–2–2. Statistics are collected only for the six activities shown, which represent over 90 percent of the department's workload related to drug distribution. There are some activities, most notably clinical activities, for which monthly statistics

are not collected. It is important to note that at this point the purpose of the collection of these statistics is to measure relevant changes in activity, not to measure total productivity. Therefore, statistics that were not readily available and those that were not expected to have a significant impact on total weighted units were not collected. This approach is consistent with the project's goals of simplicity and ease of use.

Each activity is then weighted according to its relative consumption of time. The numbers used are modifications of national standards as reported as an output of PharmaTrend and its precursor productivity monitoring systems.[13,14]

One way in which our statistics and weights differ from PharmaTrend is that new order and refill line items are counted rather than the total number of doses dispensed or charged. A new order or refill order represents one complete dispensing function, irrespective of the number of doses dispensed. Even in the unit dose drug distribution system, doses are dispensed as a 24-hour supply that often contains more than one dose and occasionally more than four doses.

For each activity the number of orders multiplied by its weight equals a number of activity units. The net total of all activity units is the basis for measuring all changes in activity and comparing them to changes in cost.

The total number of statistics is given for both the current year and the same month of the previous year. This comparison shows relevant changes in specific activities that will eventually be reflected as one net change in activity in the

Table 9–2–2 Pharmacy Department Statistics for November 1988

Activity	Weight (Minutes)	Weighted 1987 Volume	1987 Activity Units	Weighted 1988 Volume	1988 Activity Units
New orders	3.0	25,673	77,020	28,106	84,318
Refill orders	2.0	33, 375	66,750	36,538	73,076
IV admixtures	5.0	17,335	86,675	17,340	86,700
Hyperalimentation (TPN)	20.0	725	14,500	458	9,160
Chemotherapy	20.0	314	6,280	818	16,360
Peritoneal dialysis manifolds	50.0			41	2,050
Total workload units			251,225		271,664

RUC report itself. Thus this required appendix to the RUC report becomes an important backup reference document that is easily accessible in case questions arise concerning fluctuations in departmental activity.

In the example (Table 9–2–2) total parenteral nutrition (TPN) orders were significantly lower in November 1988, while chemotherapy orders were significantly higher. Non-IV new orders and refills were relatively higher in 1988, but IV orders were unchanged. The preparation of peritoneal dialysis manifolds is listed only as a current year statistic because it represents a new service initiated in August 1988. While it is appropriate to account for new services in this manner, potential users of this system are cautioned not to add statistics for services that have been provided throughout both reported years, but for which statistics are only now relevant and/or available. Statistics can be added for these activities if the previous year's data are accessible. Alternatively, statistics for these activities can be collected for one year prior to their incorporation into the reporting mechanism. Actual and budgeted costs per activity unit will decrease in both years once these statistics are added; however, this has no relevance to expense analysis. It is still the relative difference between actual and budgeted costs per activity unit from month to month that is important to monitor.

Workload Activity Compared to Budget

The next step in preparation of the monthly report is to transfer the total number of activities (orders) and weighted activity units from the statistics report (Table 9–2–2) to lines 1 and 2 of the November column of the RUC report (Table 9–2–1).

The total number of activity units in November (271,664) is divided by the budgeted monthly activity units (255,938) to produce a ratio of 1.06. (The determination of the budgeted activity units will be described later.) This ratio essentially reports that pharmacy workload was 6 percent over budget in November.

Salary Cost and Nonsalary Cost per Activity Unit

The total salary expenses ($114,100) and nonsalary expenses ($336,863) for November, as reported by the finance department, were each divided by the number of workload units (271,664) to produce a dollar cost per unit of activity ($0.42 and $1.24, respectively). These two numbers are entered on lines four and five of the RUC report. They are then compared to budgeted standards, and any difference becomes the basis for variance explanations.

There are a number of difficulties with using these gross ratios, but they can be effective indicators of expense-activity relationships in spite of their limitations. Salary expenses are typically step-variable in nature. That is, they remain fixed over a range of activity levels. Expenses are adjusted up a step or down a step by adding or subtracting FTEs if activity routinely exceeds the upper limit or falls below the lower limit of the activity range. As a result, budgeted cost per activity unit for salaries actually reflects a range that extends from a higher cost per activity unit when workload is low and a lower cost per activity unit when workload is high. This fact is frequently used as a valid explanation in the variance analysis.

At RWJUH, drug and IV costs account for 98 percent of all nonsalary costs in pharmacy. Therefore, these costs were our focus when determining an appropriate method to compare nonsalary costs to activity. The total cost per activity unit does reflect some expenses, such as advertising and travel, that are not workload volume-related and should not change at all with activity. However, these expenses are fixed and contribute so little to the total that their inclusion does not affect any interpretation or evaluation of the numbers.

Actually, on a "micro" level, changes in drug and IV costs are not directly proportional to changes in the activities that are reflected by pharmacy statistics. Changes in IV or non-IV orders can involve products that cost less than $1.00 per order or more than $100.00 per order. On a "macro" basis, however, the authors have found that changes in drug and IV costs are relatively proportional to the net change in activity. At a cost of $1.21 per activity unit, the ingredients for an average 24-hour unit dose supply would cost from $2.24 to $3.36 (weighted at 2 to 3 units per activity); the ingredients of an average IV would cost $6.05 (weighted at 5 units per activity); and the ingredients for an average TPN preparation or chemotherapy preparation would cost $24.20 (weighted at 20 units per activity). Although these numbers are not likely to be absolutely accurate, they are not bad approximations. They do provide a mechanism to account for a substantial portion of the changes in drug cost in relation to activity. The routine collection of detailed drug use data allows detection of the increased use of drugs whose cost substantially exceeds these averages. For example, a marked increase in the use of IV immunoglobulin during 1988 was cited to explain some of the excess of actual cost per activity unit over the budgeted cost per activity unit.

The last step in the preparation of the RUC form itself is to change the figures in the YTD column to reflect new averages that include the current month. After the first three or four months of the year, these YTD numbers provide a broader perspective on activity and expense trends compared to budget.

Variance Report

The last step in preparing the monthly RUC report is to document the variance analysis on the second supplementary form, the variance report. Exhibit 9–2–1 shows the variance report for November 1988. Budgeted versus actual cost per unit of activity for both salary and nonsalary costs is shown in the left-hand column. The narrative documents actual over-budget dollars but does not go any further if cost per activity unit is not over budget. If that amount is over budget, then further explanations are necessary. Significant increases in non-activity-related expenses, such as advertising or travel expenses, are exceptions and must always be explained.

The finance report, internal pharmacy drug use reports, and other available information are used to investigate increases in cost per unit of activity. The use of drug cost documentation to explain variances has already been mentioned. The pharmacy department maintains detailed monthly drug use data on 98 drug entities (16 percent of the formulary) that account for 81 percent of all drug costs. These data have been sufficient to explain all noticeable variances in actual versus budgeted drug expenses.

The finance report (i.e., expense report) can also help to explain significant variances. For example, one of the detailed line entries on the November finance report showed that the cost of sick-time buy-back payments was charged to the department in November. This figure represents an annual expense that was budgeted over the entire year. Thus this information on the finance report was used to explain a salary variance of $0.05 per activity unit in November (see Exhibit 9–2–1).

If some explanations keep appearing each month and represent permanent changes to departmental expenses, the administration may choose to establish an adjusted budget cost reflecting this change. For example, approved but unbudgeted new positions or salary increases may qualify for such an adjustment. Such an adjustment for salary unit cost appears in column 3 of Table 9–2–1. Although the original budget remains unchanged, monthly variance analysis becomes more efficient because only differences between actual cost and adjusted budget cost must be explained.

Budgeting with the RUC Report

The budgeting process takes on a new look when the data provided by the RUC report are used. Budget dollars can be projected more accurately on the basis of activity projections. For example, 1989 budget preparation materials included a projected increase of 3.2 percent in admissions for 1989. The RUC reports documented increases in pharmacy activity that were proportional to increases in admissions by factors of 1.96 in 1987 and 1.45 in 1988. Based on an average of those two results, the increase in projected

Exhibit 9–2–1 Relative Unit Cost Report Variance Analysis

DEPARTMENT: PHARMACY			

	November Budget	Actual	
Salary	0.39	0.42	Pharmacy activity was 6% over budget in November. Salary expenses are $19,028 over budget. Salary expenses for Nov. include $13,537 in sick-time buy-back expenses; this is equal to 0.05 per activity unit. Salary cost per activity unit is otherwise under budget.
		−0.05	
		0.37	
Nonsalary	1.21	1.24	Nonsalary expenses are $29,217 over budget. Of this amount, $19,000 is attributable to the increase in activity. If unbudgeted inflation (@ 7.6% = 0.09 per activity unit) and unbudgeted inventory control computer expenses (@ 0.01 per activity unit) are considered, nonsalary costs are under budget.
		−0.09	
		−0.01	
		1.14	

1989 admissions was multiplied by 1.75 to yield an estimated increase in pharmacy activity of 5.6 percent. As a result, nonsalary costs for 1989 were calculated first by multiplying 1988 activity units by 1.056. This number was then multiplied by the average cost per activity unit for 1988 ($1.27), adjusted to $1.34 to reflect an estimated inflation factor of 5.4 percent. The result was the total projected nonsalary budget for 1989. If the budget is approved, the RUC report budget column for 1989 should reflect these calculations.

An additional modification to the budget projection should be made if any drug cost increases are anticipated to be significantly higher on a cost-per-dose basis than the averages referred to previously. For example, in 1988 a budget adjustment of $100,000 was added for tissue plasminogen activator, increasing the cost per unit activity by a factor of 0.03. Similarly, if any major decreases in high-cost drug use are anticipated, an adjustment to the budget projection should be made.

The new salary cost per activity unit will be determined on the basis of the approved number of FTE positions, which may increase, decrease, or remain the same as a result of the budgeting process. The new salary cost per activity unit may also reflect an adjustment for planned salary increases in the year to come.

RESULTS AND CONCLUSIONS

The relative unit cost report took approximately six months to develop and implement. Since its implementation the report has been invaluable in correlating activity to expenses throughout all departments. Monthly variance reports have become more specific and credible. The report has also served as an educational tool. Staff members have an increased understanding of departmental operations in relation to finance, and staff confidence with respect to dealing with finance has grown as a result.

In the pharmacy department for each of the last two years, the report documented an increase in activity that was significantly different from increases as measured by patient days or admissions. Total pharmacy activity units increased by 9.4 percent from 1986 to 1987, while admissions increased by 4.8 percent and patient days increased by 6.2 percent. Similarly, total pharmacy activity units increased by 8.0 percent from 1987 to 1988, while admissions increased by 5.5 percent and patient days increased by 5.8 percent. These data confirm subjective impressions that the increase in volume at RWJUH has been concentrated in highly resource-intensive cases: cardiac surgery, trauma, cardiology, and oncology. Objective documentation of these impressions is invaluable with respect to justification of resources and expenses to the administration.

By utilizing additional available data, the system can be refined or expanded as management requires. Productivity monitors can be introduced through the addition of FTE positions or productive hours. Changes in units produced per productive hour or FTE can be an informative workload measure for the department. At RWJUH these indicators are currently being monitored and evaluated for eventual inclusion in the RUC report. Other modifications will be analyzed in an attempt to increase the sophistication of the report without jeopardizing its simplicity, its ease of interpretation, or its contribution to the efficient use of valuable administrative time.

The system described in this article has proven to be a valuable tool for management. Since it correlates relevant departmental data into a simple format, it has provided the management of RWJUH with a financial tool that reflects departmental operations more effectively than did the traditional budget variance reporting system that it replaced.

NOTES

1. A. O'Byrne. "Budget Monitoring: Understanding the Concepts." *Topics in Hospital Pharmacy Management* 3, no. 4 (1984): 33–41.

2. C. Buchanan. "Budget and Financial Reporting." *Topics in Hospital Pharmacy Management* 6, no. 3 (1986): 29–52.

3. C. Buchanan. "Selecting a Method to Forecast Drug Costs." *Topics in Hospital Pharmacy Management* 4, no. 4 (1985): 21–32.

4. R.F. Miller. "Forecasting Drug Costs." *Topics in Hospital Pharmacy Management* 3, no. 4 (1984): 42–48.

5. R.B. Williams. "Preparing the Operating Budget." *American Journal of Hospital Pharmacy* 40 (1983): 2181–2188.

6. M.L. Hunt. "Use of Financial Reports in Managing Pharmacies." *American Journal of Hospital Pharmacy* 41 (1984): 709–715.

7. E.G. Nold. "Developing a Data-Collection System." *American Journal of Hospital Pharmacy* 40 (1983): 1685–89.

8. E.G. Nold. "Financial Analysis." *American Journal of Hospital Pharmacy* 40 (1983): 1975–1979.

9. E.G. Nold. "Developing Reports." *American Journal of Hospital Pharmacy* 40 (1983): 1968–1975.

10. B. Mehl. "Indicators To Control Drug Costs in Hospitals." *American Journal of Hospital Pharmacy* 41 (1984): 667–675.

11. J.F. Coarse. "Flexible Budgeting for Hospital Pharmacists." *Topics in Hospital Pharmacy Management* 4, no. 4 (1985): 9–20.

12. Ibid., 9–10.

13. M.H. Stolar. "Description of an Experimental Hospital Pharmacy Management Information System." *American Journal of Hospital Pharmacy* 40 (1983): 1905–1913.

14. A.L. Wilson. "PHARMIS: A National Pharmacy Workload and Productivity Reporting System." *Topics in Hospital Pharmacy Management* 7, no. 1 (1987): 65–72.

Reading 9–3

Rolling Budgets and Variance Reports

Steven A. Finkler

As hospitals move aggressively to reengineer themselves to meet present and future demands, the budget process should not be overlooked. Are there elements of the way budgeting is done that do not serve the organization well? What major or minor redesign would aid managers in the planning and control process? This article considers two innovations: (1) continuous or rolling budgets and (2) rolling variance reports.

Rolling budgets require managers to draft budgets one month at a time, as each month passes. That is, once April is over, managers begin planning a budget for April of the following year. The advantage is potentially more accurate and useful budget information.

Rolling variance information refers to the information contained in the variance reports provided to managers. Generally, these reports relay information on the month just ended as well as year-to-date information. After the year is half over, year-to-date information reports on 6 months' worth of activity. However, at the end of the first month of the year, such reports provide information on only a cumulative total of 1 month. This brings into question the purpose of a cumulative variance report and whether there is a better approach.

Source: Reprinted from Steven A. Finkler, "Rolling Budgets and Variance Reports," *Hospital Cost Management and Accounting,* Vol. 7, No. 3, June 1995, pp. 1–4. Copyright 1995, Aspen Publishers, Inc.

ROLLING BUDGETS

The concept of a rolling budget is not new; however, health care organizations have not widely used this technique. As financial pressures on hospitals continue to increase, it is likely that greater managerial attention will have to be paid to improving the accuracy of budgets. Hospital profit margins have become too slim to allow room for error. The better the budget projection is, the smaller the differences between the budget and the actual results and the better off the hospital will be.

Under a continuous budgeting system, four problems exist common to budgeting: (1) accuracy, (2) time management concerns, (3) attitudes toward the budget process, and (4) improved decision-making ability.

ACCURACY

It is difficult to recall all of the events that occurred in a month that passed more than a half year ago. Yet, that is what is asked of all managers when they make up a budget for a year at a time. For example, assume that the hospital's fiscal year coincides with the calendar year. The budget for the year beginning in January might be prepared during October and November, with final approval in December.

By October, it is difficult to remember the July just past, let alone April or January. Memory dims with the passage of time. What was typical that occurred in January? What was atypical? Was there a flu outbreak among hospital staff? Was there a major traffic accident? Was there an unusual amount of snow and ice?

When budgeting is done only once a year, any outliers that occurred during the year tend to be treated as the norm. The once-in-20-years event becomes the basis for next year's budget. This assumes that the once-in-20-years event will happen 2 years in a row.

With annual budgeting, months start to run together, with July and August seeming very much alike. However, if managers could prepare a budget for next July just as soon as they have finished reconciling the variance report for the July just gone by, the chances are that the budget they prepare will be a far more accurate reflection of the events that typically happen in July.

TIME MANAGEMENT

Traditional budgeting creates a serious disruption in work patterns. By doing budgeting once a year, an intense effort must be made all at one time, and other regular activities must be set aside. Decisions that have to be made the same month the budget is prepared are generally made with less time and attention than would otherwise be the case. Cramming most of the budget work into a short time frame creates a crisis atmosphere that is not conducive to rational, thoughtful decision making.

The rolling approach suggests that one or two days be spent each month by each manager on the issue of budget planning. Instead of becoming a 2-or 3-week disruption in routine, planning can become part of the routine. Managers can be in more control of their jobs when the budget task is spread out over a longer period.

ATTITUDES TOWARD THE BUDGET PROCESS

Most people hate budgeting. The whole process tends to be associated with a variety of unpleasant events. Managers often ask for resources and are not given the resources they have requested. The process is a heavy burden in a rushed environment.

Cutting the proportions of the task down to size by requiring a smaller, although more frequent, effort can make the entire process less burdensome. By reducing the time crunch associated with budgeting, the process can only become less onerous, and managers will not enter the process with a negative attitude. If managers perceive budgeting not as an overwhelming disruption in their job, but as a normal routine part of it, there is likely to be a better effort and result.

DECISION-MAKING ABILITY

One of the great benefits of budgeting is that managers can make better decisions if they can plan for the future. When managers have a full-year horizon for decision making, they can purchase quantities at volume discounts, negotiate flexible delivery dates, and have time to shop around. Supplies can be ordered at lower prices with 6 months of lead time, instead of being acquired at high prices as rush orders are placed at the last minute.

With the general annual approach to developing operating budgets, the horizon is about 14 months when the budget is first developed. There is some perspective on the last 2 months of the current year, and the full 12 months of the coming year.

What happens as time passes? The horizon gets shorter and shorter. By the middle of the year, the perspective extends for only 6 months. By the last quarter of the year managers are suffering severe myopia. The efficiency of decision-making decreases. Decisions that would be made easily in early July must be postponed if they arise in October, because the manager lacks information about future expectations. With a rolling budget, a perspective of about a year is always maintained, and managers never suffer from a creeping myopia that gradually paralyzes their decision-making ability.

FINALIZATION

With continuous budgeting, would managers have to seek board approval every month as a new budget is developed for a month 1 year in the future? That would be unlikely. It would be more practical to simply accumulate the monthly budgets and consolidate them at the time an annual budget is normally prepared. This allows managers the benefit of monthly budgets prepared while vital information is still fresh in their mind. At the same time, the passage of time allows for rethinking the information and for modification, adjustment, or correction as new information comes to light.

By budgeting far in advance, managers can mull things over in their mind. Perhaps the budget relies on an assumption that can be changed. In the normal budget rush, there is little time to reflect and find ways to improve. Once the budget is approved, there is less pressure to find ways to reengineer the system. Rolling budgets reduce the likelihood that budgets are based on rushed decisions. Finally, the sum of the monthly budgets, revised based on what was learned throughout the year, can be presented for approval by the board.

ROLLING VARIANCE REPORTS

The monthly variance reports managers receive naturally provide information on the actual costs and budget for the month just past. Often these reports also include year-to-date information. Such information can be extremely valuable in getting a sense of how things are coming out for the year as a whole. Part of the reason for cumulative reports is to enable the manager to smooth out some imperfections in the reporting system. Perhaps supplies are reported when acquired rather than when used. For any 1 month this can cause a severe distortion. Over time, however, it should even out. Another reason for cumulative reports is to help managers determine whether there is a growing problem. A variance for 1 month may not be a problem. If the variance repeats, it causes greater concern.

The potential problem with cumulative reports is a situation similar to that described above as creeping myopia, only in reverse. Halfway through the year the cumulative variance report tells a lot about how the year is going. If there is a blip in the current month, it can be put into perspective by considering the year to date as a whole. What happens, however, when just 1 month has gone by? There is no history to use to put the month into context.

INVESTIGATION OF VARIANCES

When should a manager investigate a variance? In many situations, a variance of $100 over budget will be deemed too small to worry about. How about $200? How about $500? At some point the variance is so large that the manager will clearly feel a need to try to determine its cause. The number, however, is rarely absolute.

Some $300 variances might be investigated. However, probably all $300 variances would not be investigated. If spending was under budget by $300 for 1 month and then over by $300 the next, it might be deemed to be a random variation around the budget. On the other hand, if spending was $100 over, then $200 over, then $300 over, the last variance of $300 becomes much more significant. A pattern is developing that may get much worse if left unchecked. The manager could handle this by graphing variances to show ups and downs and trends.

Some hospitals do generate variance charts, showing graphs of variances over time. Unfortunately, most of those graphs are similar to the variance report itself. At the end of the first month of the year, the only information shown is one data point. Whether the trending information is graphed or shown on the report, if all that is shown is the current month and the cumulative year-to-date, the graph or report does a poor job providing the manager with the information needed to see this trend developing.

A better solution is a rolling variance report. Such a report would focus on the current month and the prior 3 months. Those prior months could be shown in aggregate or in average, but it would be more informative to show the value for each of the 3 months preceding the 1 month just past. As each month passes, the oldest month is dropped from the report. The key is to dissociate this reporting process from the fiscal year. From a perspective of departmental control, the process can continue, without having to start over with each new fiscal year.

For most managerial purposes throughout the year, information is needed about recent trends. What happened 9 or 10 months ago is not relevant to current problems that may be out of control and need correction. By the same token, why should a manager be deprived of historical information from 1 or 2 months ago, just because those months were in a prior fiscal year? It makes little sense to blind a manager in January (assuming a calendar fiscal year), just because a new year has begun. The variance report should show October through December information, for comparison with the January that has just passed.

REPORT FORM

What are the implications of this concept? Should year-to-date information be eliminated from variance reports? That is one possibility. For most variance reports, if it were possible to include either year-to-date or rolling quarterly information, most managers would vote for the rolling information. It is preferable to manage from a base of recent history than one of varying history ranging from just the current month through 12 months.

This is not to say that cumulative year-to-date information is not of interest. The organization is certainly interested in how close spending for the budgeted year will come to the budget. That is an important concern. However, that concern should not interfere with the ability of managers to control what is happening in their responsibility center. Organizations should strive to give their managers the best information possible with which to manage their departments.

This topic ties in closely with a broader concern of the usefulness of computer-generated reports in hospitals. Over time, reports outlive their usefulness. Circumstances change and the types of information needed change as well. Hospitals need to periodically survey people receiving reports to find out whether the reports are useful. It is important to ask, "What would you like to know, if we could generate any information you would like?" At times, it may turn out that there is more useful information that could be provided at no higher cost. Rolling quarterly variance information is one such example.

Reading 9–4

Statistical Cost Control: A Tool for Financial Managers

Terrance R. Skantz

The Medicare prospective payment system (PPS) is forcing hospital managers to reexamine their methods of cost control. Since PPS provides the same payment for any case classified in a given diagnosis-related group (DRG), this becomes a natural unit of analysis. In other words, cost control techniques will revolve around each of the 467 DRGs specified by PPS. One can expect that cost accounting techniques will be revised to provide information useful to managers in pinpointing areas that need investigation.[1] Statistical cost control is an excellent candidate for enhancing the success of the financial manager's control of resource utilization.

COST CONTROL AND CRITICAL VARIABLES

It is well recognized that success in any business endeavor depends largely on careful monitoring and controlling of critical variables. For example, in pharmaceutical firms, finding new products (drugs) is critical. Thus, careful monitoring of research, development, and clinical testing is essential.

In cost control situations, the problem is to identify the key variables that trigger cost incurrence. Two critical variables in a hospital setting are (1) patient days and (2) ancillary services.

Source: Reprinted from Terrance R. Skantz, "Statistical Cost Control: A Tool for Financial Managers," *Hospital Cost Accounting Advisor,* Vol. 2, No. 4, September 1986, pp. 1–5. Copyright 1986, Aspen Publishers, Inc.

These variables deserve careful monitoring by financial managers. It will be necessary to set standards or targets for these two variables for each DRG. Depending on the volume of cases for a given DRG, weekly or monthly reports comparing actual with standard performance should be prepared. Although this paper focuses on patient days as a critical variable, the same cost control method applies to any factor that can be classified by DRG or any other relevant unit of analysis.

INVESTIGATION OF DEVIATIONS FROM STANDARD

A key question facing financial managers is whether to investigate deviations from the targets or standards. It is costly to conduct investigations. The time of the financial manager and other personnel is a valuable commodity. It will not be cost effective to investigate all departures from standard. Some method of choosing significant deviations is necessary. Three methods are possible: (1) judgment of the financial manager, (2) an arbitrary rule such as "investigate any deviation in excess of 10 percent from standard," and (3) statistical control, a method based on the statistical behavior of the critical variable for the DRG in question.

Judgment Approach

This method requires the manager to have an intimate knowledge of each DRG. He or she would have to know if a deviation from standard is large enough to justify investigation or whether it arises from a normal situation. It is quite unlikely the manager will have this knowledge, since the DRG classification system is new, and the financial manager will have little prior experience. Indeed, as discussed in a later section, the first step in the application of the statistical cost control method is to determine the range within which the critical variable should fall under acceptable operating conditions.

Arbitrary Rule

This method probably suffers from more drawbacks than the judgment approach. It will be demonstrated later that equal deviations from standard for a critical variable may require different responses for different DRGs. Thus, a single arbitrary rule could be inferior to a judgment approach. Multiple arbitrary trigger points, e.g., 10 percent for some DRGs and 5 percent for others, is simply the judgment approach but with fewer options. Unless there is some prior experience, there is no basis for setting the cutoff points.

Statistical Cost Control

Common sense indicates that different DRGs will exhibit different frequency distributions for the values of the critical variable and that the size of the deviation from standard necessary to trigger an investigation will differ as a result. This is exactly what the statistical method takes into account. Discussed below are the two steps involved when using this method. First, one must provide a statistical description of the acceptable or "in-control" distribution of the critical variable (length of stay). Second, current results are monitored through a sampling procedure and compared with the in-control distribution in order to decide whether to investigate.

Describing the Acceptable Distribution

As a starting point, the financial manager must describe the acceptable average (or standard)

length of stay for each DRG category as well as the acceptable variation around this average. Data from a representative period, possibly the most recent six months, should be used for this phase. It is very important that only properly classified cases be included in the analysis, since the results must be representative of the DRG in question.

Table 9–4–1 demonstrates how one calculates the necessary statistics. The number of cases is small, only for illustration. As shown in equation 1, the mean (or average) length of stay for the five cases is 2.20 days. This mean, denoted $\overline{X}$, is the standard length of stay for this DRG.

Next, a valid measure of acceptable dispersion is needed. For statistical reasons, it is assumed that the typical cost control situation will involve finding the average length of stay for all cases (a sample) during some monitor period and comparing this sample average with the standard length of stay.[2] In these cases, the appropriate measure of dispersion is the standard error of sample means, not the standard deviation of the sample.

The calculation of standard error is shown in two steps.[3] First, the standard deviation is found by subtracting the mean from each case (Table 9–4–1, column c), squaring this difference, and summing these squared deviations (column d). Then, as shown in equation 2, an average of these deviations is found by dividing by one less than the original number of cases. The square root of this average is the standard deviation. Second, as shown in equation 3, the standard error is found by dividing the standard deviation by the square root of the sample size. Notice that during the analysis phase, one might find that the mean and dispersion are simply unacceptable. For the time being, however, we are taking these as measures of acceptable performance.

Table 9–4–2, Part A, provides a more realistic set of statistics for two DRGs. The mean length of stay, 1.376 days for DRG 159 and 3.695 days for DRG 160, is the goal or standard for these DRGs. The standard error is .356 days for DRG 159 and .739 days for DRG 160. The larger the standard error, the more dispersion we can ex-

Table 9–4–1 Calculation of Mean and Standard Deviation

(a) Patient	(b) (X) Length of Stay	(c) (X – X̄) Deviation from Mean	(d) (X – X̄)²
1	1.5	–.70	.49
2	2.4	+.20	.04
3	3.0	+.80	.64
4	2.3	+.10	.01
5	1.8	–.40	.16
Total	11.0	0	1.34

Equation 1.

$$\text{Mean} = \overline{X}$$
$$= \text{Sum of Observations/Numbers of Observations}$$
$$= 11.0/5$$
$$= 2.20$$

Equation 2.

Standard Deviation $= S$

$$= \sqrt{(X - \overline{X})^2 / (\text{Number of Observations} - 1)}$$
$$= \sqrt{1.34/(5-1)}$$
$$= .58$$

Equation 3.

Standard Error $= s_e$

$$= \text{Standard Deviation} / \sqrt{\text{Number of Observations}}$$
$$= .58 / \sqrt{5}$$
$$= .259$$

Table 9–4–2 Statistics for Length of Stay (Patient Days)

		DRG 159	DRG 160
Part A:	Test Period:		
	Mean (Standard), X̄	1.376	3.695
	Standard Error, s_e	.356	.739
Part B:	Monitor-Period:		
	Sample Average	2.090	4.409
	Deviation from Standard	.714	.714

two standard errors of the mean. For DRG 159, this implies that approximately 95 percent of all cases require a stay between .664 and 2.088 days from admission to dismissal, or a range of 1.424 days. For DRG 160, however, the range is 2.956 days (2.217 to 5.173). Of course, the area represented by any other range of length of stay is also known from standard statistical tables.

If this average and deviation are acceptable, then it follows that a 20 percent deviation from the standard length of stay for DRG 159 (or .275 days) is more likely than a 20 percent deviation for DRG 160 (or .739) days. For DRG 159, a .275 day deviation is equal to 77 percent of one standard error (.275/.356 = .77) while a deviation of .739 days for DRG 160 is equal to one standard error.

pect for a given DRG. More specifically, the standard error is a measure of expected dispersion in sample averages around the mean length of stay and provides a statistical basis for judging if a deviation from the standard (mean length of stay) is unusual.

Since sample averages are normally distributed,[4] the standard error and the mean length of stay allow us to describe completely the variable's distribution. Figure 9–4–1 illustrates why this is true. The familiar bell-shaped (or normal) distribution has 95.44 percent of the area within

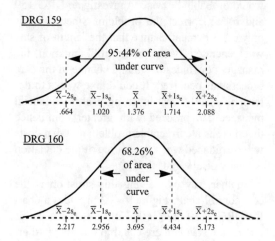

DRG 159

DRG 160

Figure 9–4–1 Distribution of Length of Stay When Conditions Are Under Control

Comparison of Actual to Standard Performance

The problem facing the financial manager is to decide whether a deviation from standard is due to random events or if there has been a real change in the process of caring for patients. A random deviation is due to the nature of the DRG. (The standard error measures in statistical terms this expected, unalterable dispersion.) On the other hand, an undesirable shift or change in the care process that increases the length of stay should be investigated and corrected.

Knowledge of the mean and standard error for a DRG gives the manager a rational basis for this investigation decision. Consider the case shown in Part B of Table 9–4–2, where there was an equal departure from standard for both DRGs during the monitor period. For DRG 159, the deviation is slightly *more than two* standard errors above the expected value of 1.376. The chance of a deviation this large or larger is about 2.3 percent *if things are running correctly*. This is the percent of the area under the distribution in Figure 9–4–1 to the right of the value 2.088. For DRG 160, the deviation is slightly *less than one* standard error above the expected value. The chance of a deviation this large or larger is approximately 16 percent.

A manager with limited time and resources would probably be wise to investigate DRG 159 and try to correct the problem. Since there is only a 2.3 percent chance that the length of stay was generated by an "in-control" situation, the manager concludes that a real change in the care process has occurred. It could take weeks to determine exactly what is wrong. But the financial manager can proceed with greater confidence that there is a correctable problem and that costs will be reduced when the source of the deviation is finally discovered.

Another way of viewing this situation is the cost control chart. Figure 9–4–2 provides a chart for DRGs 159 and 160. Notice that the bands around the standard are equal to one standard error. The upper and lower limits are set by the financial manager based on his or her judgment.

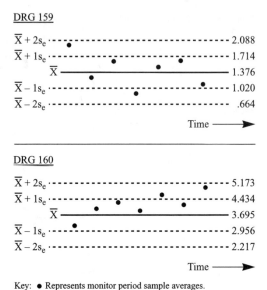

Key: • Represents monitor period sample averages.

Figure 9–4–2 Cost Control Charts

For example, the policy may be that any observation outside of two standard errors requires an investigation. The fact that there are lower as well as upper limits emphasizes that both negative and positive performance deserves investigation. Positive performance would be encouraged and could lead to a new lower standard and probably a new standard error.

An advantage of the control chart is that it allows the manager to track the performance over time. Trends might be revealed. Truly random deviations should be scattered around the standard. A trend up or down may signify a slow shift in the patient care process. Intervention may be necessary in these cases even though the pre-set limits have not been exceeded. Figure 9–4–2, for example, reveals a random scatter over time for DRG 159 but shows a disturbing upward trend for DRG 160. Notice that even with statistical methods, professional judgment is still critical.

COSTS AND BENEFITS OF ALTERNATIVES

Statistical cost control is a method for rationalizing one aspect of the financial manager's decision process. It provides an excellent basis for serious cost control/monitoring. After time, however, one additional consideration might be included in the analysis—the question of costs and benefits associated with the decision alternatives at hand.

For example, the cost of not investigating deviations (allowing them to continue) is the additional costs associated with excessively long patient stays. The hospital would need to know how costs are affected by patient days. (This illustrates why one chooses a "critical" variable for analysis, i.e., a variable tied closely to cost incurrence.) Thus, a cost-effective investigation policy would tend to investigate relatively small deviations if the cost of serving a patient day is high. A successful investigation would eliminate these high costs. Setting an effective investigation policy based on cost-benefit and statistical considerations is very complex. Most hospitals would probably find the simpler statistical model prefer-

able, since it will be much easier to implement. Once this technique was fully operational, additional cost-benefit factors could be incorporated.

NOTES

1. See Victor C. Messmer, "Standard Cost Accounting: Methods That Can Be Applied to DRG Classifications," *Healthcare Financial Management,* January 1984, pp. 44–48.

2. If the investigation decision is made on a case-by-case basis, certain assumptions about the distribution of the critical variable are necessary. These assumptions are liable to be unrealistic. The use of sample averages rather than case-by-case results avoids these assumptions.

3. Computer packages are readily available to calculate all the statistics discussed in this paper.

4. The size of the sample must be large, around 30 cases, for the normal distribution to hold. Smaller samples use the t-distribution, which approaches a normal distribution as the sample size increases.

10

Management Control

Reading 10–1

Developing a Planning and Control System for a Responsibility Unit

Steven A. Finkler

As hospitals diversify more and more, they are creating a wide variety of new responsibility units. The basic conditions that existed many years ago have changed. As a result, the systems in place for controlling the operations of routine hospital departments may not be the most appropriate systems for controlling all responsibility units. This article discusses some of the key issues to be considered in designing control systems for such units.

The role of a planning and control system is to help the manager responsible for the system to make appropriate plans for that unit as a part of the whole, and to control operations in such a way as to keep as closely to an approved plan as possible. A well-developed system should be able to generate better plans and decisions as well as to improve managerial actions during the year. Such a system should help the unit and its manager act in the best interests of the organization.

According to Dermer, a planning and control system should "(l) arouse the managers so that they are motivated to contribute to the organization's mission; (2) guide the appropriate behavior by constraining or influencing them as required; (3) help them accomplish the task requirements by either drawing attention to or helping them solve problems of planning, decision making, and controlling their sphere of responsibility; (4) provide a fair basis for evaluation; and (5) develop in them the capacity to learn and to do more. And, if the process is to be adaptive, feedback from the key variables measured must provide the input for system adaptation and evolution." [Jerry Dermer, *Management Planning and Control Systems,* Homewood, Ill.: Irwin, Inc., 1977, p. 176.]

Dermer's approach to achieve those goals for a planning and control system is based upon a series of factors that should be considered by the system's designer:

- the strategic mission of the organization
- the expectations for the responsibility unit
- the causal factors that influence success
- the key variables for the unit
- a normative system that can plan for and control the key variables
- the system gap
- organizational constraints and resources
- implementation
- evaluation based on feedback and redesign

Source: Reprinted from Steven A. Finkler, "Developing a Planning and Control System for a Responsibility Unit," *Hospital Cost Accounting Advisor,* Vol. 2, No. 12, May 1987, pp. 1, 6–7. Copyright 1987, Aspen Publishers, Inc.

Each of these factors will be discussed.

Obviously, the hospital's mission must be the starting point. Perhaps one of the key management weaknesses in hospitals is that personnel are promoted from clinical positions in a responsibility unit to management positions without hearing a discussion of the hospital's mission. It is often taken for granted that they know the mission; yet a clinician's view of the obligations, responsibilities, and goals of the organization may differ substantially from the perception of the hospital's board and top management.

A difficulty in designing a control system around the hospital's mission is that the stated mission of the hospital may well not be in terms of specific quantifiable measures. However, since hospitals tend to measure their success in quantifiable terms—revenue growth, profits, patients treated, and so on, the measurable goals used in your hospital to evaluate its overall success should be considered in designing the system of each individual unit within the hospital.

This leads into the issue of understanding the expectations the hospital has for the specific responsibility unit under consideration. In order to design a system to control the behavior of a unit in a manner that the hospital will find desirable, it is first necessary to determine exactly what behavior the hospital would find desirable. Is the unit supposed to be making a profit? Is it supposed to be capturing a growing share of the market? Is it supposed to generate high levels of patient satisfaction? Obviously the objectives will vary substantially from unit to unit. A new venture may be aimed at making profits. On the other hand, an admissions department will never generate a profit, so we must find other measures of the adequacy of its performance.

The next step in the design process is to determine the causal factors that influence the success of the unit. Causal factors are the elements which impact on a key result we hope to accomplish. For some units, dollars spent on advertising result in increased revenues and increased profits. Thus, the advertising budget would be a causal factor. But we could certainly think of responsibility centers where advertising would have little direct impact on the results of the unit.

The causal variables are often financial in nature—advertising, pay rates, bonuses; but often they are not directly financial. For example, a participatory system for a unit may increase employee job satisfaction to the point of lower turnover, resulting in lower costs. Thus issues such as the participatory setup are relevant financial management concerns, not because they are inherently financial, but because they ultimately impact on the hospital's costs of operation.

Nor do we always maximize a causal variable. For example, the amount of labor input may have a causal affect on quality, and quality may affect our reputation, which in turn affects admissions. Yet there will be a limit on the amount of labor we use, as a point of diminishing returns is reached, with the extra inputs costing more than the various benefits they generate.

Once we have a perspective on what the hospital is trying to accomplish, and what it would like a specific unit to accomplish, the causal variables can be used to establish a set of key variables for the unit. Key variables (discussed at length in *Hospital Cost Accounting Advisor,* Vol. 1, No. 6) are the most important of the causal variables. It is these variables that require planning and the highest levels of control.

The key variables are those that are measurable, that indicate critical elements in the unit's functioning, and that should be monitored to allow quick action to correct an out-of-control situation. There is some controversy over whether variables must be controllable to fit into the key variable category, but in many cases they need not be. For example, patient days and acuity are often not controllable by a nursing unit. However, they may be critical for staffing. If both patient days and acuity are falling, a nurse manager should be taking actions to reduce staffing and the associated costs. Thus, a control system would need to generate information about these variables on an extremely current basis.

As one can see, however, the focus of designing a system for a unit is first to determine the types of information that would be most useful for that unit, rather than simply supplying all units with generic information of varying levels of value to different units.

A normative system that can plan for and control the key variables represents an ideal. It is effectively the ideal system that would ensure available information about the key variables, perfect management to act in response to the information, and appropriate resources to carry out the system without glitches.

In reality, however, there will be a system gap, and it is quite important to recognize this in the system planning stage. The system gap is the difference between the ideal system and what is currently available. The difference between what currently exists and the normative ideal should be carefully evaluated. Only in that way can we move as close as possible to the ideal.

The movement toward the ideal is accomplished by considering organizational constraints and resources and redefining the system in light of them. In other words, a gap exists, and we need to see the impediments to removing the gap, as well as the resources available to us. The best possible control system, given the limitations of our organization, can be developed only if we establish an ideal system and back away from it, but only as much as is absolutely necessary.

Even the ideal system will be of little value to the unit and ultimately to the hospital unless it is implemented. The system as designed needs to have specific steps for implementation clearly laid out. Giving a system to a unit manager for implementation, without a detailed specific implementation plan, will probably result in key features of the plan never being implemented. The system will not work well as a control system, and the system itself, rather than the way it has been implemented, will be blamed. Therefore, it is vital that careful planning in developing a system not stop one step short. An implementation plan is essential to gain the benefits of the system design.

The final element in a planning and control system is feedback. Evaluation of how a system is working and redesign of the system are best done fairly soon after implementation. As time goes by, the system becomes an accepted part of life, whether it works well or poorly. The success of the system is vital in many respects. First of all, obviously, we want the system to work in the unit in which it has been installed. If it is not working properly when installed, this should be promptly corrected so that the unit can function in a controlled manner. Second, we want to evaluate the success of the planners. Systems to control the hospital's operations are crucial, and should be planned by people who can design and carry out a successful system. Third, we want to learn from our mistakes and plan future unit control systems better. Without a review of the success of our systems as we install them, we will simply repeat our mistakes over and over.

Reading 10–2

Cost Control Systems

Steven A. Finkler

All hospitals need to control costs. To help organize for such control, cost control systems can be invaluable. Barfield, Raiborn, and Dalton define a cost control system as "a logical structure of formal and/or informal activities designed to analyze and evaluate how well expenditures were managed during a period."[1] Such a system requires a specific management effort—first, to put it into place and then to monitor costs.

THE THREE STAGES OF COST CONTROL

There are three principal focal points for a cost control system: control before expenditures are made; control during the process of making an expenditure; and control after the expenditure has occurred. We can think of these three elements in terms of

- planning
- monitoring
- feedback

Planning: Before-the-Fact Control

Before-the-fact control entails the planning process. Its focus is on prevention of problems,

Source: Reprinted from Steven A. Finkler, "Cost Control Systems," *Hospital Cost Management and Accounting,* Vol. 3, No. 11, February 1992, pp. 1–5. Copyright 1992, Aspen Publishers, Inc.

rather than diagnosis or cure. In making plans for a hospital for the coming period of time, it is essential that managers focus specifically on the issue of cost control.

A focus on cost control means more than simply producing the smallest possible budget. If budget reduction is achieved by fiat—simply declaring that spending is reduced by 5 percent or 10 percent—the potential of cost control will probably not be achieved. It is more likely that there will be cost overruns.

Cost control must come about by management effort to determine places where one can reasonably spend less money. The item of expenditure that is being reduced must be identified, and the reasoning behind the assumption that the organization can live without that spending must be clear. That is why before-the-fact cost control efforts should begin before the annual budget process.

These cost control efforts should take place when managers can take some time to reflect on the way that services are provided, and can carefully assess the impacts of changes in operations. Budget time is a hectic period when new volume and patient mix information is often just translated into a new budget based on constant assumptions about the way that care is provided.

Before-the-fact planning for control of costs should not be limited to a focus on operations and budget preparation. It also requires specific input in the form of policies and specified objectives. In order to have managers make reasoned decisions about where costs can be cut and where they cannot, or even more pertinently, where they must be cut, managers must have specific organizational guidance. That guidance comes in the form of specific, well-communicated objectives, and specific formal policies. Such objectives and policies may be both quantitative and qualitative in nature.

Monitoring: Control during the Expenditure Process

All costs should be monitored as they take place. Hospitals tend to rely too heavily at times on variance reports, which are not generated until well after a result occurs. It is the job of managers to be aware of problems as they arise, and to take corrective action. In the majority of cases, by the time a significant controllable variance is reported on a management report, its cause should already have been corrected.

Managers must know that this is a direct part of their responsibility. In hospitals, with so many clinical managers, the primary focus is on the delivery of patient care. As a result, unfavorable budget variances are often dealt with only when necessary—certainly after the fact.

Hospitals need to train their management team that ongoing control will minimize unfavorable variances, and in the long run reduce the amount of effort needed, rather than increasing it. Putting a process back in control as soon as it slips out of control is easier than dealing with it after a long time period has elapsed. The result of such ongoing management is to ultimately make the managers' jobs easier, while saving the hospital resources.

Feedback: After-the-Fact Control

After-the-fact control relates to both the use of variance reports to identify quickly any problems that managers were unaware of and did not act to correct as they occurred. This form of control is also vital to the improvement of future plans and results. It constitutes the critical element of feedback.

In addition to being useful for controlling current expenditures, after-the-fact control forms the main basis for responsibility accounting. Managers are held accountable by a comparison of their expected results with those that actually occurred.

THE ROLE OF HUMAN BEINGS IN COST CONTROL SYSTEMS

It is apparent that cost control systems cannot work independently of the hospital's people. It will take changes in human behavior to make cost control a functioning, ongoing part of a hospital's management process. Barfield, Raiborn, and Dalton refer to this as a need for cost consciousness. In their words,

> Cost consciousness refers to a companywide attitude about the topics of cost understanding, cost containment, cost avoidance, and cost reduction. Individual employees, with similar goals and objectives, collectively compose the organization. The ways in which costs can be controlled by an organization inherently consider the set of attitudes and efforts of the individual employees of that organization.[2]

It is readily apparent that some of the "soft" areas of managing an organization are in fact essential. The development of team spirit and an atmosphere of community become essential if one is to create the attitudes needed to control costs.

There is no way to measure the financial benefits of a hospital employees' picnic. Nor is there any direct measure of the payback for dollars spent on most management development programs. However, there is a clear need for the hospital to design a set of programs that will instill in managers an understanding of the importance of cost control, and a desire to work for the organization to control costs.

The remainder of this article focuses on the concepts of cost understanding, cost containment, cost avoidance, and cost reduction.

COST UNDERSTANDING

In order to be able to control costs, managers must be able to understand them. Specifically, a major concern is whether managers have a good understanding of what costs are controllable, and what costs are not controllable, and of the things that are likely to cause the actual costs incurred to differ from expectations.

The most obvious causes of variations between a planned result and an actual result are changes in the work performed. If there are more patients, or sicker patients, or a different mix of the types of patients, that will impact on the cost of providing care. This assumes that some costs are variable, which is certainly the case. Hospitals should attempt to introduce flexible budgets that account for the volume of patients at a minimum. Over time hospitals should be attempting to enhance their systems by allowing them to flex for the type and acuity of patients, as well as number of patients.

In addition there are other factors that Barfield, Raiborn, and Dalton indicate can impact on an understanding of why costs might differ from expectations. These include cost changes as a result of unexpected inflation, the impact of technology, changes in supply and demand, changes in competition, changes due to seasonality, and changes in quantities purchased.

At this juncture, virtually all hospitals anticipate and plan for inflation. However, few are able to accurately prognosticate the exact impact of inflation for an organization or its departments. To the degree that inflation differs from expectations, it will be a culprit in skewing results away from plans. Of course, the most obvious and significant inflationary impact is if salary increases are granted that differ from those expected when budgets were prepared.

Hospitals are among the organizations most significantly impacted by technology change. To some extent this can be anticipated and planned for. On the other hand, some changes are so dramatic and rapid that they distort the results for the current period as compared to the plan. Managers should develop an attitude of examining each element of new technology to determine if it can in some way reduce costs. Often technology is simply a cost add-on, while the existence of the technology might allow for revisions in operating procedures that would allow for cost savings.

Supply and demand are economic concepts that certainly do affect hospitals. Prices charged for care may often not move in direct relation to the laws of supply and demand. Often, however, the prices the hospital pays for the things it acquires do change in such proportion. This is seen clearly in the cost of hospital workers. In some parts of the nation the worst of the nursing shortage has passed. In other areas there has been and continues to be a shortage of all health workers. Changes in the supply of workers, for better or worse, can have a dramatic impact on actual costs.

The health care industry has been growing increasingly competitive. Hospitals must contend not only with price pressure from HMOs and PPOs, but also with competition from clinics and free-standing surgery centers. Changes in competition should be anticipated to the extent possible. However, often there are unexpected surprises, and these may require a response from the hospital. Even if the hospital chooses not to respond, the actions of the competitor may have an impact on the volume or costs of the hospital.

Seasonality is a problem that hospitals are familiar with and tend to plan for. Hospitals are adept at knowing how many and what types of patients are likely to arrive at different times of the year. Are they equally adept at having maintenance done on equipment when it is relatively likely to be less needed? Are there formal schedules to take advantage of purchases that may be cheaper at certain times of the year? Seasonality presents a definite opportunity for cost control if managers understand its nature, and how it can impact on costs.

Quantity purchasing presents the opportunity to gain price discounts. Most hospitals will formally consider that in doing their inventory planning. But plans do go awry when something is needed on a rush basis. In those cases, given the life and death nature of hospitals, immediate, high-priced orders are often placed. Such events are likely to occur. Does the hospital have a policy regarding how large an order should be made when a rush order is placed? If the rush order includes only the specific needed item, it adds one additional purchase. If the rush order can be combined with the next scheduled normal purchase, it may only move up the date of an order, rather than adding an extra one.

The concept is that by thinking about control of costs, one can start to develop additional specific areas where costs can be controlled. In order to do that, managers must take the time to understand costs, and their behavior, to the greatest possible extent.

COST CONTAINMENT

The concept of cost containment is that increases in costs over time are constrained to the greatest degree possible. It should become a clear mission in each department to focus on each element of cost, and to plan on how the cost of that item can be prevented from increasing over time, or kept to the minimum possible increase.

There is often a presumption that if inflation is 5 percent, it is only fair and reasonable to allow budgets to rise by that amount. Such presumptions are responsible for unneeded increases in costs. Many costs of a hospital are fixed. For a relatively new building, the depreciation cost for the building itself is unlikely to increase. A presumption of a 5 percent hospitalwide cost increase would be unwarranted. Similarly, if the hospital has outstanding a substantial amount of long-term debt at a fixed interest rate, those costs would not automatically increase each year.

The same logic holds true within departments. The fact that most costs may go up each year

does not justify an assumption that all costs will rise. By granting across-the-board inflation increases, the organization is allowing each department to find some ways to expand their overall consumption of resources, without explicit justification.

On the contrary, some costs might be expected to decline each year. A manager's need for an administrative library may decline after the first few years in which a library is initially built. A department that allows a certain amount per employee for attending seminars may find that at some point it is cheaper to bring speakers to the hospital, rather than sending staff to meetings. Thus, overall training costs might be expected to hold steady or decline at some point.

Competition at times creates difficult situations for hospitals. At other times, however, it can create advantageous situations. Competition among hospital suppliers can lead to cost reductions, as price wars break out among the suppliers. Often the hospital can only take advantage of such competition by periodically pricing-out alternative suppliers.

As with understanding costs, the constraint of costs requires managers to allocate time to think about the issue of cost constraint. Managers must attack this problem at a time of the year when they can review each element of their operations and fully understand why some costs do rise over time, and why some costs might not have to rise over time.

COST AVOIDANCE

While cost containment focuses on stemming the increase in costs, cost avoidance requires managers to innovatively find ways to totally avoid spending money on some things. This is harder than simply identifying things that should not go up in cost. It requires the absolute elimination of spending on certain proposed items.

The only way to accomplish cost avoidance is with a critical review of every proposed expenditure, and a requirement that managers be able to justify the benefit received from each and every new expenditure. Not only should one be able to justify the proposed expenditure, but also to explain that there is no adequate, less expensive alternative.

Once a cost is added to a department, it becomes very difficult to eliminate. An enhancement that is nice, but that the hospital has survived for years without, becomes an inviolate essential once it has been added. Since cost reduction is the most difficult aspect of cost control, it is best to avoid costs in the first place until there is a truly pressing reason why the hospital must incur them.

COST REDUCTION

As noted above, cost reduction is probably the most difficult aspect of cost control. It is easily accepted by most managers that they must understand the behavior of costs. Cost containment—restraining the increase in costs—is something that all managers realize they must face. Cost avoidance is unpleasant, but every manager has had resource requests denied. Cost reduction, however, asks the managers of the hospital to actually find ways to make do with fewer resources.

How can a department use fewer hours of staff time per patient? How can it absolutely reduce the amount of electricity used? Is there a way to save water by shifting to restricted flow shower heads?

Cost reduction often focuses on personnel. Can the organization get by with fewer people? In most manufacturing concerns, there is a fairly direct engineered relationship between inputs and outputs. It takes just so much labor to build a certain type of machine. Hospitals are faced by a much greater challenge. There are no clearly defined appropriate amounts of labor needed for patient care.

Yet that does not justify long-time assumed relationships in terms of required personnel. As the practice of medicine keeps changing over time, there must be a continuing reassessment of how to do things differently, better, and at less cost.

One of the most difficult aspects of cost control is being tough-minded. In organizations such as hospitals, especially, it is attitude that often determines which costs cannot be avoided and which can be. On the other hand, being overly tough-minded can result in deteriorating morale. As discussed earlier, the human element is critical to the cost control equation. Cost cutting is not ruthlessness. Rather it is rational behavior in a world of competition and limited resources. Progress must constantly be made.

Managers should be trained to perceive the need for such control of costs. Unless a unified commitment from managers is made for a cost control system, attempts at cost containment, cost avoidance, and especially cost reduction are doomed to fail.

THE ROLE OF MANAGEMENT

The issue of cost control systems should make clear to every manager that it takes a lot of time to manage well. Managers can manage efficiently only if they allocate their scarcest commodity, time, carefully.

The role of management is not to do the routine, or repetitive. Managers' greatest contribution is in the area of making decisions, and doing the out-of-the-ordinary. Time must be devoted to determining how to change the current equilibrium, rather than how to maintain it.

In order for a cost control approach to be successful, managers clearly must devote a lot of time to examining, questioning, justifying, and challenging how and why money is spent in their department. One of the most difficult challenges faced by any hospital is to convince their managers to develop an approach to management that allows enough time for these activities, which require thought.

Changing the status quo is difficult. It is much easier to simply sign vacation approvals, and review purchase requisitions, than to critically review the ways things have always been done.

One must force oneself to set aside the time to take on that difficult process. But it is essential to do this for significant cost control gains, and hospitals must convey that essential nature to all of their managers.

NOTES

1. J. Barfield, C. Raiborn, and M. Dalton, *Cost Accounting: Traditions and Innovations,* West Publishing Company, New York, 1991, p. 523.
2. Ibid.

Reading 10–3

Competitive Pricing Models for Intra-Hospital Services

James D. Suver

The increased emphasis on *bottom line* results of health care providers is forcing managers to consider internal profit center concepts to improve performance. An internal profit center approach encourages managers to maximize the difference between revenues and expenses for individual departments. This approach is generally effective for services sold outside the hospital. However, dysfunctional results can occur when services are provided between hospital profit centers. What happens, for example, when a lab sells services to internal and external profit centers, when a hospital-owned HMO is evaluated as a profit center, or when a free-standing clinic is owned by the hospital? Should there be a lower price for internal users or should all services be priced based upon full cost? The price established for the service would decidedly influence the profit and performance measurements reported. Consider what happens when physicians are treated as profit centers. The revenues received from the DRGs would be compared with the costs incurred in providing the services. The costs of the resources used by the physician would heavily influence the profit reported by him. In such cases, the impacted

Source: Reprinted from James D. Suver, "Competitive Pricing Models for Intra-Hospital Services," *Hospital Cost Accounting Advisor,* Vol. 1, No. 11, April 1986, pp. 1, 3–4. Copyright 1986, Aspen Publishers, Inc.

parties would have different outlooks on what would be a fair price. A faulty internal pricing policy can result in inefficient allocation of resources, poor motivational environment, and ineffective decision making.

Basically, a problem occurs when materials or services are *sold* between profit centers in the same organization. Each manager acting in his own best interest would like to pay the lowest price for purchased items and sell his output at the highest price. A pricing policy that recognizes this conflict is essential to effective decision making.

INTERNAL PRICING TECHNIQUES

In accounting technology, internal pricing techniques are categorized as *transfer pricing policies.* An effective transfer pricing policy maximizes goal congruence. "Goal congruence" refers to a process in which an individual maximizing his own gain also maximizes the gains to the organization. This is easier said than done. All of the various techniques that have been used have deficiencies. Each of the major pricing techniques will be discussed in detail in the next section.

COST-BASED PRICES

The most commonly used transfer price is one based on cost. This can be either a full cost or a variable cost. A cost-based approach does not provide a profit margin to the selling department. Clearly, a manager of a selling division who is evaluated on bottom-line performance does not like this kind of policy. However, there are more serious problems. Services that are provided at full cost provide no incentive to the selling department to control expenses. Since the selling department cannot make a profit, it can obtain a surrogate benefit by padding overhead costs. Cost control can be achieved only through careful budget analysis and strict expenditure controls. A full-cost transfer pricing policy can also lead to passing on inefficiencies and may create a noncompetitive price for the service.

The opposite of a full-cost pricing model is one based on variable costs. Variable costs are the out-of-pocket costs incurred in providing the service. Theoretically, the use of a variable-cost pricing model will lead to an optimal decision about whether to purchase a service internally or externally. Consider, for example, the decision on whether to provide a lab test internally or purchase it from a free-standing clinic. The relevant data are:

Internal Variable Costs	$ 8.00
Internal Full Cost	18.00
Free-Standing Clinic Price	15.00

Based on a full cost of $18, it would appear that the service should be purchased externally at $15.00. A profit center manager in the health care organization would clearly prefer to buy at $15 instead of $18. But what is the impact on the entire organization? The organization is now incurring out-of-pocket costs of $15 instead of only the $8 from using internal sources. This assumes the overhead costs would be incurred by the hospital in any case. The organization would seem to have a problem in "goal congruence." The individual manager, if he has a choice, will buy externally, yet the organization from a total bottom-line approach will be worse off. Other factors, such as capacity of the producing department or product quality, can also influence the decision. These will be discussed later in this article.

MARKET-BASED PRICES

If a competitive market price exists for the output of the producing department, this price can also be used for internal pricing decisions. The use of a market price fits quite well with the profit center concept and makes profit-based performance measurement appropriate for many departments in the health care provider.

In the previous example, the buying department would pay a maximum of $15 for the internal service. With the full cost at $18, the producing department must find ways to reduce its costs or show a negative bottom line. Even with the negative bottom line, the organization as a whole is better off if the purchase is internal. Use of a market price for all internal transfers would ensure that the final price would also reflect market conditions and that internal inefficiencies are not simply passed on to the cost of the product.

The use of a market-based internal price requires that certain policies govern actions between internal divisions:

- The buying department must buy internally when the producing department meets the market price and wants to sell internally.
- The buying department is free to purchase externally if the producing division does not meet the external price.
- The producing division can reject internal sales if the manager believes there are more profitable revenues to be earned externally.
- An impartial arbitration/appeal process must be established to resolve conflicts when they occur.

NEGOTIATED MARKET-BASED PRICES

In most cases, an external market price represents the maximum amount that a purchasing department should pay for an internal service. Because of reduced administrative costs, guaranteed volume, and other cost-avoidance aspects of internal purchasing, it may be possible to justify a lower price. In such cases, the best possible approach may be a negotiated market price, with the producing and purchasing departments agreeing on the price to be established.

A negotiated market price is also the best avenue to take when there is no external market price or when there is idle capacity in the producing division. In the case of the former, the producing division must receive a price that is sufficient to encourage it to offer the internal service. When there is idle capacity, the producing division should not expect to receive full market price. A price approaching the lower limit of the variable cost will more accurately reflect the opportunity cost of not selling the service.

Opportunity costs are usually defined as the potential benefit given up when one option is selected over another. For example, when a producing department is operating at full capacity, the selling of a service internally reflects the market price given up by not selling externally. When the producing department has excess or idle capacity, there are no lost external sales, and the only costs involved would be the incremental or variable costs of producing one more service.

GENERAL FORMULA FOR TRANSFER PRICING

In most cases, the formula for transfer pricing can be expressed as:

Transfer price = variable costs per unit of service + opportunity cost per unit of service on external sales.

Given the data used earlier, the following transfer prices could be calculated:

Variable Costs	$ 8.00
Internal Full Costs	18.00
Free-Standing Clinic Price	15.00
Opportunity Costs = 15 – 8 = 7	

Case 1—Producing department has no idle capacity.

Transfer price = 8 + 7 or $15.00

Case 2—Producing department has excess capacity.

Transfer price = 8 + 0 or $8.00

It is doubtful that the producing division would want to sell at this price, but from an overall hospital perspective, the $8 would be correct. A negotiated market price approach may be the most appropriate method in this case.

NO EXTERNAL MARKET SALES

For some services there may not be an external market. In these cases, the market price approach will not be effective. Some type of cost-based approach must be used if the profit center concept is to be used. Potential methods would include variable costs plus a contribution margin or variable costs plus a flat sum equal to a share of fixed costs.

In all cases, standard costs rather than actual costs should be used in the transfer price negotiations. This can at least prevent the automatic transfer of inefficiencies to the purchasing department.

The use of a profit center concept can lead to better decision making by pushing the decisions down to lower levels in the organization. This means that the transfer of services between internal profit centers results in a keen interest in the prices paid for such services. One manager's gain is another manager's loss. Therefore, an effective transfer pricing system must be established to award sub-optimization and maximize the overall provider's gain. The concepts explained in this article offer the opportunities to establish such a system.

Reading 10–4

Transfer Pricing in the Hospital-HMO Corporation

Kyle L. Grazier

More and more hospitals are reorganizing and restructuring their operations to include alternative delivery and financing systems. The most common expansion has been the ownership or operation of an HMO. The first article in this three-part series (*Hospital Cost Accounting Advisor* 1:10) discussed the issues involved in an effective cost accounting system and the identification of fixed and variable costs within such a corporate structure. In this article, transfer pricing of goods and services between the HMO and hospital will be addressed.

GOAL CONGRUENCE

Given the decentralization of decision making inherent in a restructured hospital-HMO delivery system, there are many opportunities for the transfer of goods and services, and thus "selling" and "buying" among profit centers of the organization. Difficulties often arise from dissatisfaction among the participating managers with regard to those transfers. Properly established transfer prices increase the probability that the incentives for the managers of each division—or in this case, the HMO and hospital—will coincide with the goals of the overall organization.

Source: Reprinted from Kyle L. Grazier, "Transfer Pricing in the Hospital-HMO Corporation," *Hospital Cost Accounting Advisor,* Vol. 1, No. 11, April 1986, pp. 1, 6–8. Copyright 1986, Aspen Publishers, Inc.

FINANCIAL ACCOUNTING ENTRIES

In discussing goals and managerial incentives, it is clear that it is the cost accounting and control focus that is of interest here, not financial accounting. It should be noted, however, that in accounting for the consolidated entity, "any goods and services transferred within the enterprise and not yet sold to outsiders should be carried at cost."[1] Thus, transfer prices in excess of cost must be eliminated when periodic consolidated financial statements for external financial reporting are prepared.

TRANSFER PRICING METHODS

From a managerial and cost control viewpoint, transfer prices need to be such that they give the manager an incentive to work in the overall organization's best interests. This will occur only if the price allows the manager's part of the overall organization to be financially successful. But setting proper transfer prices is easier said than done. There are several methods, each of which utilizes a different basis for calculation, but none is considered the one and only correct method. Each has its advantages and disadvantages, and the time required to utilize the various methods must be considered to determine the practicality of a particular method for the particular management situation. Pricing on the basis of full charges, variable costs, and market prices spans a wide range of sophistication, theories, and time. As in the determination of fixed and variable costs, the manager's assessment of appropriateness is far more critical than the numerical calculation.

To illustrate the different methods, consider the following data. Hospital X, an 800-bed teaching hospital, now charges third parties $400 per day for inpatient room and board services. The hospital averages 85 percent occupancy, with few Medicare patients and about 20 percent Medicaid patients. The financial manager has determined that approximately $50 of the $400 is fixed costs and $250, variable costs; $100 is profit. Another hospital nearby (Hospital Y) charges $350 per day to its private patients and a local HMO's patients.

The new HMO manager for Hospital X has determined that she will need 1,000 patient days over the first year of operation. Although the HMO is a wholly owned subsidiary of the hospital corporation, she must procure the lowest reasonable inpatient rates for her enrollees, regardless of source. This is required if she is to break even by year's end, and if the HMO's premiums are to be competitive with other plans in the area.

TRANSFER PRICING USING FULL CHARGES

Initially, the financial manager of the hospital is likely to suggest the use of full charges as the basis for the transfer price. Charges per unit of service or product are set, and do not require additional computation or management time.

Under the full charges method of transfer pricing, the hospital would charge the HMO $400, the same as for other third party payers. The hospital operations manager would benefit from the $400,000 in increased revenues as beds are filled by the HMO's patients, but the HMO manager would be foolish to accept Hospital X's rate when her performance appraisal is based on profits. Hospital Y's rates save her $50,000 per year in inpatient charges. Thus, the corporation may stand to lose the improved occupancy and

increased revenues to its hospital from its HMO due to the incongruence in objectives.

TRANSFER PRICING USING VARIABLE COSTS

Variable costs are commonly suggested as the basis for transfer prices in manufacturing, where there has been a longer history of setting variable and fixed costs than in hospitals and HMOs. As noted in the first article in this series (*Hospital Cost Accounting Advisor* 1:10), there are inherent difficulties in calculating the fixed and variable costs in health care systems in general. But even if variable costs could be identified more easily, as in some manufacturing settings, there are difficulties in using variable costs as a basis for transfer pricing. The problems are the same as in the use of full charges: incongruence in incentives.

The "buying" manager would be pleased by a price that excluded the associated fixed costs. In our sample setting, the HMO manager would pay only $250,000 for the needed 1,000 days. However, the "selling" or producing manager would not be able to cover the fixed costs of the product through the sale of the services; if evaluated on the basis of profits, he would surely seek another buyer who could at least recover the $50,000 in fixed costs, if not contribute to profits. The results of an improperly set transfer price would be seen in a corporation that fails to reduce inventory or fill its hospital's beds, with its HMO buying services from the competition.

TRANSFER PRICING USING MARKET PRICES

The most appealing theoretical basis for transfer prices is market prices. Under this system, the buying or selling manager would determine the going rates in the community for all transfer products. These rates then become the transfer prices between divisions in the corporation. Using the data provided here, the HMO manager would obtain a market price of $350 per day from Hospital X, and still purchase in-house. The hospital's financial manager would have made a profit. The corporation would have utilized unused capacity and improved the profits of its HMO.

How often prices are changed or which markets are included or excluded is subject to negotiation among the parties. Theoretically, the managers are content: if each were buying or selling at the perfect market price, then each would be indifferent as to whether the goods or services were being provided inside or outside the organization.

Market transfer prices are not, however, without their disadvantages. Few markets are perfectly competitive; often one seller or buyer can exert an inordinate influence on supply or demand in the market. Market prices also demand the manager's time, in that the market must be assessed as to not only the going prices, but also the comparability of the products. Finally, there must also be decisions on whether to use short-run or long-run market prices as a basis; the existence of "sale" prices can pose difficult decisions as to what time period to use to "average" the market prices.

OTHER ALTERNATIVES

There are other alternatives to setting transfer prices on the basis of charges, variable costs, or market prices. Full standard costs or a full cost plus some margin are sometimes used, although deficient in their resultant incentives. Standard variable costs as transfer prices have some advantage over full costs, but have the same disincentives for the producer manager as do variable transfer costs. Standard variable costs often are modified by adding a margin based on expectations of future demand rather than actual demand. Multiple transfer prices are another alternative; here a high price might be recorded in the supplier's accounts but a lower price in the buyer's account. The managers are able to meet management objectives but the corporation as a whole risks losing the cost controls in buying and selling that the cost accounting system was designed to address.

AN INITIAL ANALYSIS

While market prices appear to be the most appealing in their ability to properly motivate managers, they are costly in time and effort. Given these difficulties, it may be time-efficient to perform an initial analysis of the total outlay costs of a product, say a bed-day from the hospital, and the opportunity costs to the corporation of transferring the product internally.[2] The opportunity costs can be viewed as the foregone profits from charges received from other payers outside the corporation.

Accountants most often record only the outlay costs (approximated here by variable costs), but transfer prices need to accommodate the opportunity costs as well. In a perfect market, opportunity costs equal market price minus outlay costs. For example, if Hospital X has no excess capacity—operations are at 97 percent occupancy—and a perfect market exists, the transfer price of the bed-day would be the outlay costs ($250/bed) + market price ($400) – outlay cost ($250)—or in other words, the market price, $400. If there were excess capacity—with occupancy only 60 percent of its 800-bed capacity—there would be almost no opportunity costs of selling internally to the HMO. In this case, the outlay costs per unit—$250—would be the appropriate transfer price.

Two final points warrant comment. First, opportunity costs are not always known or calculable; there is seldom certainty that a hospital will have a paying client. They are estimates, and benefit from sensitivity analysis (to be discussed in the next article). Second, the outlay costs and the opportunity costs change depending on the volume of bed-days requested at any point in time by the HMO. The resultant market and transfer prices, in turn, are dependent upon volume, as well; this illustrates the need to have a schedule of transfer prices rather than one transfer price that ignores timing or volume.

It should be clear from this brief discussion that determining market prices and transfer prices can take considerable time. The value of that time depends, of course, on the extent to which goal congruence among various divisions and the corporation is required for effective functioning.

The energy exerted on development of an effective transfer pricing mechanism must be governed by the goals of the overall organization. Hospital-owned and operated HMOs offer new challenges to those responsible for the financial and managerial controls of the organization. Appropriate transfer prices can enhance or undermine the goals of the organization and its managers, and for that reason deserve considerable thought and attention.

NOTES

1. C.T. Horngren, *Cost Accounting, A Managerial Emphasis,* Fifth Edition, Englewood Cliffs: Prentice-Hall, Inc. 1982, p. 643.

2. Adapted from C.T. Horngren, *Cost Accounting, A Managerial Emphasis,* Fifth Edition, Englewood Cliffs: Prentice-Hall, Inc. 1982, p. 637.

Part III

Additional Cost Accounting Tools To Aid in Decision Making

In addition to the basics of cost accounting (Part I) and the essential tools for planning and control (Part II), there are a number of additional cost accounting tools which can be helpful in generating management information for decision making. Part III examines a number of those tools.

Chapter 11 considers ratios. Most financial managers are familiar with the use of ratio analysis for financial statement evaluation. However, financial statement data are not ideal. Even when prepared in accordance with Generally Accepted Accounting Principles, financial statements are notoriously poor at recording the impact of inflation and the value of intangible assets. Further, the impact of allowable alternative accounting principles reduces the comparability of ratios based on financial statement data. These limitations in the use of ratios by managers are discussed in Reading 11–1, "Ratio Analysis: Use with Caution."

Not all ratios have to be derived from financial statement information, however. Chapter 11 in the companion text, *Essentials of Cost Accounting for Health Care Organizations, Second Edition*,[1] examines the concept of cost accounting ratios. These are ratios that are calculated from

information not contained in the financial statements. Such ratios can access data that is more detailed and more useful than financial statement information. Readings 11–2 and 11–3 provide examples of cost accounting ratios.

Productivity measurement is the topic of Chapter 12. As the need for efficiency in the provision of health care services has increased, there has been a growing focus on productivity. The companion *Essentials* book discusses specific techniques for productivity measurement. However, as is the case in many areas of cost accounting, the human role is essential in productivity. It is the action of employees that determines, to a great extent, how productive the organization will be. An article by Newton Margulies and John Duval, Reading 12–1, considers a participative management approach to productivity. Such a tack is likely to have a greater chance of success than simply designing productivity tools and imposing their use.

Chapter 13 considers cost issues related to inventory. All health care organizations tend to have some inventory. While the amount held is much less significant than in many other industries, there are a number of important inventory issues in health care. One of the most important issues related to inventory is the decision of how much to buy at one time. This affects storage costs, ordering costs, capital and other costs. These issues are addressed in Reading 13–1, "In-

---

[1]Steven A. Finkler and David M. Ward, *Essentials of Cost Accounting for Health Care Organizations, Second Edition*, Aspen Publishers, Inc., Gaithersburg, MD, 1999.

ventory Management System Reaps Savings for Department."

Uncertainty is a problem for most health care organizations. Even using sophisticated forecasting and cost estimation techniques, we are unlikely to have a perfect prediction of the future. Chapter 14 addresses the problem with several tools aimed at improving decisions under conditions of uncertainty.

Readings 14–1 and 14–2 utilize decision analysis techniques to look at two very different problems. In Reading 14–1, Donald Chalfin considers a capital budgeting problem, in light of the uncertainty concerning the future number of patients to be treated. This article, "Decision Analysis and Capital Budgeting: Application to the Delivery of Critical Care Services," notes that "Decision analysis is based upon the explicit stipulation of all possible events along with their associated probabilities of occurrence." The article deals with the creation of a decision tree (outlining possibilities and their probabilities), expected value calculations, selection of the optimal alternative, and sensitivity analysis. The expected value technique is also employed in Reading 14–2, "Expected Value Technique Useful in HMO Negotiations." As the title indicates, this article focuses on getting the information needed to prepare appropriate price bids to use in managed care contracting.

In contrast, Reading 14–3 looks at a very different approach to decision making under uncertainty, linear programming. Linear programming is a mathematical technique (made relatively less complex with the use of computer software) that optimizes the value of an objective, subject to a variety of constraints. For example, a health care organization might be interested in maximizing the number of patients treated, while still making a profit of at least a certain amount. Or it might be interested in maximizing profits, as long as certain levels of services are maintained. In this article Jennifer Rosenberg explains the linear programming approach and provides an example.

The last decade has seen a revolution in the capabilities of computer systems. Chapter 15 considers information systems and cost accounting. Computerized cost accounting systems can be very costly. As health care organizations pour millions of dollars into new information systems, we should not lose our common sense. Information should never be collected if the cost of obtaining that data exceeds the value of the information. Reading 15–1 by Arthur Keegan considers issues related to the cost of cost accounting information systems.

Computerized cost accounting systems tend to be very complex. In some cases, however, even complex systems do not respond to the needs of managers throughout the organization. In addition to being concerned about cost, one must try to assure that the system will be responsive. This requires taking time before the system is designed to determine exactly what you want from the system. The design of new cost accounting systems is discussed by Randall Stephenson in Reading 15–2, and by Raco and VanEtten in Reading 15–3.

The final chapter in Part III is Chapter 16. That chapter is concerned with performance evaluation and incentive compensation. Performance evaluation is addressed in Reading 16–1, "Measuring Segment Performance: New Ventures of Today's Innovative Hospital Systems Pose Evaluation Challenges." Creating compensation incentives is the major focus of Reading 16–2, "The Impact of Motivation and Incentive Programs on Financial Budgets," by Janice Alger.

11

Cost Accounting Ratios

Reading 11–1

Ratio Analysis: Use with Caution

Steven A. Finkler

Health care management literature has recently contained a number of articles extolling the virtues of ratios and exhorting the health care manager to use ratio analysis to compare the institution over time with itself and with its peer group.[1–3] It is time to step back and question the serious limitations of ratio analysis when removed from the textbook and put into use. In some ways it is almost sacrilegious to be critical of ratio analysis for health care management. Recent years have seen a constant effort to develop the use of modern management techniques in the health care area. Ratio analysis is certainly used in industry in general. In fact, few managers would consider ratios to be a controversial topic—they are merely one more tool for the aware manager.

Yet ratios can be misleading. They can obscure relationships and confuse the manager if they are used without a full understanding of the implicit assumptions made by ratio analysis. Two of the principal problem areas that have led numerous managers to draw incorrect conclusions from ratio analysis results are: (1) inflation, which significantly distorts ratios and makes

their interpretation highly questionable; and (2) trends, which in themselves are not important, although the underlying cause of trends should concern the manager.

An extra degree of understanding is needed so that ratios may be used with enough care to be of value to managers. Note, however, that given financial information currently available in the health care field, reasonable comparisons among institutions are quite difficult and in many cases not possible.

That is a strong assertion and one that will not be likely to please those individuals and groups with a vested interest in ratio analysis. Many health care consultants provide a ratio analysis service. Is the product they sell something of value to the health care manager? If the ratio analysis consultants cannot overcome the difficulties raised below, they must either attempt to hide these limitations from their clients or disclose them and risk the loss of substantial amounts of lucrative business.

RATIOS AND INFLATION

Inflation creates a complicating factor in the use of ratio analysis. It distorts the ratios themselves and, without the exercise of some care, can distort the interpretation of observed trends.

Source: Reprinted from Steven A. Finkler, "Ratio Analysis: Use with Caution," *Health Care Management Review,* Vol. 7, No. 2, Spring 1982, pp. 65–72. Copyright 1982, Aspen Publishers, Inc.

Cause of the Distortion

Financial statements prepared in accordance with Generally Accepted Accounting Principles (GAAP) are primarily oriented toward historical cost information. Balance sheets based on GAAP must show assets at their cost, as opposed to some measure of their current value. If the hospital owns a piece of vacant land that doubles in value, the financial statements will show it at its old cost, rather than its new market value. This tends to make financial statements misleading. Yet to show the assets at their market value would require an appraisal. Because appraisers generally cannot agree exactly on an asset's value, accountants show the assets at their cost (less accumulated depreciation) until they are sold or otherwise disposed of.

The accounting profession has been studying this problem and is beginning to establish new rules. The process is a difficult one, and the debate consumes volumes. There are two principal alternatives, both of which have weaknesses. The price level adjustment approach would take the historical cost and adjust it upward based on the increase in a representative price index. Unfortunately, individual assets rarely change in value by the same amount as any price index, which is a broad average. The second alternative is replacement cost, which would value an asset at the cost to replace it. The problem there is a return to subjective estimates of what it might cost to replace the asset.

The advantages of the methods have been discussed.[4] However, for the present and the foreseeable future, hospital financial statements will remain on a historical cost basis. Given that the financial statements are used for preparing the ratios, if the statements are distorted, the ratios are distorted. Given the inflation of the last 15 to 20 years, there are significant distortions on the balance sheet.

The Current Ratio Example

Hypothetical data are presented in Tables 11–1–1 and 11–1–2 for a hospital for two years,

1980 and 1975. The current ratio is the most commonly used ratio to assess the liquidity of the firm, a key measure of financial viability.

Using the Table 11–1–1 data, the current ratio is as follows:

$$\text{current ratio} = \frac{\text{current assets}}{\text{current liabilities}}$$

$$\textbf{1980 current ratio} = \frac{10,363,274}{10,055,417} = 1.03$$

$$\textbf{1975 current ratio} = \frac{7,187,753}{6,518,896} = 1.10$$

The use of ratios to signal trends flashes a warning. The current ratio has fallen significantly from 1975 to 1980. Or has it?

Consider the effect of the last-in first-out (LIFO) method of inventory accounting. Briefly, LIFO is an acceptable form of valuing inventory at cost, but it assumes that the more recent purchases of inventory are consumed prior to older purchases. During inflation, this method funnels recent, higher-priced purchases into the income statement (thus maximizing cost and therefore reimbursement), but at the same time it leaves older, lower-priced purchases on the balance sheet.[5]

The result is that the balance sheet inventory figure stated at cost for a firm on a LIFO system will become more distorted each year that inflation persists. Assume that at the start of 1977 the hospital owns 1,000 bags of saline solution purchased for $5 per bag. In 1977 an additional 20,000 bags are purchased at $6 apiece, in 1978 an additional 20,000 bags are purchased at $7 apiece, in 1979 an additional 20,000 bags at $8 apiece, and in 1980 an additional 20,000 at $9. Each year consumption equals 20,000 bags. At the end of 1980 the balance sheet would show inventory of 1,000 bags worth $5 each. However, the value is really $9 each. Thus inventory is stated at $5,000, but is actually worth $9,000, a significant understatement in the value of the inventory.

Table 11–1–1 Hypothetical Consolidated Balance Sheet for Hospital *A* for the Years Ended 1980 and 1975

	1980	1975
Current assets		
Cash	$ 506,226	$ 557,240
Short-term investments	485,995	443,980
Accounts receivable net of uncollectable accounts	8,078,653	4,825,104
Estimated retroactive receivables—third party	83,883	139,428
Due from other funds	89,455	218,770
Inventories at cost	589,387	498,001
Prepaid expenses	152,549	87,746
Other accounts receivable	251,919	379,016
Other current assets	125,207	38,468
Total current assets	10,363,274	7,187,753
Noncurrent assets		
Board-designated investments	3,822	200,728
Property, plant and equipment, net of accumulated depreciation	20,498,986	17,053,958
Marketable securities and investments	2,494,769	2,973,426
Estimated reimbursement—due from third parties		
Long-term investments	308,353	
Deferred expenses	28,088	64,000
Construction in progress	269,032	712,678
Funds held for expansion	—	268,775
Total noncurrent assets	23,603,050	21,273,565
Total assets	$33,966,324	$28,461,318
Current liabilities		
Accounts payable	$ 3,883,148	$ 2,872,733
Accrued expenses	2,362,883	1,442,125
Current portion of long-term debt	393,665	191,258
Demand note payable	452,753	1,060,468
Due to other funds	2,051,046	312,897
Due to third-party agencies	869,973	573,549
Other current liabilities	41,949	65,866
Total current liabilities	10,055,417	6,518,896
Noncurrent liabilities		
Deferred revenue	99,038	94,500
Due to other funds	303,091	303,091
Reserve for self-insurance	477,448	—
Long-term debt due after one year	6,053,618	3,270,364
Other noncurrent liabilities	156,900	107,324
Total noncurrent liabilities	7,090,095	3,775,279
Fund balance	16,820,812	18,167,143
Total liabilities and fund balance	$33,966,324	$28,461,318

Table 11–1–2 Hypothetical Operating Information for Hospital *A*

	1980	1975
Total operating revenues	$97,290,300	$68,169,100
Total operating expenses	98,406,850	69,995,000
Total operating income	$(1,116,550)	$(1,825,900)

This is a byproduct of the historical cost method. Under LIFO, the historical cost of the inventory is $5,000, even though its value is $9,000 and even though the 1,000 saline bags on hand may actually have been purchased in 1980, and even though the bags purchased for $5 were physically consumed years ago. This perfectly allowable accounting system is sometimes referred to as accounting magic, or creative accounting.

Consider the implication for the current ratio. Assume that the hospital in Table 11–1–1 records inventory on a LIFO basis and that inflation in the prices of inventory items has been 15 percent per year for the five years from the end of 1975 to the end of 1980. On a compounded basis, that means that an inventory item purchased in 1975 for $1.00 would have cost $2.01 in 1980. The inventory value shown for 1980 could be understated by almost 100 percent. If this were approximated by adding the 1975 inventory cost to the stated 1980 inventory cost, it would yield an approximation that is not unreasonable given some of the effects of LIFO accounting. In that case the 1980 current ratio would be 1.08; that is, it would be almost the same as 1975, and there would be much less impression that any deleterious trend had developed.

Should downward trends in the current ratio be ignored? No. However, users of ratios should adjust for the current value of the inventory if it is based on the LIFO method.

The Rest of the Iceberg

In a sense the current ratio is the tip of the iceberg, because it makes use of only one asset that is likely to be distorted, inventory, and then only for a firm on the LIFO method. The full iceberg comes into view when one begins to look at ratios that include noncurrent assets as well as current assets.

Exhibit 11–1–1 defines a number of commonly used ratios that are likely to be affected by the impact of inflation. The noncurrent assets are likely to distort a great deal. The value of land,

Exhibit 11–1–1 Financial Ratios Most Distorted by Inflation (besides the current ratio)

Capital Structure

$$\text{Percentage of assets financed by total liabilities} = \frac{\text{total liabilities}}{\text{total assets}}$$

Activity

$$\text{Total asset turnover} = \frac{\text{total operating revenue}}{\text{total assets}}$$

$$\text{Fixed asset turnover} = \frac{\text{total operating revenue}}{\text{net fixed assets}}$$

$$\text{Current asset turnover} = \frac{\text{total operating revenue}}{\text{current assets}}$$

$$\text{Inventory turnover} = \frac{\text{total operating revenue}}{\text{inventory}}$$

Profitability

$$\text{Return on assets} = \frac{\text{operating income + interest}}{\text{total assets}}$$

Other

$$\text{Viability} = \frac{\text{total liabilities}}{\text{total assets}} \times \frac{\text{operating expense}}{\text{operating revenue}}$$

buildings, equipment, and investments becomes radically altered during periods of inflation. These ratios are not a comprehensive listing of all ratios distorted by inflation, but they can serve as examples of the problems to be encountered. Table 11–1–3 calculates the ratios displayed in Exhibit 11–1–1 for 1975 and 1980, based on the hypothetical information in Tables 11–1–1 and 11–1–2.

Percentage of Assets Financed by Total Liabilities

The purpose of this ratio is to show the extent to which the hospital has to borrow to finance its asset base. The ratio should be as small as possible, inasmuch as it is preferable for liabilities to be small, relative to the value of the assets. In Table 11–1–3 the ratio has increased from .36 to .50. Is this indicative of an unfavorable trend? Not necessarily.

The largest single asset group is property, plant, and equipment, net of depreciation. In both years, it represents well over half of total assets. This category is also likely to represent costs far different from the current value of the assets.

A better ratio to use here would compare the current value of assets to liabilities. Although accounting rules prevent reporting the financial statements on a current value basis, they do not prohibit the use of current value estimates for internal management uses. Assume that the replacement value of the property, plant, and equipment in this example was approximately $42 million in 1980 and $22 million in 1975. This ratio would then become .31 in both 1980 and 1975. No change in the ratio would have occurred over the five-year period. The implications of this ratio, adjusted for the effects of inflation by using current values in both years, are far different from those cited above when using an unadjusted ratio.

A ratio similar to percentage of assets financed by total liabilities is the debt-to-equity ratio. This ratio compares total liabilities to total fund balances. Although financial statements rarely say so explicitly, the total fund balance is simply total assets minus total liabilities. Therefore the equity, or fund balance, is calculated from balance sheet historical-cost asset information. This ratio

must therefore be adjusted by subtracting liabilities from assets adjusted to current value to get an appropriate fund-balance value for the equity portion of the ratio.

Total Asset Turnover

This ratio indicates how much revenue is generated relative to the assets used; thus the more revenue per dollar of assets, the better the financial position of the hospital. Table 11–1–3 shows that a favorable trend exists, with the ratio having increased from $2.40 of revenue per dollar of assets employed in 1975 to $2.86 of revenue per dollar of assets employed in 1980.

However, assets are unadjusted for the distortions of inflation. Assume once again that property, plant, and equipment have current values of $22 million in 1975 and $42 million in 1980. This adjustment alone would show that when revenue is compared to the value of the assets that are being employed, the ratio is 2.04 in 1975 and 1.75 in 1980. That means that the trend is an unfavorable one, not favorable as indicated by the unadjusted figures. Once again, other assets such as inventory and investments would have to be adjusted as well as plant, property, and equipment to be able to calculate meaningful ratios.

Fixed Asset Turnover

This activity ratio seeks to focus on how well the hospital employs its noncurrent assets. Together with the current asset turnover ratio below, they provide a detailed breakdown of the total asset turnover ratio. Because property, plant, and equipment is a much greater proportion of noncurrent assets than it is of total assets, the distortion will be even greater here. Making the same adjustment as before, to bring property, plant, and equipment to current values, this ratio changes from 3.20 and 4.12 in 1975 and 1980, respectively (a favorable trend), to 2.60 and 2.16 in 1975 and 1980, respectively (an unfavorable trend).

Current Asset Turnover

The principal current asset that requires adjustment for inflation is inventory. The current

---

Table 11–1–3 Ratios Based on Hypothetical Example

	1980	*1975*
Percentage of assets financed by total liabilities	.50	.36
Total asset turnover	2.86	2.40
Fixed asset turnover	4.12	3.20
Current asset turnover	9.39	9.48
Inventory turnover	165.07	136.88
Return on assets	–.03	–.06
Viability	.51	.37

asset ratio, intended to compare the amount of current assets needed to generate revenue, will be affected by the inventory distortion, if there is any. For a firm on a first-in first-out (FIFO) inventory accounting system, the inventory will be only slightly undervalued, and the ratio will be approximately correct without current value adjustment, although such adjustment will improve the accuracy of the ratio by at least some small amount. If the inventory is maintained on a LIFO basis, the same distortions will occur here as did in the current ratio.

Using the same inventory adjustment that was used for the current ratio, the current asset turnover ratio changes from 9.48 and 9.39 in 1975 and 1980, respectively (almost no trend), to 9.48 and 8.96 in 1975 and 1980, respectively. Thus an unfavorable trend is exposed, which would have otherwise gone undetected.

Inventory Turnover

The implications of adjusting the current asset turnover ratio are even more greatly magnified when ratios designed to focus on inventory activity are considered. The inventory turnover ratio compares current revenues to investment in inventory. Unadjusted, a favorable trend is clearly apparent. Each dollar invested in inventory supported $165.07 of revenue generation in 1980, as compared to $136.88 in 1975. But this may be a fiction of the accounting system used. If the firm were using LIFO, making the same correction as earlier, the ratios would be 89.47 in 1980 and 136.88 in 1975.

Note how misleading ratio analysis can be. If two firms were identical according to the financial statements, but one used a LIFO system and the other a FIFO system (something only noted in the footnotes to the financial statements), their inventories could in fact have widely differing values, and their true financial trends could be totally opposite from each other. In other words, for the LIFO firm one could totally misinterpret the ratios unless they are adjusted to reflect the current value of the inventory instead of the historical cost.

Return of Assets

Obviously, if assets are understated the return on assets will be overstated. The key to be aware of here is that the return measured by this ratio is the return on the amount originally invested in assets, unless adjustment to current value is made.

Viability

Using the viability index defined here, a low ratio is desirable. A low ratio implies high assets relative to liabilities and/or high revenue relative to expenses. An adjustment for inflation is required to avoid undue alarm. Of the four factors, assets are the most largely affected by inflation without automatic adjustment. That is not meant to imply that the other three factors are not severely affected by inflation. They are. However, as most revenues, expenses, and liabilities increase due to inflation, their inflated amounts are channeled directly into the financial statements. Assets, however, are locked in at their historical cost. Thus the financial information concerning assets is the most out of date and therefore misleading.

If the data are adjusted to reflect the assumptions made above about inventory and property, plant, and equipment values, the viability index ratio for both years can be recalculated. The results are ratios of .31 and .32 for 1980 and 1975, respectively. Thus the impression of decreased viability given by the unadjusted ratios in Table 11–1–3 may simply reflect the fact that the ratio acknowledges inflation's impact on three factors considerably more than on the fourth. The value of the ratio as a tool is considerably weakened by the impact of inflation unless that fourth item, assets, is brought closer in line with the other three by adjusting to some estimate of current value before calculating the ratios.

Implications for Internal Ratio Analysis over Time

The problems caused by inflation are not insurmountable when it comes to evaluating one given institution over time. An effective manager should have a good idea of the replacement value of the resources of the organization. Certainly, fire insurance must be based on replacement cost rather than historical cost. And the manager knows at least roughly the current price of inventory, the current value of land and so forth.

If the manager makes an annual practice of preparing a set of financial statements based on replacement cost, then it is a relatively simple matter to determine ratios over time that are comparable. Simply use these internal financial reports based on replacement cost, instead of the official GAAP-prepared statements when the ratios are calculated.

Implications for Interorganization Comparison

The problem of comparison among organizations is much more severe. Rarely is sufficient information given in an annual report for a manager to make a reasonable estimate of the current value of items on the financial statement of other organizations.

For large publicly held corporations in for-profit industries, this problem has been overcome. Such corporations are now required to include price level adjustment and replacement cost information in their annual reports. Given this information and a bit of numerical manipulation, the ratios—adjusted for the impact of inflation—can be calculated for a variety of companies over time and used for reasonable comparison of those companies.

Most health care organizations do not fall under the rules requiring that disclosure. That means that it probably is not possible to make reasonable comparisons across institutions. Frequently that comparison has been the major thrust of attention on ratio analysis. Is your institution in trouble? Compare yourself to the industry average and find out!

It is not clear, however, how there can be a benefit from a comparison of pears with an average of apples and oranges. If the ratios are not inflation adjusted, they make no sense for interim comparison. This is a problem for which a solution has not been presented by proponents of ratio analysis.

An Example Not Given

It might seem desirable at this point to take Tables 11–1–1 and 11–1–2 and restate them based on adjustments for inflation that occurred during that period. Then a new set of ratios could be calculated, and the reader would be dazzled by the substantial difference between the Table 11–1–3 ratio comparisons and the resulting new ratios reflecting the impact of inflation.

The logical way to restate Table 11–1–1 would be to use price-level adjustments. Using government indexes, one could restate numbers in current terms, but that contains the strong assumption that all assets related to health care are equally affected by inflation. If the medical-care component of the consumer price index rises 75 percent over that five-year period, then it must be assumed that land, buildings, inventory, investments, and so forth have all increased at a 75 percent rate. This is obviously not the case, since the index is based on a weighted average of different rates of price increase for different items.

Even if it were possible to separate the index into a separate rate for each various type of asset, one would not be much better off, since land has increased in price by different percentages in different geographic locations—even from one town to the next.

Replacement cost information is a much more reasonable approach to the problem. However, only the managers of an institution can get a reasonable estimate of replacement costs. The balance sheet simply does not give an external user the detailed information about specific individual assets that is needed to make an informed estimate of replacement costs. To restate, Tables 11–1–1 and 11–1–2 would imply that the reader can adequately make an adjustment to the financial statements of any organization. Because these data are generally not available, except for the manager's own institution, Tables 11–1–1 and 11–1–2 have not been restated.

TREND ANALYSIS

One of the principal uses for ratios is to compare an institution with itself over time. Trend analysis can be quite useful in discovering potential problems in their early stages. Ratios based on a manager's own institution over time can be adequately adjusted for inflation.

In general, this analysis can be quite helpful, but its principal limitation is that it focuses on how much relationships change, instead of how or why they change. For example, consider a hospital with a current ratio, adjusted for inflation, of 1.7 in 1975, 1.9 in 1976, 2.1 in 1977, 2.4 in 1978, 2.8 in 1979, 2.4 in 1980, and 1.8 in 1981. What does this trend tell us? The hospital had growing liquidity and therefore improving financial health from 1975 through 1979. In 1980 liquidity started to fall, and it dropped severely in 1981. Is the hospital in trouble? Has something gone wrong?

Not necessarily. Consider a hospital raising funds for a major expansion and putting those funds in a short-term money market fund until construction is to begin. In 1980 construction starts, and in 1981 the bulk of the construction takes place. The current ratio merely showed the accumulation of current assets in anticipation of the project, followed by their planned expenditure.

On the other hand, consider a current ratio pattern as follows: 2.4 in 1975, 2.2 in 1976, 2.0 in 1977, 1.9 in 1978, 1.7 in 1979, 1.6 in 1980, and 2.2 in 1981. This trend might indicate a health care organization with increasing liquidity problems. Was 1981 a turnaround year? The ratio increased sharply in 1981. Perhaps cost-cutting measures had been undertaken, and the situation turned around. Or perhaps things have become so desperate that the organization is selling off some of its fixed assets to generate sufficient cash to survive a little while longer.

Of course these examples are so extreme that one would anticipate that the organization's manager would know what was happening. The point, however, is that the ratios can lead one to draw a conclusion exactly opposite from what really happened. And presumably ratios are most useful when they tell about something not already known.

What if the stability of these two hospitals relative to the industry norm was assessed? If the industry average was 2.0 in 1981, it can be concluded that the healthy institution that just laid out a substantial amount for expansion (ratio 1.8) is in trouble and that the hospital really in trouble but selling off assets (ratio 2.2) will look healthy. At the very least, one will not be able to distinguish the extent to which the latter hospital has turned around a viability problem and is improving versus the extent to which the problem is worse and has led to a fixed asset liquidation for temporary survival.

The problem is the simplistic approach of how much things have changed instead of why they change. A current ratio, inflation adjusted, that hovers at 2.0 year after year would provide no signal to the manager. But if every year there were $100,000 transferred from endowment fund income to the general fund and this year the endowment fund is only earning $10,000, there is a problem.

One way to overcome this problem is to be sure to use a broad enough variety of ratios. If long-term assets are being sold to improve the current ratio, then the total-liability-to-total-asset ratio will become worse. Unfortunately, some ratios tend to carry more weight than others, and even though many things affect the current ratio and can mask underlying problems, it remains a key focus. Also, it is not clear which ratio could inform the manager that endowment income was crucial for a safe current ratio and that endowment income was down this year.

A second approach to this problem is greater reliance on the statement of changes in financial position (often called the statement of sources and uses of funds, the statement of sources and uses of working capital, or the statement of changes in working capital). This statement must be included along with a balance sheet and statement of revenues and expenses (income statement) to receive an opinion from a Certified Public Accountant on an organization's financial statements. It focuses on the sources and uses of current assets. Unlike the current ratio, which only gives an indication of the amount of change in current assets and current liabilities, this financial statement details what caused the change in these items. For example, one major source of current assets listed would be endowment fund income. A manager would quickly see that this number must be carefully monitored during the year because of its ultimate impact on working capital.

Any manager concerned enough to be interested in the current ratio should take the next step and carefully review the statement of changes in financial position, not only to see what has happened in the past, but as a better indicator of the future.

Ratios are a useful managerial tool, but their value has been substantially overstated. Especially during inflationary periods, their use requires a great deal of caution. In general, ratio analysis has been offered without qualification regarding its limitations. The risks and dangers of using ratio analysis evoke the cliche about the danger of a little knowledge.

At the very least, users of ratios should be aware of two points. First, ratios describe relationships between numbers, but not how those relationships came about nor whether there is reason to believe the relationship will persist. The focus is on how much, rather than how or why. Second, ratios are generally calculated from financial statement data prepared with GAAP. This implies use of historical cost rather than current cost. Therefore all distortions inherent in financial statements during inflationary periods will be inherent in the ratios, although perhaps not as obvious. These distortions are probably great enough that the usefulness of ratios based on GAAP financial statement numbers must be seriously challenged.

NOTES

1. R. Caruana and G. Kudder. "Seeing Through the Figures With Ratios." *Hospital Financial Management* 8:6 (June 1978) pp. 16–26.

2. R. Caruana and E.T. McHugh. "Comparing Ratios Shows Fiscal Trends." *Hospital Financial Management* 10:1 (January 1980) pp. 12–28.

3. W.O. Cleverley and K. Nilsen. "Assessing Financial Position With 29 Key Ratios." *Hospital Financial Management* 10:1 (January 1980) pp. 30–36.

4. B.R. Neumann and A.L. Friedman. "Should Financial Statements Disclose the Cost of Replacing Hospital Assets." *Health Care Management Review* 5:1 (Winter 1980) pp. 49–58.

5. S.A. Finkler. "LIFO Inventory Accounting." *Hospital Financial Management* 10:1 (January 1980) pp. 38–44.

Reading 11–2

Hospital Industry Cash Flow Ratio Analysis: A Sufficiency and Efficiency Perspective

Thomas L. Zeller
Brian B. Stanko

Financial ratios play a central role in hospital financial analysis. The objectives of hospital financial ratio analysis are, for instance, performance evaluation; liquidity and capital structure analysis; profit estimation; comparative analysis; and prediction of hospital success, closure, and failure. Creditors, donors, management, community leaders, and others combine and group key financial ratios over time, by location and across the industry, with qualitative measures for predictive, explanatory, and descriptive purposes.

Cash flow ratios that capture hospital industry sufficiency and efficiency measures are useful for predictive, explanatory, and descriptive purposes when combined with existing financial ratios. *Sufficiency*[1] describes the adequacy of operating cash flow in meeting an organization's needs. *Efficiency* describes how well an organization generates cash flows relative to service revenue and productive assets.

AUTHORITATIVE ACCOUNTING REGULATIONS

According to Financial Accounting Standards Board (FASB) Statement of Financial Account-

Source: Reprinted from T.L. Zeller and B.B. Stanko, "Hospital Industry Cash Flow Ratio Analysis: A Sufficiency and Efficiency Perspective," in *Hospital Cost Management and Accounting,* S.A. Finkler, ed.,Vol. 5, No. 10, pp. 5–8, Copyright 1997, Aspen Publishers, Inc.

ing Concepts No. 1, para. 48, reliable accounting information is defined as: information that is reasonably free from error and bias and faithfully represents what it purports to represent.

The reliability of cash flow information for financial ratio analysis improved in the 1990s as a result of two major changes in hospital cash flow reporting.

First, hospital cash flow reporting became standardized when the American Institute of Certified Public Accountants (AICPA) provided authoritative guidance to cash flow reporting in *Audits of Providers of Health Care Services (1990).* With this guide, the AICPA recommended that not-for-profit (NFP) health care entities apply the provisions of Statement of Financial Accounting Standards (SFAS) No. 95, Statement of Cash Flows.

Second, as of December 1995, hospital cash flow reporting became mandated by SFAS No. 117, Financial Statements of Not-for-Profit Organizations. SFAS No. 117 requires that NFP organizations, which include NFP hospitals, follow SFAS No. 95 in cash flow reporting.

Although SFAS No. 95 was widely followed before SFAS No. 117, these changes ensure that cash flow information is reliable and comparable because the reporting framework is mandated and standardized according to authoritative accounting literature. For example, SFAS No. 117 changes one component of cash flow reporting. The format of cash flow reporting for restricted donations and income earned by restricted funds is now standardized. Prior to SFAS No. 117, this cash flow activity was reported as an operating cash flow. Now under SFAS No. 117, this cash flow activity is to be reported as a financing activity.

A SUFFICIENCY DIMENSION OF HOSPITAL FINANCIAL ANALYSIS

Exhibit 11–2–1 summarizes the hospital industry's cash flow ratios. The two *sufficiency cash flow ratios* are important to hospital industry creditors and general stakeholders. These ratios are designed to measure a hospital's: (1) adequacy in generating cash flows, and (2) ability to meet recurring obligations—both stated objectives of SFAS No. 95.

The first sufficiency measure, *cash flow adequacy ratio,* is defined as:

$$\frac{\text{Total debt}}{\text{Net cash flows from operations (CFFO)}}$$

(Net cash flows from operations [CFFO] can be drawn directly from the statement of cash flows. It represents the net cash flow generated from day-to-day operations and unrestricted contributions.)

The cash flow adequacy ratio signals the time required to repay all debt, regardless of maturity, and focuses attention on the availability of funds from operations. This is important because recent evidence indicates that hospital management has been utilizing short-term financing sources for long-term purposes.

A hospital with a high debt to CFFO ratio could experience debt repayment problems due to insufficient cash flow from future operations. Continual increasing values of this ratio indicate that the hospital's financial position is weakening, while decreasing values indicate that the hospital's financial position is improving.

Exhibit 11–2–1 Hospital Industry Cash Flow Ratios

Ratio	Defined Measures
Sufficiency Ratios	
Cash Flow Adequacy	= **Total debt/Net cash flows from operations (CFFO)**[*] *(Measures the time required to repay total debt.)*
Cash Flow Coverage	= **(CFFO + interest expense)/(Current portion of long-term debt + interest expense)** *(Measures the coverage of current debt from cash flow from operations.)*
Efficiency Ratios	
Quality of Revenue	= **CFFO/Total unrestricted revenues, gains, and other support** *(Measures percent of net revenue that results in dollars generated.)*
Cash Recovery from Assets	= **CFFO/Total assets** *(Measures "cash recovery" from asset utilization.)*
Quality of Earnings	= **CFFO/Net change in unrestricted assets**[†] *(Measures percent of net change in unrestricted assets that results in dollars generated.)*

[*]As defined according to SFAS No. 95 and indicated (CFFO).

[†]Unrestricted net assets generally result from revenues from providing services, producing and delivering goods, receiving unrestricted contributions, and receiving dividends or interest from investing income producing assets, less expenses incurred in providing services, producing and delivering goods, raising contributions, and performing administrative functions (SFAS No. 117, par. 16). An increase in unrestricted net assets must be adjusted for the net gain or loss from sale of investments and equipment.

The second sufficiency ratio, *cash flow coverage ratio,* is defined as:

$$\frac{\text{CFFO + interest expense}}{\text{Current portion of long-term debt + interest expense}}$$

This ratio measures the necessary cash flow from operations to cover the current portion of long-term debt plus interest. A major caveat associated with this ratio rests in the definition of CFFO. This ratio, traditionally, is calculated using a proxy for CFFO defined as net income plus depreciation expense.[2] However, empirical analysis provides ample evidence that this ratio with the traditional definition of CFFO follows an unexplained random variability making its interpretation and value in hospital financial analysis very questionable.

With a standardized definition of CFFO, the reliability of this ratio should improve. This means that the reliability improves in measuring the coverage of debt payment and interest expense with CFFO defined according to SFAS No. 95. Increasing values of cash flow coverage mean an improved debt position, while decreasing values mean a weakening debt position.

In summary, sufficiency ratios offer two perspectives of performance that traditional hospital ratios fail to capture. A cash flow adequacy ratio measures the time required to satisfy a hospital's obligations. An increasing trend in this ratio represents a weakening financial position, and a decreasing trend represents an improvement in a hospital's financial position. A cash flow coverage ratio measures the ability of a hospital to cover its current portion of long-term debt and interest obligations.

Generating cash in excess of current debt and interest obligations means the hospital is generating sufficient cash to fund current and future operations. Failure to generate enough cash to meet current obligations means cash is being taken from savings, debt, or outside contributions in order to fund current operations. This can be characterized as a short-term solution to a potential long-term problem.

Including this information among traditional ratios should provide a greater understanding of

a hospital's financial position and future performance potential. A strong financial position is required by a hospital to respond to the changing competitive health care environment.

AN EFFICIENCY DIMENSION OF HOSPITAL FINANCIAL ANALYSIS

Efficiency cash flow ratios provide valuable insight regarding a hospital's cash recovery. With NFP hospitals following SFAS No. 95, it is now possible to develop comparable and reliable cash flow efficiency measures. This is an important contribution to performance evaluation because a cash recovery perspective represents the true economic consequence of management's decision making.

The first efficiency ratio, the *quality of revenue ratio,* measures the CFFO generated from each dollar of total unrestricted revenues, gains, and other support. The quality of revenue ratio equals:

$$\frac{\text{Net cash flow from operations (CFFO)}}{\text{Total unrestricted revenues, gains, and other support}}$$

This ratio represents a quality of revenue measure of performance and signals the immediate economic consequence of operational decisions. For instance, assume in early 1996 management loosens the hospital's credit policy and expands the number of services offered to encourage greater asset utilization. The economic impact of this decision, measured by a traditional return on revenue ratio (change in net assets/total unrestricted revenues, gains, and other support—defined to reflect terminology of SFAS No. 117), would likely indicate an improved performance by year end 1996.

An improvement can be explained by a larger percentage increase in change in net assets than total unrestricted revenues, gains, and other support. However, it is not clear whether the measured benefit is in fact an improvement in true economic performance.

The improvement in the traditional ratio, for example, may simply reflect an increase in accounts receivable. However, the quality of revenue measure may signal a reduced operating cash flow from loose credit standards due to the costs associated with expanded services and a likely increase in receivables in 1996. This brief scenario shows the advantage of a quality of revenue ratio.

The true cash recovery of management's decisions becomes readily apparent with this ratio. This type of information should be useful to management in balancing the need to: (1) generate the necessary cash to operate a hospital long-term, and (2) meet its institutional mission.

The second efficiency ratio measures the cash recovery from the utilization of a hospital's assets. The *cash recovery from assets ratio* equals:

$$\frac{\text{Net cash flow from operations (CFFO)}}{\text{Total assets}}$$

This ratio represents the cash recovery from assets that is entrusted to management. Although generating cash flow from operations may not be the primary mission of a hospital, it is vital for survival because the majority of funds used to finance the organization are generated from operations.

Typically, government and philanthropy support are small for NFP hospitals. Therefore, management must invest in assets that generate operating cash flow to survive long term, regardless of its mission. An increasing (or decreasing) trend in this ratio suggests that management is (or is not) responding to the competitive nature of the health care industry in cost control and resource allocation to plant and equipment.

A cash flow recovery from assets ratio also reflects a measure of risk to all stakeholders that is not readily available under traditional hospital ratio analysis. A traditional return on assets measure (net change in unrestricted assets/total assets—defined to reflect terminology of SFAS No. 117) may be relatively stable over a period of time. Stability in this measure is a desirable financial characteristic because a common assumption is that a business enterprise with stable earnings carries less risk than one in which the

return pattern is largely variable. This is important because the greater the variability in earnings, the greater the cost of capital. Thus, if management can show stable earnings, they can reduce the cost of operating performance.

Applying this concept to the hospital industry would suggest that management has an incentive to smooth earnings with various accruals and deferrals. The stability, however, may be the result of true performance or management's use of accounting accruals and deferrals to smooth performance. However, a cash flow recovery ratio exposes this type of management behavior. A greater variability in CFFO/total assets would indicate a greater risk for the hospital than that signaled by return on assets. This suggests that management can no longer hide true hospital economic performance behind accounting accruals and deferrals when including CFFO/total assets in financial analysis.

The third efficiency ratio measures the CFFO generated from each dollar of net change in unrestricted assets. The *quality of earnings ratio* is defined as:

$$\frac{\text{Net cash flow from operations (CFFO)}}{\text{Net change in unrestricted assets}}$$

(Net change in unrestricted assets generally results from service revenues, producing and delivering goods, receiving unrestricted contributions, and receiving dividends or interest from investing income producing assets, less expenses incurred in providing services, producing and delivering goods, raising contributions, and performing administrative functions [SFAS No. 1 17, para. 16]. For this ratio to be meaningful, the net gain or loss from sale of investments and equipment must be removed from the net change in unrestricted assets.)

The quality of earnings ratio represents a quality of earnings perspective of hospital performance. Over time, this measure should be slightly greater than 1 because depreciation expense is an annual noncash charge against net change in unrestricted assets. Furthermore, it is likely to revolve around the value of 1 over time because of noncash charges and accrual based operating expenses included in net change in unrestricted assets.

Therefore, if a trend develops where this measure is continually greater than or less than 1, this may suggest that net change in unrestricted assets is not a representative value of true operating economic performance. This would be an important signal to management because several ratios incorporate the net change in unrestricted assets measure as a key component in hospital financial ratio analysis. (We assume hospital financial ratio analysis will adjust to the terminology of SFAS No. 117.)

If it is determined that net change in unrestricted assets does not accurately measure true economic performance, any analysis using such a measure should be questioned. Further, this type of trend should force management to investigate why there is a difference over time between net change in unrestricted assets and CFFO.

CONCLUSION

The operating cash flow ratios outlined in this article can be incorporated into traditional financial ratio analysis to gain a better understanding of hospital performance and financial position. The impetus behind these cash flow ratios stems from two authoritative accounting releases: (1) the AICPA guide *Audits Of Providers Of Health Care Services (1990),* and (2) SFAS No. 117, where NFP hospitals must now follow SFAS No. 95 in reporting cash flows.

Sufficiency cash flow ratios were proposed as a means to gain a better understanding about a hospital's ability to meet its long-term obligations and fund future operations. Efficiency cash flow ratios were proposed as a means to measure a hospital's cash recovery from operations. The primary contribution of cash flow ratio analysis is that the true economic financial position and performance of a hospital becomes more readily apparent.

Thomas L. Zeller and **Brian B. Stanko** are assistant professors, Department of Accounting, Loyola University Chicago. They may be contacted at 312/915-7626.

REFERENCES

1. The sufficiency and efficiency perspectives employed in this article extend the work of Giacomino and Mielke (Cash Flows: Another Approach to Ratio Analysis, *Journal of Accountancy,* March 1993, pp. 55–58) to hospital cash flow ratio analysis.

2. *The Comparative Performance of US Hospitals: The Sourcebook.* Health Care Investment Analysis, Inc., and Deloitte & Touche. Baltimore, MD. 1993. p. 228.

Reading 11–3

Ratio Analysis for the Development Office of Health Care Institutions

Mei Yee Lam

It is common for the board of trustees and management to measure the success of the development office in a health care organization by its fundraising results only. Achieving the annual fundraising target draws all the focus of development staff and managers. As long as the target is met, cost issues tend to be disregarded. Besides, the development office is viewed as an important revenue center that brings resources from outside. Even in a tight budget situation, there is more spending leeway for the development office. However, this leads to unnecessary waste such as a high level of return mail from the annual appeal.

Why is anyone interested in measuring the cost-effectiveness of the development office? It is in the hope that fundraising efforts will be maximized by minimizing costs. Profits raised from each activity should be maximized to the largest extent for patient care. In addition, studying cost-effectiveness helps to determine the best activities in which to invest our time and money. We will do better if we focus our resources on those activities.

We will approach the issue of cost-effectiveness in the development office from four perspectives. They are:

1. assessment of efficiency;
2. assessment of effectiveness;
3. assessment of timeliness; and
4. assessment of capital investment.

Specific activities in the development office are described to further explain these approaches.

ASSESSMENT OF EFFICIENCY

Evaluation of the Development Office

The size of development offices varies from institution to institution. A large and well-funded medical center may have a small development office, whereas a small health care center may have a large number of development staff in support of fundraising campaigns to sustain the existence of the organization.

How can we address the efficiency of the office? One way to approach the question is to analyze the direct costs of the office and conduct a trend analysis. It is useful to measure the organization's control over direct costs by comparing ratios of these costs with ratios from past years and ratios of other organizations in the same industry. The number of fundraising staff has a significant impact on the direct costs of the development office, and it varies in different organizations. Ratio analysis provides information for comparison.

A large part of direct cost consists of the salaries of the fundraisers. We can measure the effi-

Source: Reprinted from M.Y. Lam, "Ratio Analysis for the Development Office of Health Care Institutions," in *Hospital Cost Management and Accounting,* S.A. Finkler, ed., Vol. 9, No. 5, pp. 1–6. Copyright 1997, Aspen Publishers, Inc.

ciency of raising funds by using the following ratios. The larger the ratios are, the better, because they indicate that larger amounts of funds are raised per salary dollar or per fundraiser.

$$\text{Return on each dollar of salary} = \frac{\text{Total revenue}}{\text{Total salaries of fundraisers}}$$

$$\text{Return on an FTE fundraiser} = \frac{\text{Total revenue}}{\text{Number of FTE fundraisers}}$$

Furthermore, we can examine if the experience of fundraisers and their years with the organization have any impact on revenue. A system should be built to track the fundraising records of each fundraiser, their years of experience, and their years with the organization. This information will help management to hire appropriate personnel for different types of campaigns. The following ratios can be applied:

$$\text{Return on years of experience} = \frac{\text{Revenue raised by a fundraiser}}{\text{His or her years of experience}}$$

$$\text{Return on years with the organization} = \frac{\text{Revenue raised by a fundraiser}}{\text{His or her years with the organization}}$$

The same concept can be used to create a ratio analysis for fixed, variable, and total costs. A high ratio indicates that a dollar of cost has been maximized to the largest extent to generate revenue. Fixed costs in the development office include the cost of fax machines and computers, the salary of the fundraising supervisor, etc. Variable costs in the office consist of the salaries of temporary staff for special projects, the salaries of permanent staff, mailing costs, etc. Comparing these ratios with past ratios and with industry comparison ratios will provide us with key information for improvement.

Suppose we wish to assess the return on fixed cost for the newly established development office of ABC Hospital. The total amount raised by the office is $1,000,000. All equipment is purchased this year at the cost of $100,000 and will

last for five years. The residual value of this equipment is $2,000. In addition, rent of the office is $3,000 per month, and salary of the fundraising supervisor is $100,000 per year. Fixed costs of the office are calculated as follows:

Equipment	($100,000 – $2,000)/5 years	$ 19,600
Rent	($3,000 × 12 months)	36,000
Salary		100,000
Total Fixed Costs		$155,600

$$\begin{aligned}\text{Return on fixed cost} &= \text{Total revenue/Fixed cost}\\ &= \$1,000,000/\$155,600\\ &= 6.43\end{aligned}$$

Suppose that variable costs of the office are $300,000. The total cost of $455,600 is the sum of the fixed cost and variable cost ($155,600 + $300,000). The return on variable cost and the return on total cost are calculated as follows:

$$\begin{aligned}\text{Return on variable cost} &= \text{Total revenue/Variable cost}\\ &= \$1,000,000/\$300,000\\ &= 3.33\end{aligned}$$

$$\begin{aligned}\text{Return on total cost} &= \text{Total revenue/Total cost}\\ &= \$1,000,000/\$455,600\\ &= 2.19\end{aligned}$$

Evaluation of Special Event

Raising money by holding special events is a common practice in health care organizations. Theater openings, auctions, cocktail parties, carnivals, and tennis and golf tournaments—any activities that generate donations—are held to benefit almost everything from general operation funds to the establishment of a special unit.

Some of the events raise thousands of dollars, with very little cash outlay or financial risk. Others, however, barely break even or wind up in the red. Sometimes, a project's failure may be caused by a failure to establish a budget. Cost was greater than revenue because event expenses were not calculated in advance.

The use of ratio analysis to evaluate past projects can identify problems and point out the direction for improvement. The following ratio will show how well we do in a special event. If the ratio is equal to or greater than one, revenue covers total cost: The event breaks even or makes profit. We should track this ratio for different events because it indicates which type of event is a winner and which one is a loser.

$$\text{Return on cost of a special event} = \frac{\text{Total revenue}}{\text{Total cost involved in the event}}$$

It is not unusual to look for financial support from individuals, businesses, and corporations in the form of expense underwriting. Many firms support such activities because it gives them exposure and recognition in the community. We can compare the total amount of underwriting to the total expenses. The higher ratio of underwriting means the lower our expenses.

$$\text{Ratio of expense underwriting to total expenditure} = \frac{\text{Total expense underwriting}}{\text{Total expense}}$$

Moreover, the efficiency of various activities in a special event such as ticket sales, charity sales, and sponsorship packages can be assessed by using ratio analysis. It will indicate which type of activity raises more funds. For instance, we can compare the profitability of ticket sales to charity sales.

$$\text{Percentage of ticket sales to total revenue} = \frac{\text{Ticket sales}}{\text{Total revenue}} \times 100\%$$

$$\text{Percentage of charity sales to total revenue} = \frac{\text{Charity sales}}{\text{Total revenue}} \times 100\%$$

$$\text{Percentage of sponsorship package to total revenue} = \frac{\text{Sponsorship package}}{\text{Total revenue}} \times 100\%$$

Most organizations will hold several special events a year. Knowing the average labor cost, supply cost, and total cost per event will help us to prepare a better budget for next year.

$$\text{Average labor cost per event} = \frac{\text{Total salary}}{\text{Total number of events}}$$

$$\text{Average supply cost per event} = \frac{\text{Total supply cost}}{\text{Total number of events}}$$

$$\text{Average total cost per event} = \frac{\text{Total cost}}{\text{Total number of events}}$$

The contribution margin of a special event should be calculated and compared with that of a similar event held by other organizations. Trend analysis for contribution margins of similar kinds of events can highlight improvements and spot downfalls.

ASSESSMENT OF EFFECTIVENESS

We have mentioned that the development office is usually allowed to have a greater budget than other departments. Focus has historically been drawn to the amount raised by the department. The cost-effective issue of raising funds has seemed unimportant to management. As financial constraints become more severe in health care organizations, we should be more conservative in evaluating resource consumption by the development office and ensure that resources are not wasted.

Resources devoted for a fundraising effort should produce expected results. Ensuring expected results requires building up a tracking system, providing careful analysis, and changing the ways of doing things. Ratio analysis can help us assess the effectiveness of activities such as direct mail campaigns and grant applications.

Direct Mail Campaign

When the development office completes a direct mail campaign, it should analyze the result, decide what changes should be made, and use this information for the next campaign. We can measure the result by using ratios. For example, the return on the cost of direct mail indicates the effectiveness of our campaign. The higher the return rate, the more revenue was generated with the limited resource. A lower return rate may indicate that we should alter the ways of doing the mailing. Varying the headline, the photographs, and the copy style and tone may bring different results. The ratios should be compared with past records to evaluate the effectiveness of return.

$$\text{Return on cost of direct mail} = \frac{\text{Revenue from direct mail}}{\text{Cost of direct mail}}$$

$$\text{Revenue per piece of mail} = \frac{\text{Revenue from direct mail}}{\text{Total pieces of mail}}$$

$$\text{Revenue per thousands of mail} = \frac{\text{Revenue}}{\text{Total pieces of mail}} \times 1{,}000$$

$$\text{Cost per piece of mail} = \frac{\text{Cost of direct mail}}{\text{Total pieces of mail}}$$

$$\text{Cost per thousands of mail} = \frac{\text{Cost of direct mail}}{\text{Total pieces of mail}} \times 1{,}000$$

Reaching the right person on the right list is an important approach to fundraising. It is much more efficient and usually much more productive if the development office aims more carefully at a selected target audience and talks specifically to them. It is important to conduct research on a target audience prior to the direct mail campaign. However, it is also significant to evaluate whether the campaign is targeted to the right group of people.

The following percentage can be applied to measure responses. Comparing this information with other direct mail results and results from prior years can help us evaluate the efficiency of the mailing.

$$\text{Percentage of responses} = \frac{\text{Total number of responses}}{\text{Total pieces of mail}} \times 100\%$$

$$\text{Amount donated per responses} = \frac{\text{Total amount donated}}{\text{Total responses}}$$

Sometimes, the development office purchases mailing lists that may consist of people whose addresses have already changed. Because of staff shortage, direct mailing lists may not be updated regularly and could lead to a large number of pieces of returned mail. This cost should be measured and added to the total cost of direct mail. In addition, a control system should be established to prevent further waste of resources. For example, if the percentage of return mail reaches a certain level, the development office should research mailing lists and make appropriate corrections in a timely fashion. The number and cost of return mail can be measured by the following percentage:

$$\text{Percentage of return mail} = \frac{\text{Number of return mail}}{\text{Total number of direct mail}} \times 100\%$$

$$\text{Percentage of return mail cost} = \frac{\text{Cost of return mail}}{\text{Total cost of direct mail}} \times 100\%$$

Proposal/Grant Application

Many fundraisers of health care organizations spend a lot of time researching private foundations, putting together grant proposals and requests, and communicating with foundations that are interested in supporting their particular projects. However, the success of obtaining funds relies on many elements:

- The health care organization needs to have a project the foundation is interested in supporting.
- A proposal must be properly submitted and meet its deadlines.
- The organization has to show that it is capable of providing the service it is proposing.
- The organization has to build a strong case for support and show that it deserves support.
- The organization should ask for an amount that is consistent with the support levels of the foundation.
- The organization should be willing to maintain a relationship with the foundation and report regularly on its progress after the grant is received.

- The organization should show that it knows the project's budget, time constraints, staffing needs, and other details.

Annual grants and general endowment awards of foundations are usually a large amount of money, which can impact the financial situation and program development of the awarded organization. In order to obtain money from a foundation, a proposal must be submitted. Analyzing the effectiveness of grant application will benefit the organization in the long run.

If the successful rate of grant application is low, appropriate actions can be taken to improve the situation. For example, hiring a professional grant writer may enhance the chance of receiving foundation support. Some ratios can be used to measure the successful rate, revenue, and cost of grant applications. These ratios should be compared with ratios of prior years and ratios of other health care organizations.

$$\text{Successful rate of grant applications} = \frac{\text{Number of successful grant applications}}{\text{Total number of grant applications}} \times 100\%$$

$$\text{Return on proposal applications} = \frac{\text{Total revenue from proposals}}{\text{Total number of proposals}}$$

$$\text{Cost of proposal applications} = \frac{\text{Total cost devoted to generate proposals}}{\text{Total number of proposals}}$$

$$\text{Return on cost of applications} = \frac{\text{Total revenue}}{\text{Total cost of applications}}$$

ASSESSMENT OF TIMELINESS

Knowing the timeline of activities helps managers to efficiently plan the work schedule and properly allocate staff for different projects in the following year. For instance, we can estimate the average time for preparation of a grant application and the average time for coordinating a special event. The assessment of timeliness helps managers make reasonable projections of the fundraising target and better estimate the budget

of expenses for next year. For example, we should examine the revenue and cost of grant applications per day spent on preparing proposals.

$$\text{Average time for preparation of a grant application} = \frac{\text{Days spent on grant applications per year}}{\text{Total number of applications}}$$

$$\text{Average time for coordinating a special event} = \frac{\text{Days spent on special event preparation per year}}{\text{Total number of special events}}$$

$$\text{Revenue received per grant preparation day} = \frac{\text{Revenue received from proposals}}{\text{Days spent on preparing proposals}}$$

$$\text{Cost per day spent on preparing grant applications} = \frac{\text{Cost spent on preparing proposals}}{\text{Days spent on preparing proposals}}$$

ASSESSMENT OF CAPITAL INVESTMENT

Capital investment is essential for the development office. In their quest to be better informed, fundraisers sometimes spend excessive amounts on data collecting systems. This trap can be avoided by deciding exactly what an information system must do for the office, such as track pledges, produce mailing labels, compare actual contributions with goals, research potential donors, and update donor records. Then, the office can acquire a system to do those things, in addition to meeting some long-term needs.

Software vendors generally are willing to modify databases to meet an organization's special requirements. These changes are often far less costly than having a data system specially designed. Purchasing a new information system is a major expenditure that needs to be explained to board members, especially in terms of cost-effectiveness. Ratio analysis will help the board understand the importance of acquiring the system by comparing the cost and benefit. For example, a high return on the new information system indicates that a dollar of cost to acquire the system is maximized to generate revenue and savings.

Revenue generated from the information system includes benefit from research by using the system, reduction of staff time for tracking donor records, and others. An example of savings includes the elimination of salaries for filing clerks or temporary staff who conduct manual recordkeeping. Costs of the system consist of purchasing cost, installation cost, consultation fees, maintenance fees, additional work force to update the system, etc.

$$\text{Return on information system} = \frac{\text{Revenue and savings caused by the new system}}{\text{Costs of the system}}$$

After the computer system is installed, managers of the development office should assess the productivity improvement of the department, including comparing the speed of tracking pledges before and after the system is installed. The following ratios can be used to evaluate the timeliness. The smaller the ratio, the less time was spent on the same kind of activities after the system was installed.

$$\text{Improvement of timeliness for tracking pledges} = \frac{\text{Time spent on tracking pledges after the system is installed}}{\text{Time spent on tracking pledges before the system is installed}}$$

$$\text{Improvement of timeliness for researching donors} = \frac{\text{Time spent on researching donors after the system is installed}}{\text{Time spent on researching donors before the system is installed}}$$

CONCLUSION

Measuring the cost-effectiveness of the development office may be considered ineffective by some people because funding decisions are not going to be based on that analysis. In fact, this statement is not accurate. Measuring the cost-effectiveness of the office is important because it will improve the effectiveness of fundraising efforts. Knowing its spending and revenue patterns can help the office better plan and budget limited resources. It will also help the office maximize its ability to raise funds.

Ratio analysis is a vital tool to evaluate the efficiency, effectiveness, timeliness, and capital investment of the development office. It is also a powerful managerial tool for understanding and improving the financial performance of the office. Ratios are generally used as a basis for comparison. The development office should track its own ratios over time and should compare itself to a specific close competitor or to firms in the fundraising industry.

NOTES

Campbell, B. "A Powerful Analysis Technique." *Fundraising Management,* Vol. 25, No. 5, July 1994, pp. 16–18.

Cook, J. "Why Nonprofits Don't Measure Cost-Effectiveness." *Foundation News.* Vol. 33, No. 5, Sept./Oct. 1992, pp. 35–38.

Cook, J. "Cost Effectiveness: First the Grantmakers Must Do Their Job Right (Part 2)." *Foundation News.* Vol. 33, No. 6. Nov/Dec. 1992, pp. 34–38.

Finkler, S.A. "Cost Accounting Ratio." *Essentials of Cost Accounting For Health Care Organizations,* pp. 228, 232, Gaithersburg, MD: Aspen Publishers.

Goodale, T. "Computers—Our Servants or Our Masters?" *Fundraising Management,* Vol. 19, No. 1, March 1988, pp. 78, 80.

Grasty, W.K. & Sheinkopf, K.G. "Successful Fundraising: Handbook of Proven Strategies and Techniques," pp. 19, 126, 159, 262. Copyright © 1982, the Bern Convention.

12

Measuring Productivity

Reading 12–1

Productivity Management: A Model for Participative Management in Health Care Organizations

Newton Margulies
John F. Duval

In recent months the issue of improving the productivity of America's work force in both the service and the manufacturing sectors has received considerable attention. In the health care area, the pressures of spiraling medical costs, the problems associated with government-sponsored reimbursement, and the high costs associated with labor and labor-intensive industries have prompted management within the health care community to investigate various approaches to improving productivity.[1,2]

Since 1965 there have been many attempts to slow the upward spiral of health care costs. Professional standards review organization legislation, certificate-of-need legislation, and congressional mandates for an ongoing appropriateness review of existing services are all attempts of government-imposed limitations on reimbursement.[3] These programs, however, have not been targeted at the largest single cost to hospitals—labor. In spite of the high technology associated with modern health care delivery systems the industry remains labor intensive. A full 60 percent of hospital costs are labor related.[4]

LACK OF COMMITMENT TO PRODUCTIVITY THINKING

The principal difficulty encountered by hospitals in addressing the question of productivity is that productivity analysis in health care stands as a relatively underdeveloped management tool.

Productivity analysis is a relatively new idea in the health care field. Prior to 1965, and the enactment of Medicare and Medicaid legislation, productivity improvement received minimal attention. However, the current cost of inflation in the health care industry, contributed to in part by the Medicare and Medicaid legislation, has created concerns for productivity that can no longer be ignored by health care administrators.[5] Despite these concerns and in the face of increasingly scarce resources, many hospitals have not yet established productivity tracking systems or methods for measuring and analyzing potential areas for productivity improvement.[6]

Multiplicity of Activities

Within the hospital environment, the flow of services administered to the patient comes from a variety of disciplines: professional, allied pro-

Source: Reprinted from Newton Margulies and John F. Duval, "Productivity Management: A Model for Participative Management in Health Care Organizations," *Health Care Management Review,* Winter 1984, Vol. 9, No. 1, pp. 61–70. Copyright 1984, Aspen Publishers, Inc.

fessional, technical, and nonprofessional. In many instances, in order to provide one service several other services must be integrated and co-ordinated. The complexity of the situation serves to complicate the organizational environment, thus making the job of identifying a specific work unit as a focus for productivity analysis an extremely difficult task.

Product Search

Many of the activities in health care are ser-vice related and have no readily measurable product. An example would be the social ser-vices component. It is difficult to measure a product in a department where not only the needs of the client are changing, but where the nature of the client is changing also. However, the intangible quality of the output may not pre-clude some productivity analysis. It has recently been argued that productivity measures are not only possible but necessary.

Units of Work Activity

Difficulty in defining units of work activity follows the problems encountered with measur-ing a physical product forthcoming from a given service. In order to quantify output, one must first be able to define it. This problem seems to be an ongoing one in many health care service departments.[7]

In an effort to resolve this problem, many pro-ductivity measures have been developed, but they may not reflect the product or service. Med-ical record labor hours per discharge unit, nurs-ing labor hours per patient day, radiology labor hours per patient day, radiology labor hours per procedure, and laundry labor hours per 100 pounds are just a few examples. A common problem exists in many of these measures. For example, nursing labor hours per patient day are aggregate statistics that yield no information on the amount of productive, relative to nonproduc-tive, time that is being spent on the job. Because of this the statistic is of limited value. In radiol-ogy, if the number of procedures and total labor hours is known, the productive time per paid la-

bor hour (or something proportional to it) can be computed.

A number of traditional methodologies have been used to evolve viable work standards in de-veloping the various productivity measures. Most of the methodologies are derived from his-torical data standards, estimated standards, time standards (stopwatch studies), and standard data standards (College of American Pathologists standards).[8] All of these methodologies are used to arrive at work standards through which indi-vidual or group productivity can be measured.

These traditional methodologies make some common assumptions about the worker, most of which are closely aligned to McGregor's mana-gerial philosophy, which he labeled Theory X.[9] Theory X and its counterpart Theory Y were identified by McGregor as being the two basic sets of assumptions on which managers base their style. Theory X assumes that the worker is lazy, self-seeking, motivated only by monetary incentives, and must be controlled by manage-ment in order to work toward organizational goals. Theory Y assumes that the worker is capa-ble of self-direction and self-control and will in-tegrate his or her efforts with organizational goals. Theory X's approaches to productivity analysis tend to view the worker as being inci-dental to the study; therefore, little attempt is made to involve the worker in the decision-mak-ing processes that guide the study or interpret its outcome. These approaches are clearly less than ideal because they do not make use of the wealth of information about the workplace that is avail-able from those who perform the work functions directly.

Although there is still a good deal of merit in the traditional approaches to developing produc-tivity/work measurement systems, the value po-sition reflected in the Theory X assumptions may be detrimental to the development of viable and useful productivity improvements.

PARTICIPATIVE MANAGEMENT

Over the last decade, and more recently due to the publicity of the Japanese participative management success, there has been a tendency for American management to more seriously consider the merits of participative management.[10–12] Many organizations have initiated, in a variety of forms, approaches to facilitate greater participation among workers. To be sure, not all organizations have met with instant success but enough have experienced significant increases in morale and productivity to support the notion of participative management. There is a growing body of empirical research that supports the premise that the success of these approaches may rest with the quality and abilities of management and not with the employee.[13] The core issue may simply be education in the broadest sense. It is not realistic to expect employees (or managers) to enthusiastically participate in management processes when, for the most part, they do not have the necessary skills to perform such activities. The success of participative programs rests in management's commitment to educate themselves and their employees in how to participate and how to engage with employees in collaborative problem identification and resolution.

AN APPROACH TO PRODUCTIVITY MEASUREMENT

In developing a cohesive approach to the development of participative productivity measurement systems, management must not only commit itself to supporting such efforts, but must also commit itself to the careful mapping of strategies by which to accomplish them. Figure 12–1–1 represents the theoretical construct that provides the framework for the development of participative management systems. The model is described in two phases. *Phase I* represents the necessary education and management support needed to prepare the worker to participate in such an effort. This phase identifies the critical components required to develop an environment that facilitates participative management activities. *Phase II* represents a means by which participative methods can be put into operation in developing productivity tracking systems. Specifically, those steps and components are identi-

fied that facilitate the development of accurate activity standards to be used in the tracking and evaluation of productivity.

PHASE I: PREWORK

Management Support

The initial ingredient, and perhaps the most significant factor, in developing any participative system is the strong program support of key management personnel. Enthusiasm and encouragement of management can provide the impetus for initiating and sustaining the program. Participation is often threatening to many managers. This subtle resistance can provide obstacles for the implementation of participative mechanisms.

Financial Support

Participative management practices cost money, primarily in terms of invested worker and management time. Remember that management time is spent in both active participation and administration of the program. An example of how quickly participation time can accrue is reflected in the use of quality circles—a participative quality control technique.[14] Quality circles generally consist of eight to ten members representing a cross section of their respective organizations who meet for one hour a week. The purpose of quality circle meetings is to discuss ideas and problems affecting the workplace. For a group of ten members, the cumulative time consumed by group meetings equates to 13 personnel weeks a year. Thus management must be aware of the magnitude of the commitment that it is making. Such commitments are generally based on the assumption that the long-term benefits provided to the organization by worker participation will outweigh the costs encountered in initiating and maintaining participative programs.

Attitudinal Support

In order to successfully implement participative management programs, managers must learn

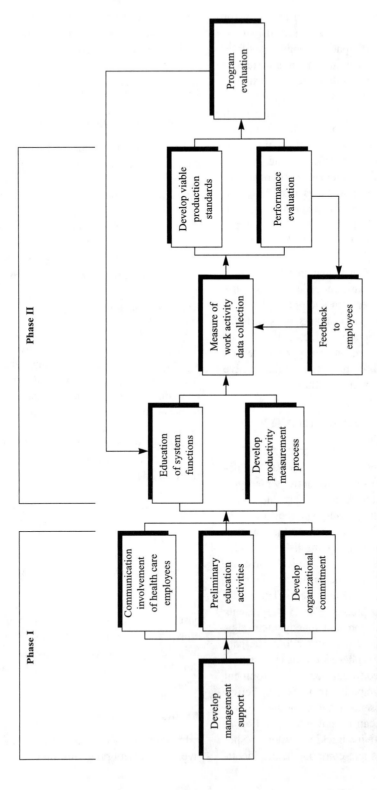

Figure 12–1–1 Phasal Model for Productivity Improvement

to participate with the employee and encourage the rank and file to participate in the organizational decision-making process. Management must demonstrate an active willingness to work toward participation and to leave old management styles behind. The core of a participative management program, whether aimed at productivity problems or any other workplace difficulty, can only further the improvement of management–worker relations.[15–16]

Structural Support

The final element required to support the worker in the implementation of participative programs is structural in nature. Management must make provisions for the necessary organizational structural changes required to facilitate the participative process. Provisions may include changing official lines of communication, worker participation in various meetings, establishing internal resources to facilitate the process, or they may include the actual restructuring of the physical environment, for example, where people sit and the types and location of offices.

Educational Support

The role of education and training in participative management is usually underemphasized. Because of the newness of the participative approach, few workers or managers have had the opportunity to be exposed to participative skills. Bluntly stated, management and workers alike must develop the appropriate participative skills before they can be expected to participate effectively. Of particular importance is the inclusion of middle managers in retraining and educating in participative skills. Since middle management is the critical interface in linking the organizational goals established by top management with the participation of workers, adequate training of these individuals is almost requisite for program success. This need is underscored by the fact that many middle managers have developed their management skills and styles in authoritarian work environments.[17]

Marketing of Participation

The implementation of participative management styles, independent of their long-range goals, generally requires the expenditure of additional effort on the part of both management and workers. The added responsibilities coupled with the stresses introduced into the workplace by the changing of roles can generate a good deal of resistance to participatory programs.[18] For this reason it is critical that a well-planned marketing program be developed to inform and educate the participants in participative management programs on the use of such programs and the potential benefits that might be reaped by all involved.

Marketing support of participative productivity measurement, like any participative program, is important because it helps provide momentum to such programs. While this fact may be obvious, it is important to note that these programs are not self-perpetuating. In order for participative programs to be successful, they must be nurtured and supported by ongoing educational and marketing efforts, which are necessary to effect attitudinal changes in the workplace.[19]

PHASE II: APPLICATION

Phase II of the model specifically addresses the application of the arguments made in Phase I to the development of a productivity tracking system.

As shown in Figure 12–1–1, Phase II employees have already been provided with the necessary skills to prepare them to participate in the program. Theoretically the worker now has a sound enough knowledge base and appropriate communication channels to permit the introduction and implementation of the factual phase of the program.

Introduction of the Productivity Measurement System

The introduction of the productivity tracking system is a critical step in the flow of the model with respect to the means by which the introduction is handled. Throughout Phase I, management has taken steps to develop a foundation of trust and communication to support worker participation. In the introduction of the productivity measurement system to the worker, this trust must be maintained by openly communicating the processes and methods by which the system will be developed, what the system will ultimately measure and what the goals of the system are. The authors' experience has been that the participants must have a comprehensive knowledge of what it is they are participating in in order to be effective. Too much information may be better than too little.

Education on System Function and Worker Responsibilities

Following the introduction of the system, the employee–manager discussions help to develop the specifics of how the participative program will be designed. Early formulation of roles, responsibilities, employee–manager interaction, schedules for meetings, and relevant others who need to be involved provide important formulations of the program format.

Measurement of Work Activity

The actual measurement of work activity is where all the previous activities identified are molded into a cohesive effort. Employees are asked for their substantive input into developing the method and measurement system. By identifying and measuring the time to complete the various tasks in their respective workdays, the employees are providing data on work activities that reflect a quality and depth not readily available to management.

If program development has progressed smoothly to this point, the data collection phase generates a "sense of mission" that contributes to the enthusiasm and quality of the measurement. Participants now regard the program as a joint venture between management and employees, and this commonality of purpose can ensure the accuracy and adequacy of the data forthcoming from the productivity analysis. Once the participants have developed a sense of involvement, participation, and "ownership" of the program, the more accurate the information will be and the more likely that even better productivity criteria will be formulated.

The measurement of work activity and the source via the process described previously provides the basis for the evolution of viable worker productivity standards. The substantive data provided by the employees allow for the informed establishment of a system of activity standards against which individual and departmental performance can be tracked and evaluated.

Feedback

Finally the model incorporates the necessary feedback loop. Feedback essentially follows two routes; both routes flow back to the employees, one route being performance evaluation and appraisal of the function, and the other being feedback on how well the individual is functioning within the framework of the work unit.

As experience with the implementation of quality circles has shown, commitment on the part of management to worker participation can be a motivating force to maintain system viability.[20] This two-channel communication facilitates the expansion of the management–worker dialogue into other facets of the organization's performance. It also fosters a climate of trust and collaboration throughout the organization.

HOW THE MODEL WORKS

To illustrate how the model (Figure 12–1–1) operates to use participative methods to develop productivity tracking systems, the following section describes a specific case in which the fundamental principles and many of the mechanics of the model were used.

Background

The University of California Irvine Medical Center (UCIMC) is a large acute care facility in

Orange, California. In addition to providing general acute and psychiatric care, the hospital serves as a poison, burn, and trauma center and provides other services for central Orange County.

In May 1981 top management targeted the Department of Respiratory Therapy at UCIMC as the unit within the hospital where productivity tracking measures would best be initiated. Respiratory Therapy, a unit of the Department of Medicine, Pulmonary Division, employs 45 full-time equivalents, inclusive of support and clerical personnel, and provides approximately 30 different services to the patient population. Patient service areas within the department are divisionalized by medical specialty and are geographically dispersed throughout the hospital's grounds. Reflecting this fact, the department's structure is organized around its patient mix with the major structural divisions being adult and neonatal respiratory therapy. In addition, there is a small ancillary materiel management group that supports the other divisions. With patient care being the primary mission of the department, the focus of the productivity study was specifically on the adult and neonatal divisions.

The Environment

At the time of the productivity study, three major destabilizing factors were at work that adversely affected the environment within the department. First, the manager of the department was relatively new and on arrival had instituted a variety of different and generally more stringent policies that created dissatisfaction among department personnel. Second, the department was working under relatively high workloads. This, coupled with a relatively understaffed condition, contributed to a stressful, low-morale climate within the department. Finally several members of the department's rank and file were active in union activities and continually attempted to recruit new members, which generally created significant peer pressure adding to an already stressful situation.

All of these factors contributed to the destabilization of the environment into which the productivity study was to be launched. The principal impact of this destabilization was that a general sentiment of mistrust was widespread among employees and among the management personnel ranks.

Groundwork

Prior to the initiation of the actual program development, a good deal of time (four weeks) was invested in studying the number of both the inputs into and the products forthcoming from the department activities. Careful identification of the flow, types, and number of services was also carried out in order that instruments could be designed to effectively measure the therapists' activity levels.

Additionally, during this period careful observation and documentation were made of potential destabilizing factors so that when the actual work activity measurement segment of the productivity study was introduced, the marketing program could target those specific problems most likely to impact data gathering and program development.

Throughout the preliminary and operational periods of the productivity study, strict neutrality was maintained by the study coordinator so as not to be identified with either management or labor. Given the existing environment in the department, it was felt that this approach would be most expeditious in bridging the gap between the various participants.

Work Activity Measurement Inventory

Based on the information gathered during the preliminary phase, the Work Activity Measurement Inventory (Exhibit 12–1–1) was designed as the productivity study's principal data collection vehicle. The inventory measured the time required for procedure delivery, inclusive of cleanup and charting, and was filled out by all line therapists on a daily basis during the productivity study period. The format of the inventory

Exhibit 12–1–1 Worksheet Productivity Tracking

Date: _____   Current Classification: _____

Work Period: DAY,   PM,   NIGHT   Start Time _____   "S" If done with Student
(circle one)   Stop Time _____   Work Area Code

PROCEDURE	TIME REQUIRED*								COMMENTS**
	1	2	3	4	5	6	7	8	
Aerosol									
Aerosol Continuous									
Bedside Spirometry									
Blood Gas Analysis									
Blood Gas Puncture									
Bronchoscopy— Biopsy									
Bronchoscopy— Diagnostic									
C.P.A.P. (Check)									
Incentive Spirometry (Check)									
Incentive Spirometry (Set-up)									
Hydro Room									
I.P.P.B.									
Optimal PEEP Study									
Postural Drainage									
Therapist Stand-by									
Ventilator— Continuous (Check)									
LB-3									
CPR									
Volumes & Capacities									

* Please enter time at beginning of set-up and at end of clean-up or charting.

** Please note any incident or peculiarity that affects time required for completion of a procedure or that affects patient care.

Work area codes:

Burn ICU	1	Surgical ICU	
CCU	2	Tower	
Clinics	3	3rd Floor	
Emergency Room	4	4th Floor	
Mental Health	5	5th Floor	
Out Buildings	6		

also allowed the documentation of shift-to-shift variations in completion time, the effects of teaching responsibilities on procedure completion time, and any effects caused by the geographical constraints of particular work areas within the hospital.

The introduction of this data-gathering instrument to department personnel followed a two-step format. In order that imperfections in the instrument, and the marketing program designed to introduce it, could be identified and corrected, the inventory was first tested with the working supervisors. This test introduction lasted two weeks. During the two-week period the supervisors completed the inventory daily and closely monitored the effectiveness of the marketing activities and the quality of the data forthcoming from the inventory. Additionally, feedback on the inventory was continually solicited in order that needed changes could be effected prior to implementation of the department-wide study.

In general, this approach to developing productivity standards was well received by the supervisors. An unforeseen benefit was that the data gathered from the supervisors provided an excellent baseline against which the line therapists' responses could later be compared for accuracy.

The second step in the format was the marketing and introduction of the inventory to the line therapists. Because of the number of persons involved, and in order to maintain consistency of information, the marketing of the productivity study took the form of several large group meetings during which the basic philosophy behind the study, the role of the therapists in the study and the potential long-range impacts of a productivity tracking system in the department were discussed. Because of the limited amount of resources available for use in support of the study, continuing education of the therapists in the various aspects of participative management skills was handled on an informal basis. This approach proved to be inadequate because it was extremely difficult to meet with all the therapists, individually or in groups, due to the constraints of their normal workday. The lack of formal training in participative methods had adverse effects on the process: in essence participants had to learn by trial and error, which presented a serious obstacle to program implementation.

Data Collection

Following the introduction of the inventory, the study moved into a six-week data collection phase. During this period the therapists completed and handed in the inventories daily. The data were then compiled in a central log to be used later in the development of time standards. Incoming data were compared with the preliminary test study results and with stop-watch measurements, which were carried out for selected procedures. Although some variations did occur, possibly due to individual measurement differences or other unidentified factors, on the whole the data compared quite favorably.

Time Standard Development and the Activity Reporting System

Following the data collection phase, the time data for all the procedures provided by the department were compiled and their respective means computed. The mean completion time for a given procedure was then adopted as the time standard for that procedure.

The time standards developed in the productivity study were incorporated into a computer-assisted, three-step, productivity tracking system. Daily activity was documented by the individual therapists at the end of their shifts. The data were then compiled by the shift supervisor. Totals for each 24-hour period were then entered into the computer (PDP 1134, Digital Equipment Corporation). The computer compiled daily and monthly personnel power use reports that documented total department activity and productive time (time spent in delivery of procedures for which the medical center would be compensated) in terms of minutes worked per paid personnel hour by the therapists (Table 12–1–1).

Table 12–1–1 Computer Summary: Productivity Tracking

*** DEPARTMENT OF RESPIRATORY THERAPY ***

WORK FORCE UTILIZATION STATISTICS
MONTHLY REPORT FOR JAN

Treatment	Total Treatments	Total Work Minutes
(1) Aerosol	1774.0	30158.0
(2) Aerosol Continuous	2598.0	20056.6
(3) Bedside Spirometry	158.0	1422.0
(4) Blood Gas Analysis	2051.0	15382.5
(5) Blood Gas Puncture	405.0	5670.0
(6) Bronchoscopy—biopsy	3.0	507.0
(7) Bronchoscopy—diagnostic	8.0	560.0
(8) C.P.A.P.	37.0	185.0
(9) C.P.R.	20.5	1230.0
(10) Hydro Room	6.5	390.0
(11) Incentive Spirometry—check	1460.0	9373.2
(12) Incentive Spirometry—set-up	194.0	2677.2
(13) I.P.P.B.	792.0	15285.6
(14) LB- End Tidal CO_2	84.0	789.6
(15) Optimal PEEP Study	4.0	240.0
(16) Postural Drainage	1269.0	18527.4
(17) Therapist Stand-by	84.5	5070.0
(18) Ventilator Continuous	2033.0	16894.2
(19) Volumes and Capacities	247.0	2544.1

Total Treatments Delivered—	13228.5	
Total Minutes Worked—	146962.39	
Minutes Worked per Paid Hr. This Period	34.39	

KEY LESSONS TO DATE

In reviewing and reflecting on the experience of the productivity study approach, when used in an actual work environment, the following important learnings emerged.

1. The need for a formal training program in participative skills, involving both management and workers, to support the activities in the study was clear. In the case study formal training was substituted with informal group meetings. Although these proved useful, the episodal nature of the contacts did not provide adequate reinforcement to ensure an optimal response from the workers.

2. Effective marketing of the program through discussion and supported by formal education and training is critical.

3. Successful change programs must rely on informed and motivated persons within the organization if the results are to be maintained. Although outside consultants are often useful in the preliminary stages of analysis, designing the program and executing the initial efforts of organizational change, consultants cannot sustain the organization's efforts over time. The maintenance of change falls on the internal resource persons within the organization. Those internal resources do not develop spontaneously; individuals must be trained,

developed, and given the legitimacy to perform required tasks.

4. Organizational change is more likely to meet with success when key management persons are involved and support the change process. Planned change must have the support and understanding of management and other key personnel if it is to proceed smoothly and produce enduring effects. Although there may be exceptions, change without support of key management is generally at a great disadvantage. Basically there is no substitute for the positive boost that an informed and sophisticated management can provide.

5. Organizational change is best accomplished when persons most likely to be affected by the change are brought into the process at its inception. Change is generally threatening, but much of the anxiety and uncertainty can be reduced by early involvement of participants.

For the most part, sudden and unexpected change creates and intensifies resistance to it. Involving persons early in the change process not only acclimates them to the idea of change, but permits them to influence those changes that will affect their jobs, relationships, and personal satisfactions.

6. Given the feelings of threat and paranoia brought on by organizational change, honest and open communication about change plans is imperative for the overall and ultimate success of the program.

The experience described in this article rekindles and supports the notion of participative management as a vehicle for productivity improvement. It seems abundantly clear, however, that management support, organizational preparation, and a long-term perspective are necessary for successful implementation of this approach.

NOTES

1. J. Maron-Cost, "Productivity: Key to Cost Containment." *Hospitals* 54, no. 18 (1980):77–79.

2. W.A. Michela, "Numerous Productivity Indicators Analyzed." *Hospitals* 52, no. 23 (1981):62–69.

3. M.C. Burkhart and M. Schultz, "Management of Health Service Delivery and Professional Productivity: A Case Study Model." *Public Health Reports* 94 (July–August 1978):326–331.

4. Maron-Cost, "Productivity: Key to Cost Containment."

5. Ibid.

6. M. Mannisto, "An Assessment of Productivity in Health Care." *Hospitals* 54 (September 16, 1980):71–76.

7. Ibid.

8. Maron-Cost, "Productivity: Key to Cost Containment."

9. D. McGregor, *The Human Side of Enterprise.* New York: McGraw-Hill, 1960.

10. "The New Industrial Relations." *Business Week* 2687 (May 11, 1981):84–98.

11. "A Try at Steel Mill Harmony." *Business Week* 2694 (June 29, 1981):132–136.

12. C. Deutsch, "Trust: The New Ingredient in Management." *Business Week* 2695 (July 6, 1981):104–105.

13. C.G. Burck, "What Happens When Workers Manage Themselves?" *Fortune* 104 (July 27, 1981):62–69.

14. E. Rendall, "Quality Circles—A 'Third Wave' Intervention." *Training and Development Journal* 35 (March 1981).

15. "The New Industrial Relations."

16. Deutsch, "Trust: The New Ingredient in Management."

17. Burck, "What Happens When Workers Manage Themselves?"

18. "The New Industrial Relations."

19. Ibid.

20. Rendall, "Quality Circles."

13

Inventory

Reading 13–1

Inventory Management System Reaps Savings for Department

Simone M. Turner, Karen Lopienski, Rahsaan Gammon, and *Robert Broderick*

CASE STUDY: DEVISING A SYSTEM TO ORDER, TRACK, AND STOCK INTRAOCULAR LENSES

The administration of the Manhattan Medical Center (MMC)[*] has contracted with us to study the current inventory method used in the Department of Ophthalmology for obtaining intraocular lenses (IOLs) for cataract surgery.

Currently, the hospital is ordering 700–1800 units per year for use among the 16 surgeons on staff.

Due to the specific preferences of each surgeon, the administration has allowed the surgeons to order from various vendors of these lenses. There has been a recent increase in the number of cataract surgeries, which has resulted in clerical staff spending excessive amounts of time trying to best accommodate the ordering practices of all 16 surgeons.

---

[*]Note: This following case study is based on actual analysis. The name of the hospital, its location, and the names of vendors have been changed for reasons of confidentiality.

Source: Reprinted from S.M. Turner et al., "Inventory Management System Reaps Savings for Department," in *Hospital Cost Management and Accounting,* S.A. Finkler, ed., Vol. 8, No. 4, pp. 1–7. Copyright 1996, Aspen Publishers, Inc.

The current stock of lenses is comprised of a group of generic lenses and is used only in emergencies. There is also another group of lenses in storage that have become technically obsolete.

Presently, there is no system for tracking inventory and orders. It is often necessary to have lenses delivered by Federal Express Overnight if there are any shipping and/or ordering errors. This has resulted in an increase in the department's shipping and ordering costs. Furthermore, if the unit cannot be delivered on time, it results in a delay of surgery.

Because of this sporadic, haphazard system of formal order and tracking, the department does not receive quantity discounts, does not establish a working relationship with one vendor, and has no idea of its total inventory at any given time.

At present, the MMC is being reimbursed the cost of each lens, regardless of the lens price. The administration is concerned that in light of the vast changes in health care and the push toward managed care, the current system will not be able to cover the department's costs.

Typically, managed care companies will reimburse a specific, predetermined amount for lenses, and the MMC needs to control its inventory costs in order to remain competitive with other facilities.

The administration has asked us to devise a systematic method of ordering, tracking, and stocking the units. Our proposal as consultants with the Wagner Group is as follows:

- Using 1994 data, study the historical cost of each IOL and the quality of each implant used. Identify the most cost efficient and most widely used vendor.

- Survey the surgeons about their manufacturer preferences to identify how the surgeons' needs for specific lenses can best be accommodated. By reducing the number of vendors used, ordering costs may also decrease and the department will qualify for quantity discounts.

- From the information provided by the surgeon survey, allow the two most popular vendors to bid for contracts with the Department of Ophthalmology. One vendor will be awarded the contract to be the sole distributor to the department, based on its ability to provide high quality, reasonably priced lenses. It is expected that this vendor will meet the needs of all the physicians, while appeasing the majority of them.

- As the present inventory system is inefficient, determine the optimal number of lenses required to be in stock by using the economic ordering quantity (EOQ) technique.

- Explore the just-in-time (JIT) approach to ordering to determine whether this method would work for the department and the cost implications of this approach.

- Explore the periodic vs. perpetual inventory tracking systems to determine which of these systems will work best for the department's needs. In addition, designate specific employees to be responsible for ordering and maintaining the inventory.

At this time, the inventory and ordering process for IOLs at MMC's Department of Ophthalmology is chaotic and costly. An adequate inventory system will reduce time spent by employees' tracking piecemeal orders and will also reduce costs related to overnight deliveries. In addition, by reducing the inefficiencies in the system, the number of postponed or delayed surgeries due to shipping errors will be reduced.

BACKGROUND

The MMC's Department of Ophthalmology, which was opened in 1973, provides outpatient cataract surgery, which involves the implantation of an IOL. This lens is a plastic device that is inserted into the eye to focus light rays on the retina once the cataract has been removed.

Cataract surgery has become increasingly common, and MMC performs approximately 800 surgeries per year. Because of the high number of surgeries, MMC needs to keep a large inventory of IOLs in stock.

Problems with the Current Inventory System

Presently, the system at MMC has provided the surgeons with "carte blanche" in respect to ordering IOLs. The 16 surgeons can order an IOL from any vendor, regardless of the price, given that the lenses are approved by the Food and Drug Administration.

Currently the clerical staff is spending excessive amounts of time trying to accommodate the ordering practices of the various surgeons. The staff is now making small quantity orders in an ad hoc, informal manner.

Additionally, there is no formal system of tracking the inventory, and it is often necessary to have the lenses delivered by Federal Express Overnight. This haphazard system has resulted in extremely high shipping and ordering costs, and surgeries are often delayed due to shipping errors, costing the department more.

Since inventory represents only a small part of the year-end balance sheet in comparison to labor, many health care organizations have not been cost effective in their inventory practices.

The MMC is no exception. Past invoices from the department revealed that the prices of lenses ordered ranged from $145 to $495, with virtually no difference in quality. The department needs to design a system that is more cost effective and efficient so that they can avoid being in an unfavorable position when it comes time to negotiate contracts with managed care companies.

It became evident to the team that the present inventory system was costly and inefficient. Streamlining the IOL ordering and inventory process would result in substantial savings.

RESEARCH AND DATA COLLECTION

The goal of our research was to identify the vendor that would most effectively meet the needs of our surgeons and patients, while providing the most cost efficient mechanism to purchase and stock the lenses.

The following objectives were pursued: examination of IOL ordering trends for 1994 (vendors used, types of lenses ordered, quantity, and prices); obtaining of surgeons' preferences in regards to lens characteristics and manufacturers; and examination of 1994 operating room trends to collect data on loss of operating time due to shipping delays.

1994 Ordering Trends

Research showed that the Ophthalmology surgeons were ordering from four different vendors *(Opticon, Fundop, Retinar, and Oculus)*, in no organized fashion. IOL orders were placed in extremely inefficient ways. One example of this inefficiency occurred during the month of July 1994. During this time, there were a total of 50 lenses ordered from Retinar. These lenses were ordered on 17 separate occasions, on an average of every 1.8 days. On only three of these occasions, more than three lenses were ordered at the same time. Orders placed to all of the vendors followed a similar pattern throughout the year.

The prices charged for the lenses also varied greatly among the four vendors. Exhibit 13–1–1 shows 1994 prices charged by each vendor for IOLs.

Exhibit 13–1–1 IOL Prices in 1994

Opticon	$250
Fundop	$396
Retinar	$200
Oculus	$495

Surgeon Preferences

We surveyed the 16 surgeons using a questionnaire to ascertain what their preferences were (see Exhibit 13–1–2). There was a 100 percent response rate to the questionnaire.

There was not a great variety of lens type in the market. The main types were plastic or silicon. The trend appeared to be toward silicon (small incision) lenses. These lenses are flexible and require a smaller incision at the insertion site. Most of the surgeons (97%) preferred the silicon lenses. The questionnaire revealed that Retinar and Opticon were the two most popular vendors among the 16 surgeons.

1994 Operating Room Trends

Operating room schedules for the year were analyzed. Data showed that a moderate amount of operating room time was lost in the Department of Ophthalmology. Sixty-eight percent of the surgeons encountered some loss of operating room time due to shipping and ordering errors, or late orders throughout the year (see Exhibit 13–1–2). This resulted in an 11 percent overall loss of operating room time.

COMPONENTS OF CONTRACT NEGOTIATIONS

Data revealed that Retinar and Opticon were the two most reasonably priced vendors among their competitors, at $200 and $250 respectively. Retinar and Opticon also proved to be the most popular vendors among the surgeons (see Figure 13–1–1.) Because MMC would use the services of one vendor exclusively to annually stock an inventory of 800 lenses, Retinar and Opticon

Figure 13–1–1 Surgeon Preferences among Vendors

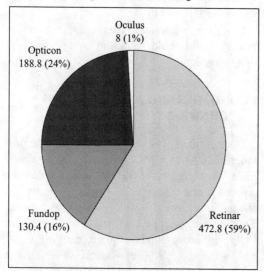

Exhibit 13–1–2 IOL Questionnaire

1. What lens characteristic do you require for a high quality transplantation?
   - Silicon: 98%
   - Plastic: 2%
2. Besides the material of the lens, are there any other characteristics that are considered when choosing lenses?
   - No: 100%
3. How many lens manufacturers do you do business with?
   - Only 1: 31%
   - 1–2: 56%
   - More than 2: 13%
4. If you had to choose one vendor, who would it be?
   - Retinar: 59%
   - Opticon: 24%
   - Fundop: 16%
   - Oculus: 1%
5. Are there any differences in the lenses among the vendors that you use (if you use more than one vendor)?
   - No: 100%
6. Would you be willing to select your IOLs from a vendor other than the one (or the variety) you deal with now if lenses of equal quality could be provided to you?
   - Yes: 19%
   - No: 81%
7. Approximately how many cataract surgeries do you perform per year?
   - Total: 800
8. Are the IOLs always available at least one week prior to surgery?
   - Yes: 12.5%
   - No: 87.5%
9. If no, list some of the reasons that lenses are not available:
   - Shipping errors: 35%
   - Late orders: 29%
   - Errors in orders: 35%
10. Do you ever find it necessary to cancel or postpone a procedure due to errors/failure of lenses to arrive on time?
    - Yes: 68%
    - No: 32%
11. Approximately how many procedures do you cancel per year because of lens errors?
    - Total: 88
12. Would you be interested in a centralized inventory system to stock the IOLs?
    - Yes: 75%
    - No: 25%

were given the opportunity to bid for the contract. Retinar proposed the most cost effective deal, offering MMC 800 lenses at $150 per lens. Opticon followed closely at $175 per lens. Retinar was given the contract.

In addition to quantity and price of lenses, we negotiated that Retinar would be responsible for shipping and handling costs, and for stocking the lenses on a consignment basis. Retinar was very flexible and met our demands with ease. Retinar also agreed to make any reasonable provisions throughout the year (e.g., quantity changes, specialty lenses) if needed.

THE FEASIBILITY OF JUST-IN-TIME

The JIT system of inventory is a system in which products are delivered precisely at the time they are needed. Many organizations benefit from the implementation of this system because the total cost of each unit decreases with the reduction of storage costs, handling costs, and interest costs. Organizations that use JIT can also benefit by using storage space in new, more lucrative ways. Finally, JIT systems can reduce the risk of products becoming obsolete before they are used.

To determine the feasibility of a JIT system for MMC, it was necessary to determine the total cost of the current inventory system. The Department of Ophthalmology's total costs included a portion of an employee's salary, storage costs, interest costs, and ordering costs. These costs will be explained in detail in the following section, Economic Ordering Quantity Technique. Each component of total cost needs to be compared to the total cost of implementing a *perfectly* working JIT system.

Many health care professionals are skeptical about the feasibility of a JIT system in the health care industry. The system works best in factory-type organizations where events are more predictable and errors will not result in the loss of human life. However, cataract surgeries in the Ophthalmology Department are performed on a scheduled, elective basis. Under these circumstances, we examined JIT to determine if the department would benefit from its implementation.

We first looked at the storage space. The units were quite small and currently stored in a locked cabinet located in one of the operating supply rooms. The department could not necessarily increase revenue by finding another use for the current storage space, so few benefits, if any, would be found in storage costs using the JIT system.

IOLs have a shelf-life of approximately five years. Obsolescence occurs because of technological advances. Since the department does not plan to stock the lenses for a long period of time, obsolescence was not a factor that needed to be considered.

Normally, interest costs would have to be investigated, but they do not apply when units are provided on a consignment basis. Since Retinar has agreed to stock the units on a consignment basis, interest costs will not exist for the department.

Taking the above factors into consideration, instituting the JIT system would have few benefits. The system would require time and effort in the early stages that would cost more than it is worth for the results that would be achieved.

Therefore, we do not recommend that MMC institute the JIT system.

It was our opinion that the most savings on inventory costs could be found by applying the EOQ technique.

ECONOMIC ORDERING QUANTITY TECHNIQUE

Once Retinar was chosen to be the sole provider of IOLs to MMC, we used EOQ to determine what quantity of the 800 lenses should be ordered at one time. We also needed to determine at what intervals the inventory should be ordered. Three factors must be known in order to measure EOQ: inventory purchase price, carrying costs, and ordering costs. (See Exhibit 13–1–3 for a breakdown of the costs that follow.)

Purchase Price of Inventory

The inventory purchase price in MMC's situation was zero, because of Retinar's consignment agreement. Because MMC will be charged as each unit is used, inventory costs are driven down.

Exhibit 13–1–3 Economic Ordering Technique, IOL Inventory

Purchase price of inventory	$0
Carrying costs	
Capital costs	$0
Out-of-pocket costs	
Cost of annual inspection	
1 hour per month at $15 per hour	720 (sic)
Obsolescence	0
Damage, loss, theft	
1/150 lenses are damaged	1,200
Total carrying costs	$1,920
= $1,920/800 lenses	
= $2.40 (cost to carry each unit)	
Ordering Costs	
Labor of employees	$40
Error in orders	2
Other costs per order	8
Total ordering cost per order	$50

Carrying Costs

There are two major categories of carrying costs: *capital costs* and *out-of-pocket costs*. Capital costs represent the resources spent for inventory that could otherwise have been earning interest. MMC had zero capital costs because Retinar committed to stock the IOLs free of charge. Out-of-pocket cost includes annual inspection assigned to one employee spending approximately one hour per month at $15 per hour ($720 (sic) annually); obsolescence ($0); and the cost of lost, damaged, or stolen lenses—approximated to be $1,200 because according to 1994 data, one out of every 150 lenses fell into this category.

After gathering the above data, we then estimated the cost to carry one unit to be $2.40 ($1,920 total carrying costs/800 total units). This figure was used later to calculate the optimal quantity to be ordered at one time.

Ordering Costs

Ordering costs are the third factor used in calculating the EOQ. Ordering cost consists of employee labor costs of $40 of labor per order. Ordering errors average an additional cost of $2 per order. Other ordering costs total $8 per order. Therefore, the total cost per order is $50 (based on 1994 data).

Once we gathered the information necessary to calculate the carrying costs, we were almost able to calculate the total costs. But first, the optimal quantity is required. To calculate the optimal quantity, we took the square root of two times the annual number of lenses multiplied by the cost per order, divided by the carrying cost per lens (see Exhibit 13–1–4). The EOQ was found to be 183 lenses.

Since the need would be for 800 lenses annually, the 183 lenses ordered at a bulk rate will last only a few months. In order to avoid supply shortages, we calculated the number that would serve as an indicator to the clerk that a new order needed to be placed. At 800 lenses per year, an average of 2.2 lenses would be used per day (800/365 days in a year). Multiply 2.2 by the number of days from placing an order until receipt to find the time to reorder. Assuming 10 days for receipt from the order, we should reorder when 22 lenses are left (2.2 × 10). Due to possible shipment delays or errors, we have decided to carry a safety stock of an additional 20 lenses so that a new order should be placed when stock reaches 42.

Now that the optimal quantity was known, we could calculate the total cost, which is equal to the carrying costs plus the ordering costs. These two factors of the total cost should be equal when the optimal quantity is reached. At 183 lenses, our total cost was $438, which represents the optimal quantity to be ordered at the lowest total cost (see Figure 13–1–2). As you move away from the optimal quantity in either direction, the total cost steadily increases.

In summary, we recommend that MMC take the following actions:

- Place IOL orders in bulk of 183 lenses.
- Place a new order when stock reaches 42 lenses.
- Keep a safety stock of 20 lenses at all times.

Exhibit 13–1–4 Calculating the EOQ

$$Q^* = \sqrt{2(A)(P)/S}$$

$$Q^* = \sqrt{2(800 \text{ lenses})(\$50)/\$2.40}$$

$$= 183 \text{ lenses (Ordered approximately every 3 months)}$$

Total Cost = Q* (S)/2 + A(P)/Q*
carrying   ordering
costs   costs

$$TC = \frac{183 \times 2.40}{2} + \frac{800 \times 50}{183}$$

$$= \quad 219.60 \quad + \quad 218.60 = \textbf{\$438}$$

Q^* = optimal ordering quantity
A = quantity ordered each year
P = cost to place each order
S = cost to carry one unit

Figure 13–1–2 Cost Curve TC = Q(S)/2 + A(P)/Q

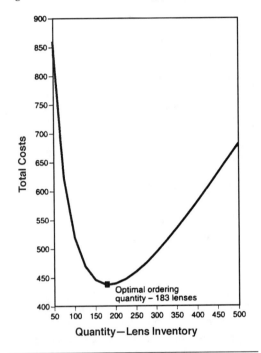

PERPETUAL VS. PERIODIC
INVENTORY TRACKING

When considering the type of inventory tracking system to use to follow the IOLs, perpetual and periodic inventory methods were considered. A periodic inventory tracking system is less time consuming and requires less resources. However, a perpetual inventory system is recommended due to the nature of the department.

Although a perpetual inventory tracking system is more time consuming, it is important to know the exact amount of lenses available at all times. The lenses are small and take very little time to track, so the employee responsible can allot a minimal amount of time per month (approximately 60 minutes) to check the stock.

Since there is a certain number of lenses that will serve as an indicator when to reorder, it is important for personnel to know the status of inventory, as delays and improper timing could mean a loss of revenue.

**SUMMARY AND
RECOMMENDATIONS**

The MMC's Department of Ophthalmology inventory system was decentralized, costly, and inefficient. After our consultation with this entity, we suggest the following changes:

- Retinar will be the sole vendor for providing IOLs.

- 183 lenses will be available in stock effective January 1, 1996.

- Stock will be reordered when the supply reaches 42 lenses.

- 183 lenses will be ordered at intervals of approximately every three months.

- A perpetual inventory tracking system will be used to follow stock.

- Specific employees will be designated to maintain, audit, and inventory stock on a monthly basis.

- Re-evaluate system in one year.

Savings are expected to exceed $77,000 per year from reduced purchase of lenses alone. Also, it is anticipated that there will be profits earned from cases that in prior years would have been turned away due to stock-outs.

14

Dealing with Uncertainty

Reading 14–1

Decision Analysis and Capital Budgeting: Application to the Delivery of Critical Care Services

Donald B. Chalfin

Rising health care costs, prospective payment and diagnosis-related groups (DRGs), along with the growing concern over the inability to deliver high quality care, have forced clinicians and administrators alike to examine the ways in which we allocate scarce resources and budget limited expenditures. In light of this heightened cost consciousness, a great deal of attention has been focused on the disproportionate share of resources used in intensive care units (ICUs). Specifically, ICUs account for only 5 percent of all hospital beds, yet they consume nearly 20 percent of all hospital budgets.[1,2] At the same time, many issues have been raised concerning the cost-effectiveness and the efficacy of intensive care. In view of this and in view of the growing national proliferation of ICUs, hospitals are now exploring alternative solutions to the treatment of the critically ill.

Recently, hospitals have explored the use of intermediate care ("step-down") units in lieu of ICUs.[3] Step-down units (SDUs) can be viewed as hybrids between ICUs and the standard hospital beds or wards, both in terms of the scope of

services provided and the severity of illness of the patients who are treated. SDUs usually exist in conjunction with ICUs and are reserved for patients who require less intervention than the standard ICU provides but who nonetheless need closer monitoring and more therapeutic support than is available on the general medical or surgical floor. SDUs (or similar variants) have become popular because of the perception that many patients who are admitted to ICUs can be treated just as effectively in less aggressive and thus less costly settings. Thus, the issue of whether or not a hospital should build an SDU represents a timely and important capital budgeting decision that is well suited to formal modeling techniques.

METHOD OF MODELING: DECISION ANALYSIS

Formal decision analysis and its systematic approach to the "quantification of uncertainty" provides a valuable framework to study the general issue of capital budgeting and the specific question of whether or not to build an SDU. Decision analysis originated from the fields of operations research, economics, and mathematics and was first applied to military and business problems.[4] Over the past decade, decision analysis techniques have been used with increasing frequency

Source: Reprinted from Donald B. Chalfin, "Decision Analysis and Capital Budgeting: Application to the Delivery of Critical Care Services," *Hospital Cost Management and Accounting,* Vol. 2, No. 9, December 1990, pp. 1–8. Copyright 1990, Aspen Publishers, Inc.

in clinical medicine and have also been applied to problems involving cost-effectiveness and cost-benefit analysis.[5–8] Decision analysis is based upon the explicit stipulation of all possible events along with their associated probabilities of occurrence. A complete discussion of the methods and techniques of decision analysis is beyond the scope of this article and can be found elsewhere.[9,10] In general, however, decision analysis models provide both a quantitative and a qualitative assessment of the problems under study along with an accurate estimation of expected outcome and, thus, an optimal and logical solution. The assessment is quantitative because it incorporates a precise "valuation" of the underlying utilities (e.g., dollars, years of survival) for each of the possible outcomes, given a specific course of action. Additionally, every valid and viable model yields significant qualitative insight with respect to each individual process that comprises the "structure" of every problem. In order to effectively formulate a model and determine the appropriate "heuristic" approach, each component of every situation, along with all underlying assumptions about every possible alternative, must be rigorously reviewed prior to its inclusion into the model.

DECISION ANALYSIS: STRUCTURE AND STEPS

The basic component of any decision problem structured under formal decision analysis is the decision tree. The decision tree, essentially, is a method in which all alternatives for any problem under analysis are explicitly stipulated, along with each of the possible subsequent outcomes. From this, quantitative expected values for each of the problem options can be determined, thereby leading to an informed choice.

Several sequential steps are crucial in the construction of every decision analytical model:[9]

1. *Creation of the decision tree.* Includes the actual formulation of the decision problem, assignment of probabilities, and determination of appropriate outcome values or measures.

2. *Expected value calculations.* A numerical determination for each of the decision alternatives.
3. *Selection of the alternative with the highest expected value.*
4. *Sensitivity analysis.* Testing the conclusions and the "robustness" of the model in terms of how variations in the underlying assumptions (e.g., probability and utility assessments) would alter one's choice among the alternatives.

The following case study involving capital budgeting illustrates the basic science and steps of decision analysis and its direct application to budgeting problems. It focuses on whether or not a particular hospital should build a brand new SDU or expand its ICU. SMLTREE, a commercial software package specifically developed for medical decision analysis, will also be used to demonstrate one of several invaluable decision analysis computer programs.

CASE STUDY: CASHEN MEDICAL CENTER

For this case study, several facts and assumptions must be noted prior to construction of the formal model. It is also important to note that all of the figures and statistics represent hypothetical values, as the purpose of this example is to demonstrate the appropriate use of decision analysis in long-term capital budget preparations.

Cashen Medical Center (CMC), a 500-bed community hospital, has decided that a dire need exists to expand its critical care services, because its current 10-bed ICU is always completely full. It has determined that only two possibilities are feasible:

1. expansion of the current 10-bed ICU to 15 beds
2. construction of a new 10-bed SDU

Either of these two options is acceptable to the medical and nursing staffs.

The annual fixed maintenance costs for either alternative that CMC has projected (in present dollars) are as follows:

ICU expansion	$2,500,000
SDU construction	$4,000,000

Both of these projected costs include all expenditures for all equipment associated with a properly functioning unit (monitors, ventilators, etc.). For the purposes of simplicity, we will assume that the initial construction costs for both of these options are insignificant.

CMC receives all of its reimbursement according to DRGs for its particular state. Like most other hospitals in the nation, CMC has determined that it loses significant amounts of money on all patients who require special services such as ICUs or SDUs. Because of economies of scale, CMC has determined, based upon state-wide data, that projected losses for the expanded ICU or the new SDU will be directly linked to each unit's occupancy rate over the course of a one-year period. The projected losses are as follows:

Expanded ICU. CMC will lose $1,500,000 if the average annual ICU occupancy falls below 80 percent of capacity, or below 12 beds. If occupancy falls below 60 percent, or below 9 beds, CMC will lose $2,500,000. Above 80 percent occupancy, losses will amount to $150,000.

Step-down unit. CMC projects that if SDU occupancy falls below 80 percent, or 8 beds, they will lose $500,000. If occupancy falls below 60 percent, or 6 beds, they will lose $1,250,000. Above 80 percent occupancy, losses will amount to a mere $75,000.

CMC has determined that each scenario has an associated probability of occurrence:

Occupancy rate	*Expanded ICU*	*New step-down unit*
80% or greater	0.30	0.15
Between 60% and 80%	0.20	0.45
Less than 60%	0.50	0.40

(Note that the sum of all probabilities for all events must equal 1).

To simplify matters, CMC expects that the losses and the resultant probabilities will remain constant from year to year.

The Decision Tree Structure for Cashen Medical Center

In the initial step of the problem, the two decision alternatives, along with all possible chance events, are carefully delineated in the basic tree structure with the appropriate decision tree notation (see Figure 14–1–1).

This figure carefully illustrates the choices that are available to CMC. The box in the figure is the conventional symbol for a *decision node,* which is the point in the tree where a choice among the possible alternatives must be made. Each alternative is represented by a line that is attached to the box.

As previously stated, both decision alternatives—the expansion of the ICU or the construction of the SDU—are subsequently associated with three unique and mutually exclusive possible outcomes that are controlled by chance, or probability. Thus each alternative is termed a *chance node,* which is depicted in decision trees as a circle. All possible chance events, in this case the three possible rates of occupancy, are connected to the chance nodes by lines (see Figure 14–1–2).

At this juncture in the creation of the decision tree, the appropriate probabilities are assigned to each of the chance events (see Figure 14–1–3). It is important to reiterate that the sum of all probabilities for all chance events must add up to 1.

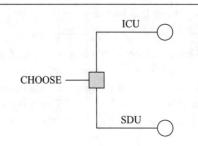

Figure 14–1–1 Basic Decision Tree

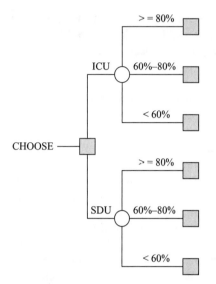

Figure 14–1–2 Decision Tree with All Chance Events

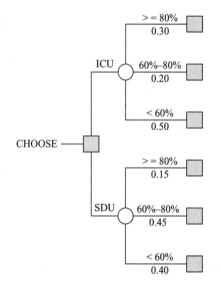

Figure 14–1–3 Decision Tree with All Probabilities

The final aspect in the construction of any decision tree is the assignment of valid "utility" measures to each of the possible outcomes. Very often, this is one of the most difficult steps in decision analysis because of multiple subjective influences that are often present. For this problem, the outcome measures will be the sum of all

costs and expenditures for each of the projected rates of occupancy.

Table 14–1–1 shows the specific outcome values that were used. The costs consist of the sum of the annual maintenance costs ($2,500,000 for ICU expansion and $4,000,000 for SDU construction) plus the projected losses for each of the three occupancy rates.

Figure 14–1–4 thus consists of the final decision tree, complete with all of the probabilities and associated costs for each respective branch.

The Baseline Analysis and Solution

The next step in decision analysis is to determine the expected value for each possible choice. In this step, the tree is "averaged out" or "folded back"[9,10] by sequential multiplication of the outcome measures and their respective probabilities. The resultant values are then summed and then the alternative with the highest expected value is ultimately chosen.

In the case of CMC, since the medical and the nursing staffs find the ICU and the SDU option equally acceptable, the administration wants to opt for the cheapest choice: the one that will minimize expenditures and losses. The expected values for the total expected costs for each alternative are as follows:

1. ICU Expansion:
   Expected costs =
   $$(0.30 \times 2,650,000)$$
   $$+ (0.20 \times 4,000,000)$$
   $$+ (0.50 \times 5,000,000)$$
   $$= 795,000 + 800,000 + 2,500,000$$
   Expected costs = \$4,095,000

Table 14–1–1 Outcome Values

Choice	Outcome (Occupancy)	Costs ($)
ICU expansion	80% or greater	2,650,000
	60% to 80%	4,000,000
	less than 60%	5,000,000
SDU construction	80% or greater	4,075,000
	60% to 80%	4,250,000
	less than 60%	4,500,000

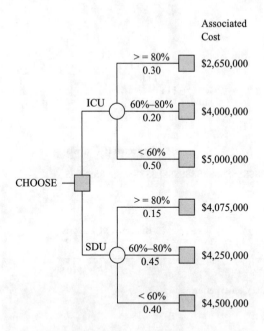

Associated
Cost

ICU

>= 80%
0.30 — $2,650,000

60%–80%
0.20 — $4,000,000

< 60%
0.50 — $5,000,000

CHOOSE

SDU

>= 80%
0.15 — $4,075,000

60%–80%
0.45 — $4,250,000

< 60%
0.40 — $4,500,000

Figure 14–1–4 Decision Tree for Cashen Medical Center

2. SDU Construction:

Expected costs =
$$(0.15 \times 4,075,000)$$
$$+ (0.45 \times 4,250,000)$$
$$+ (0.40 \times 4,500,000)$$
$$= 611,250 + 1,912,500 + 1,800,000$$

Expected costs = $4,323,750

Given the indifference of the medical and nursing staff with regard to the alternatives, and seeing that the costs of a new SDU exceed the costs of an expanded ICU by $228,750, the CMC administration should elect to expand the current ICU.

Sensitivity Analyses and Threshold Determinations

The final phase in any decision analysis is perhaps the most crucial, for it establishes the strength and "validity" of any particular model, especially in situations where the underlying probability and outcome measures are subject to

considerable variation. Sensitivity ("what-if") analyses allow one to vary the underlying assumptions and to study how one's choices may be altered. Threshold determinations show points, for any variable or set of variables, where no meaningful difference exists between any two choices. Many methods, such as multiway analyses and Monte Carlo simulations, are available for sensitivity and threshold analysis, but these are beyond the scope of this article. For the CMC example, it is obvious that all of the probabilities, along with all of the costs, can be varied. Additionally, some of the underlying assumptions, such as the stipulation concerning the negligible construction costs for both units, further lend themselves to rigorous sensitivity analysis. To illustrate the basic concepts and their application to capital budgeting, sensitivity analyses and threshold analyses will be performed on two variables: (l) the annual maintenance costs of the ICU and (2) the annual maintenance costs of the SDU.

One-Way Sensitivity and Threshold Analysis

Often enough, analysts are interested in how a change in just one variable affects a final decision, both in terms of the magnitude of change and the ultimate choice. One-way sensitivity analyses permit an analyst to test conclusions by calculating the expected value over a wide range for the variable under question.

ICU Annual Maintenance Costs

The baseline value that the CMC administrators assigned to the expanded ICU was $2,500,000. However, some of the administrators questioned this value because it relied upon several conditional assumptions. As a result, CMC believes that the decision should be tested over a wide range of costs for the expanded ICU: for $0 to $10,000,000. Figure 14–1–5 displays this analysis over this range.

As the figure shows, the threshold for the value of the annual ICU maintenance costs is

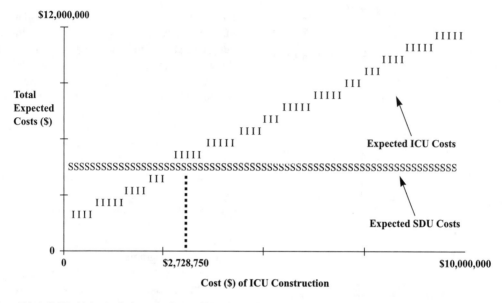

Figure 14–1–5 Sensitivity Analysis on the Costs of ICU Expansion

$2,728,750. At this value, with all other variables being held constant, there is no difference between expanding the ICU or building a new SDU (assuming that the decision makers exhibit risk averse behavior). Above this value, the costs for ICU expansion will exceed the costs for a new SDU; hence CMC should proceed with plans to construct a new SDU. Below this value for ICU maintenance costs, it is cheaper to expand the ICU and thus CMC should shelve the SDU plans.

SDU Annual Maintenance Costs

In the second one-way analysis, SDU maintenance costs will also be varied from $0 to $10,000,000, as shown in Figure 14–1–6.

In this analysis, with ICU maintenance costs and also other variables held constant, the threshold for SDU maintenance costs is $3,771,250. Above this value, CMC should expand the ICU because it represents the less expensive option. Below this, CMC should elect to build a new SDU because of the lower total expenditures.

Two-Way Sensitivity Analyses

One-way analyses are helpful in analyzing isolated changes. However, they often do not depict realistic situations, for most problems and decisions involve multiple concurrent variations. Hence multiway analyses serve the purposes of determining the change in decisions when several underlying variables are simultaneously altered. For this case study, a simplified two-way analysis will be performed, as changes in both ICU and SDU costs will be studied. Table 14–1–2 and Figure 14–1–7 show the results of this analysis. Note, in Table 14–1–2, that for each of

Table 14–1–2 ICU Cost Threshold

SDU Costs ($)	Threshold of ICU Costs ($)
0	Not found
2,000,000	728,750
4,000,000	2,728,750
6,000,000	4,728,750
8,000,000	6,728,750
10,000,000	8,728,750

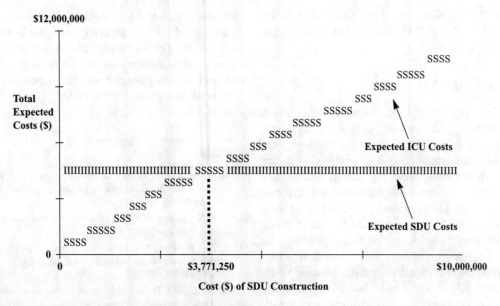

Figure 14–1–6 Sensitivity Analysis on SDU Maintenance Costs

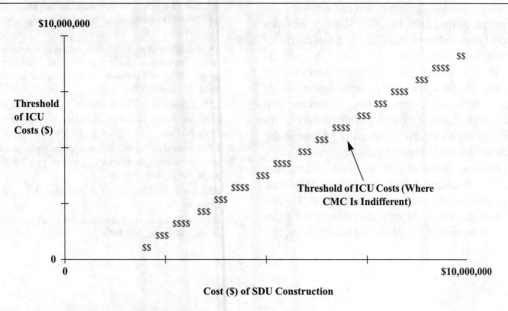

Figure 14–1–7 Two-Way Sensitivity Analysis

the last five alternatives the SDU cost exceeds the ICU cost threshold by $1,271,250.

Two-way sensitivity analyses implicitly involve threshold determinations, for they show, given the value of a certain variable, what the value of another variable would be at the threshold, or the point of indifference between two decision alternatives. In this case study, CMC should proceed with the SDU construction if the SDU costs are less than the ICU costs plus

$1,271,250. Similarly, they should elect to expand the ICU if ICU costs fall below SDU costs by the same amount.

CONCLUSIONS

The purpose of this article was to demonstrate how formal, quantitative decision analysis can be used in problems of capital budgeting and how commercial decision analysis software, which generated all of the graphs and studies, can be used for these purposes. For the case study that was presented, the baseline analysis showed that both the expanded ICU and the new SDU would lose money. Yet given the underlying assumptions and constraints, budgetary losses would be minimized with the expansion of the current ICU from 10 to 15 beds. It must be reiterated, however, that this example was greatly simplified in order to illustrate the usefulness of decision analysis for important and timely health care problems. Specifically, it did not incorporate future value or inflation, and assumed that initial construction costs for both of the projects were equal and negligible. Dollar losses for each of the occupancy rates were simplified into only three strata. Furthermore, the assumption that the medical and the nursing staffs would be indifferent with regard to the choice between the alternatives is perhaps unrealistic.

Accurate decision analysis involves a significant investment of time and human resources. Painstaking attention must be given to the collection of data in the determination of the baseline probabilities for all chance occurrences, and

appropriate outcome measures must be rigorously sought. More generally, decision analysis models must closely represent the way in which people solve problems and search for solutions if its methods and conclusions are to become invaluable aids in the capital budgeting and other decision-making processes.

NOTES

1. C. Bekes et al., Reimbursement for intensive care services under diagnosis-related groups. *Crit Care Med* 1988; 16:478.

2. M.R. Chassin, Costs and outcomes of medical intensive care. *Med Care* 1982; 20:165.

3. R.C. Bone and R.A. Balk, Noninvasive respiratory care unit: A cost effective solution for the future. *Chest* 1988; 93: 390–394.

4. J.P. Kassirer, The principles of clinical decision making: An introduction to decision analysis. *Yale J Biol Med* 1976; 49:149.

5. D.F. Ransohoff et al., Prophylactic cholecystectomy or expectant management for silent gallstones. *Ann Int Med* 1983; 99:199.

6. J.P. Hollenberg et al., Cost-effectiveness of splenectomy versus intravenous gamma globulin in treatment of chronic immune thrombocytopenic purpura in childhood. *J Pediatr* 1988; 112:530.

7. S.D. Roberts et al., Cost-effective care of end-stage renal disease: A billion dollar question. *Ann Int Med* 1980; 92:243.

8. J. Tsevat et al., Cost-effectiveness of antibiotic prophylaxis for dental procedures in patients with artificial joints. *AJPH* 1989; 79:739.

9. H.C. Sox et al., *Medical decision making.* Boston: Butterworths, 1988.

10. M.C. Weinstein et al., *Clinical decision analysis.* Philadelphia: WB Saunders, 1989.

Reading 14–2

Expected Value Technique Useful in HMO Negotiations: Tool Helps Managers Consider Potential Outcomes of Bidding Process

Steven A. Finkler

The pressures inherent in negotiating managed care contracts have spread nationwide, and are now faced by managers in hospitals throughout the country. There are many factors that must be taken into account in negotiating with managed care organizations, and much has appeared in print on the topic. A controversy rages over when to make bids based on marginal costs and when to stick with average costs. However, little information has been provided to help managers deal with some of the uncertainties involved in making their bids. The *expected value technique* is one tool that can aid managers faced with tough, critical decisions in negotiating managed care contracts and in making other complex decisions.

FINANCIAL ESTIMATES

The first step in preparing for negotiations is to gather financial information. Estimates must be made regarding profitability given a variety of alternative prices and volumes (based on capitated members or discounted rates).

Once you have that information, you must still make many decisions without knowing exactly

Source: Reprinted from S.A. Finkler, "Expected Value Technique Useful in HMO Negotiations: Tool Helps Managers Consider Potential Outcomes of Bidding Process," *Hospital Cost Management and Accounting,* Vol. 8, No. 11, pp. 1–8. Copyright February 1997, Aspen Publishers, Inc.

what will happen after your decision is made. You may be able to determine your profits if you keep your price high and attain a certain patient volume. You also can determine your profit (or loss) if you lower your price and achieve a certain patient volume. However, when you make the decision to charge a high or low price, you often cannot be assured of the exact volume of patients that the hospital will have at that price.

For example, it is possible that if you keep your HMO contract bid relatively high, other hospitals in the area will do the same. If so, then managed care organizations may be forced to pay higher rates, helping the financial viability of all hospitals in the community, including yours. On the other hand, if a close competitor cuts their price, and you haven't, you might suffer a severe financial setback as patient or member volumes fall.

However, if you cut your prices substantially, you also are not assured of one particular result. Competition may or may not cut prices to meet your low bid. Competitors' actions will again have a dramatic impact on whether you come out in great shape, okay, or in poor shape. Strategic decision making becomes an essential element in the process. And one key to that strategic decision making is recognition of the uncertainties you must consider.

Given that you don't *know* what your competitor will do, how can managers work to achieve the best outcome for their organization? Expected value is a management science technique that is frequently used in situations of uncertainty. It is a simple tool to understand, and a practical tool to use. It can be a powerful one as well.

Expected value has the capacity to inject clarity into situations where uncertainty exists. Using expected value cannot ensure a favorable outcome. Sometimes, such outcomes are not achievable. However, the technique can improve the quality of management decisions. Thus, users of the technique are more likely to make the decision that will achieve a good outcome.

THE EXPECTED VALUE CONCEPT

The underlying basis of expected value analysis is the fact that alternative events might occur. Management can take actions to affect outcomes or results, but *events* are defined as occurrences that are beyond the control of managers. For that reason events are sometimes referred to as *states of nature* in operations research or decision sciences literature.

In negotiating contracts, hospital managers often know that there are different possible events that may occur—however, they cannot know for sure in advance which event will happen. Your main competitor may bid high or low, as indicated above. In such situations decisions are often made based on a gut instinct of what to do.

Gut instincts are valuable. A manager's raw intuition can be based on years of experience and solid judgment. Expected value does not ignore the manager's intuitive feel for the situation. Rather, it takes that instinct and combines it with mathematics to improve the ultimate decision made by the manager.

Expected value is based on the mathematical concept of weighted averages and probabilities. Without using expected values, managers often decide which event is "more likely" and make their decision based on that. However, most decisions are further complicated by the fact that the payoff for the more likely event may not be the same as the payoff for the less likely event.

To consider an extreme example, sometimes lotteries have a $40 million dollar payoff for a $1 ticket. Are you more likely to win the $40 million or not if you buy a ticket? We know that you probably will lose. However, that does not mean it is automatically a mistake to buy a ticket. The payoff is great if you win. We will return to this example later.

Let's consider a somewhat less ambitious example for a moment. Suppose that a hospital is considering trying a new type of cleaning agent in the housekeeping department. The old chemical costs $10 a pound and the new chemical, highly touted by a sales representative, costs only $3 per pound. The states of nature that are possible are that the new chemical is good enough to do a satisfactory job, or that it is not. The manager's decision to try the new agent or not try it cannot change the underlying true quality of the new cleaning agent. Either it is good enough or not, but we don't know which unless we try it. If we try it and it is not good enough, we will incur a loss. If we try it and it is good enough, we will be financially better off. However, the potential loss and gain related to the decision are not likely to be equal, and the chance that the new cleaner is adequate is not necessarily fifty-fifty.

Assume that the hospital uses 10,000 pounds of cleaner per year, and that we can buy a 10 pound box to try the new chemical. What if the manager believes that the new chemical probably won't work? In fact, the manager believes that there is a 99 percent chance that the new chemical will be inferior to the old one, and unsatisfactory for the hospital's purposes. Given such a strong intuition, the manager might just not bother with the new chemical.

But that would probably be a bad decision. What if we buy one box for $30, and it turns out not to be an adequate product? The hospital will have lost $30. However, what if it is an adequate product? Then the hospital could buy 10,000 pounds a year, at a savings of $7 a pound. The potential benefit is $70,000. An investment of $30 is small relative to the potential benefit. Even though there is a very high chance it will be inadequate, it might be worthwhile to try it.

The expected value technique, explained in detail below, allows one to calculate specifically whether it would or would not pay to try that new cleaning agent. Similarly, it can provide managers with an ability to improve the outcomes of their decisions in managed care negotiations.

EXAMPLE

There are many examples of situations where alternative events might occur. Let's consider a situation where a hospital is considering contracting to provide heart surgery services to an HMO at a substantially discounted price per treatment. Although the discount is steep, if we can get enough HMO patient volume to help spread fixed costs, we expect the contract to be profitable.

Assume that if the HMO sends all of its heart surgery patients to us, we expect to increase volume by 500 patients per year. However, there is the possibility that a nearby competitor will also offer a deep discount to the HMO. In that event, demand at our hospital would probably increase by only 350 per year. Because there would be fewer patients, it is determined that money would be lost if that occurs.

Certainly, one could make arguments for making the deal even if it loses money. It might enhance the hospital's reputation to increase open heart surgery volume by even 350. Or it might allow the hospital to meet the broader demands of gatekeeper physicians who might otherwise refer all of their patients to specialists at another facility, not just those patients who need heart surgery.

Here, however, we simply want to focus on the financial calculation with respect to the HMO heart surgery patients themselves. Other factors can be taken into account in making the final decision, but the decision maker must have a reasonable idea regarding whether the new contract will directly make or lose money.

Should the manager assume 500 patients, or 350 patients? Some managers might tend to be

conservative, making the calculation assuming the most unfavorable event will occur. In this case, the manager might use the 350 estimate. Other managers might look to the most likely result. What if there is only a 25 percent chance that the other hospital will offer a similarly low price and also get a contract with the HMO? In that case, the manager might use 500 for the calculation, since that is what will probably happen. Neither of these approaches is optimal.

Expected value finds a middle ground between the two extremes. It does not rely on either event, but rather on a combination, or weighted average of the two. And the weighted average to be used must be based on a combination of the likely gain or loss in each event, and the probability of that gain or loss occurring. One might at first object to this. We are fairly certain that one or the other event will occur, not somewhere in between. Either the other hospital will be the sole contractor or it won't. Volume will be very close to 500, or close to 350, not somewhere in between.

That is true. However, from the viewpoint of maximizing the financial results of decisions, in the long run it still makes sense to undertake the weighted average approach. The reason for this is that over the course of time, any hospital will make a large number of decisions. It can never predict totally what events will occur, but it must make decisions anyway. The best strategy is to approach the decisions so that *on average* over the long run, the financial results are maximized. To understand this we must consider some basics of the laws of chance.

THE LAWS OF CHANCE

The laws of chance, or probability theory, govern uncertain events. Consider a coin flip. It might come up heads or tails, and there is an equal chance. You can bet heads or tails and in the long run should come out even. However, not all gambles have fifty-fifty probabilities like a coin flip.

For instance, consider dice. The typical six-sided die can land with any one of its six surfaces face up. The chances of any particular side coming up are only one-sixth. If you bet on any one number a large number of times, you would usually lose. Since each side will be face up an even number of times, any one side would land face up only one time out of six.

In fact, if you frequently bet six times on number six, you would win once and lose five times out of every six bets, *on average*. We say on average, because in just six rolls of the die, all six *could* come up number six, or number six might *never* come up. However. with a larger number of rolls, and a balanced die, you would win one time out of six, on average.

What if you bet $1 per roll of the die. If the payoff for a win was $1, you would lose $4 for every six bets on average. That is because you would lose $1 five times and win $1 once, for a net loss of $4. It certainly does not seem to make sense to ever bet on dice under those circumstances.

However, those are not necessarily the circumstances you are faced with. Suppose that when you lose, you lose your dollar. However, when you win, what if you win $500? This changes the game entirely. Now, the chances are that you will lose $1 five times, and win $500 once, for a net win of $495. The amount that you can benefit if you are successful is extremely important, and must be taken into account. That is why it might pay to try the new cleaning agent, even though we know there is a 99 percent chance that it is inadequate. The problem with the conservative approach of assuming that there will be 350 heart surgery patients, or the optimistic alternative of considering that 500 patients is most likely, is that it ignores the payoff. How much will we lose if we wind up with just 350 patients, and how much profit would we make at 500 patients?

Equally important is the likelihood of each event occurring. Earlier we noted that if the amount you win just equals a $1 bet, you would lose $4 on every six rolls of the die, on average. Suppose, however, that the die we use has three sixes, one two, one three, and one four. The probability of a six occurring has risen to three-sixths. Fifty percent of the time the die should

land with a six up, since half of the sides have a six. If you bet $1 six times on number six, and the payoff was $1 for a win, then you should lose three times and win three times, and just break even. You no longer expect to lose $4 even though the payoff is the same as the bet. The probability of winning has changed, and must be taken into account.

Since both the amount you win or lose, and the chances of winning and losing are variables, the decision of whether or not to make a bet is complex. Simple decision rules such as avoiding the heart surgery contract if there is a possibility of the 350 patient volume, or offering the HMO the low price because there would probably be 500 patients, are poor. They do not consider the payoffs or the probability of each event occurring.

USING EXPECTED VALUE

The expected value approach takes into account both the likelihood of each outcome and the payoffs for each outcome through its weighted average approach.

In order to compute the expected value, it is first necessary to establish a listing of the possible states of nature. For example, suppose that if we offer the HMO a low price on heart surgery, there is only a one-third chance that our competitor will also do so. This might be because once they know we have a contract, they will realize that they will probably lose money on the deal if they offer a very low price.

Further, suppose that the profits from 500 patients are expected to be $100,000, while the loss related to 350 patients will be $200,000. We can restate this as follows:

HMO Heart Surgery Contract

Probability	Payoff
.333	($200,000)
.667	100,000
1.000	($100,000)

Note that the total of the probability column must always equal 1.0.

The expected value of this proposed project can be measured by multiplying each probability by the expected payoff, and summing the results:

$$.333 \times (\$200,000) = (\$66,667)$$
$$.667 \times \quad 100,000 = \quad 66,667$$

$$\textbf{\textit{Expected Value}} = \$ \quad 0$$

The large potential loss is so great that it just offsets the benefit from the probable gain, and the expected financial result is zero. In this case there is not expected to be a financial gain or loss from the HMO contract.

Bear in mind, however, that it is *not* expected that the contract will result in no financial impact. Either there will be a $200,000 loss, or there will be a $100,000 profit. However, over a large number of contracts with similar characteristics, we can expect on average to just break even—losing on some and gaining on others.

What about the housekeeping example?

Probability	Payoff	Expected Value
.99	($30)	$ (.30)
.01	70,000	700.00
	Expected Value	$699.70

Here we see that there is a positive expected financial benefit from taking the risk, even though the probable success is low, since the payoff is so large.

RISK

One problem with the expected value approach is that it assumes that managers are risk neutral. That is, you don't mind losing if you are likely to win an equal amount, and the potential size of the loss is not a major concern.

Some managers are averse to taking any risks. They would rather forgo a profit than risk a loss. Further, many managers will always try to avoid the risk of a large loss. In the above HMO contract example, the potential loss is $200,000 while the potential gain is only $100,000. It

would not be unusual for some managers to be reluctant to take such a large potential loss when the expected value is zero. However, as the expected value rises, they may be more willing to risk the loss. Expected value information can help even risk averse managers to make decisions.

While large possible losses are often avoided, small possible losses are often taken even if the expected value is negative. Earlier we used the example of a lottery ticket that costs $1 and has a $40,000,000 payoff to the winner. Assume that the lottery (usually the state) keeps half of all proceeds. Only half of all sales are returned in the form of prizes. The expected value of a lottery ticket must be negative. For every dollar bet, only 50 cents is returned in prize money.

However, people still buy lottery tickets even though the expected value for each ticket is minus 50 cents. The reason is that the total risk, $1, is small, while the potential gain, $40,000,000, is great. People are willing to make a bad bet (i.e., go against the odds) in such a situation. The size of the potential loss affects how you respond to risk and expected values.

In our HMO contracting example, what if the chances of the HMO contract being profitable were three-quarters, rather than two-thirds? The expected value would then be positive, as follows:

$$.25 \times (\$200,000) = (\$50,000)$$
$$.75 \times \quad 100,000 = \quad 75,000$$

$$\textbf{\textit{Expected Value}} = \$25,000$$

Even in this case, some managers will choose to avoid the contract because of the large potential loss of $200,000. They exhibit "risk-aversion." Even though we would expect to make a profit of $25,000 per contract, on average, what if we have bad luck at the beginning? If we lose $200,000 several times in a row, we may not have an opportunity for the law of large numbers to average things out. In real life we cannot flip the coin or roll the dice an unlimited number of times, waiting for the laws of probability to work.

Given that perspective, it may make sense to demand a risk premium. That is, rather than be-

Exhibit 14–2–1 Original HMO Contract Alternatives and Expected Value

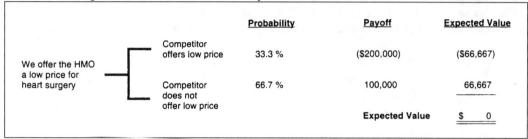

		Probability	Payoff	Expected Value
We offer the HMO a low price for heart surgery	Competitor offers low price	33.3 %	($200,000)	($66,667)
	Competitor does not offer low price	66.7 %	100,000	66,667
			Expected Value	$ 0

ing neutral, one might decide that a project must have a positive expected value to be accepted. This will represent a reward for being willing to accept the risk of losses.

The size of the risk premium should be determined after considering the magnitude of the potential loss, in comparison with the magnitude of the potential gain.

THINK INCLUSIVELY

In making decisions based on expected value, one should also attempt to consider all possible events that might occur. In our HMO heart surgery contract example, we have treated the problem as if the only possible events are that we offer the HMO a low price or not, and then if we do the competition may or may not also offer a low price. See Exhibit 14–2–1 above for the options we have considered.

We have implicitly assumed that if we do not offer a low price to the HMO, there is no change from our current status. However, if our hospital does not offer the HMO a low price, there are still two possible outcomes. The competition also may not offer the low price, or the competition may offer the low price.

SUBJECTIVE ESTIMATES

What are the chances that the other hospital in town will make a deal with the HMO at a low price if we don't? We can only guess at that. However, we have also guessed at the probability that they would follow suit if we offered a low price. We must recognize the fact that all of these estimates are based on *subjective probability.*

When we flip a coin or roll a die, we know that there is a fifty-fifty chance of heads or tails, and that there is a one-sixth chance of each side of the die landing face up. Assuming it is a "fair" coin or die, the probabilities are known with certainty. In situations facing managers, we often do not know with certainty what the probabilities are.

There may be situations in which we know with a high degree of confidence what will happen. Past history may provide information that convinces us that there is a 30 percent chance of one event, and a 70 percent chance of another. We may have seen this type of situation before and our experience tells us how often it tends to wind up one way or another. More often than not, however, managers must use their knowledge, experience, and judgment to make a best guess about the likelihood of each event.

One reason that risk aversion is common, and that managers often demand a risk premium, is because of the nature of subjective probabilities. We might have the odds wrong. The probabilities are based on the manager's gut feel or intuition discussed earlier. Managers often have a good sense of how likely events are to take place. However, they are not infallible. They may have the odds or payoffs wrong.

There is always the risk of unknown negative factors that were not taken into account in determining the probabilities or payoffs. Unexpected negative surprises are often more painful than unexpected positive surprises are pleasant. Therefore many organizations demand a substantial positive expected value to move forward.

In the HMO example, suppose that we believe that if we do not offer a very low price to the HMO, there is a 60 percent chance that the other hospital will. Perhaps we think that they might not be willing to offer a low price to compete directly with us, since we will both have low prices and low volume. However, if they can get the HMO business for themselves, it is more likely to be profitable for them. Therefore, they are more likely to make the low price offer.

This complicates the expected value calculation, but also makes it more realistic and accurate. Suppose we calculate that if they offer a low price and we don't, the HMO will shift some of our current patients to our competitor. As a result, we will have lower profits by an amount equal to $30,000. On the other hand, if neither hospital makes a low price deal with the HMO, there will be no shifting of patients and no financial effect. In that case, the options and expected values would appear as in Exhibit 14–2–2.

Note that this figure provides a more comprehensive look at all of the possible events that might occur. In looking at Exhibit 14–2–1, we were blinding ourselves to a possibility that might occur and might have negative impacts on the hospital.

While it is true that Exhibit 14–2–1 indicates there is no expected profit from making a low price deal with the HMO, the expected value analysis in Exhibit 14–2–2 reveals that the hos-

pital may still have a clear financial interest in doing so. It turns out that if the hospital does not enter into the HMO contract, it has a *negative* expected value.

In other words, if we enter into a contract, we might make money or lose money. If we do not, Exhibit 14–2–2 reveals that we will either have no financial effect or have a loss. The expected value is a loss of $18,000. It is easy see why it is necessary to try to be inclusive in considering all alternative events that might occur.

Preparing a decision-tree of the possible outcomes, such as appears in Exhibit 14–2–2, can help to visualize whether all alternative possibilities have been considered.

RESULTS

Sometimes appropriate decisions result in favorable outcomes. Sometimes they do not. In this situation, we are not faced with very pleasant alternatives. If we don't sign a low price contract, we have a negative expected value. If we do, our expected value is neutral, but we have the possibility of losing $200,000.

However, those results are based on one set of probabilities and payoffs. What if instead the probabilities were expected to be as follows:

Exhibit 14–2–2 Expected Values If We Do or Do Not Offer the HMO a Low Price

		Probability	Payoff	Expected Value
We offer the HMO a low price for heart surgery	Competitor offers low price	33.3 %	($200,000)	($66,667)
	Competitor does not offer low price	66.7 %	100,000	66,667
			Expected Value	$ 0
		Probability	Payoff	Expected Value
We do not offer the HMO a low price for heart surgery	Competitor offers low price	60%	($30,000)	($18,000)
	Competitor does not offer low price	40%	0	0
			Expected Value	($18,000)

	Competitor does	Competitor does not
We offer low price	10%	90%
We do not offer low price	80%	20%

Based on this, we can recalculate our expected values. (See Exhibit 14–2–3.)

In this situation, we find that if we make the low price offer to the HMO, there is an expected increase in profits by $70,000. This expected value has increased from the zero value that we calculated earlier, because the example now assumes that there is an even smaller chance of the competitor making a low price offer if we do.

On the other hand, if we don't make the offer, the expected value is a loss of $24,000. This is because we have increased the likelihood that they will if we don't.

What would the correct decision be for our hospital? We expect to make a profit if we contract with the HMO at the low price, and to lose money if we don't. The analysis clearly indicates that it is a good decision to offer the low price. What if we do, and our competitor does as well?

In that case, we will not attain our volume of 500 patients. There will be only 350 patients, and we will lose $200,000. The good decision will

have yielded a very bad outcome. Nevertheless, it was the right decision to make.

If managers worry too much about bad outcomes, they will become frozen, unable to make decisions. There will invariably be some bad outcomes. Failing to act is not an insurance policy against bad outcomes. In this example, failing to contract with the HMO would have likely resulted in the competitor doing so.

Failure to act would probably have cost the organization $130,000. This is based on the $100,000 profit we will probably make if we contract, vs. the $30,000 loss we will probably incur if we don't. True, if we contract and they do too, we will lose $200,000. However, that will be a relatively rare event, given the probabilities in this hypothetical example. In the long run, if our ability to make subjective estimates is reasonable, the good results will outweigh the bad ones by a substantial amount.

This raises the question, however, of whether we have the ability to make reasonable predictions. Managers should be capable of making subjective estimates. These are not really wild guesses, but rather are founded in experience.

The actual likelihood that our competitor will offer a very low price for heart surgery is unknown. However, from past experience, we prob-

---

Exhibit 14–2–3 Expected Values Based on New Probability Estimates

		Probability	Payoff	Expected Value
We offer the HMO a low price for heart surgery	Competitor offers low price	10%	($200,000)	($20,000)
	Competitor does not offer low price	90%	100,000	90,000
			Expected Value	$70,000

		Probability	Payoff	Expected Value
We do not offer the HMO a low price for heart surgery	Competitor offers low price	80%	($30,000)	($24,000)
	Competitor does not offer low price	20%	0	0
			Expected Value	($24,000)

ably do know how often our competitor has acted independently as a leader at cutting prices, how often they have followed our lead in cutting prices, and how often they have retained high prices. Thus, based on even subliminal knowl-edge, managers are generally good judges of subjective probabilities. Taking those probabilities and combining them with the expected value method can enable those managers to make im-proved decisions.

Reading 14–3

Decision Making under Uncertainty: A Linear Programming Approach

Jennifer L. Rosenberg

The management process is in essence a process of decision making. Rarely is a decision made with an outcome already known. Under certain conditions predictions can be made, but these predictions are assumed to be imperfect. More often decisions are made in uncertain times. Horngren defines uncertainty as the "possibility that an actual amount will deviate from an expected amount" (p. 615). Uncertainty means that an organization will be faced with multiple and often conflicting objectives, some conflicting with the objectives of the organization itself.

A decision model is a formal method used by organizations for measuring the effects of alternative actions that will be made in uncertain conditions. A cost-volume-profit model is the most obvious example of a decision model used to make decisions for planning and control as it relates to the interrelationships of factors affecting profits, particularly cost behavior at various levels of volume.

Generally, decision models contain each of the following:

- objective function (also called choice criterion)—some quantity that the decision maker would like to either maximize or minimize

Source: Reprinted from Jennifer L. Rosenberg, "Decision Making under Uncertainty: A Linear Programming Approach," *Hospital Cost Management and Accounting,* Vol. 1, No. 3, June 1989, pp. 1–5. Copyright 1989, Aspen Publishers, Inc.

- a set of actions to be considered
- a set of all possible relevant events that can affect the outcomes (also known as states or states of nature)
- a set of possible outcomes that measure the predicted consequences of the various possible combinations of actions and events

Decision models usually fall under the larger category of constrained optimization models. Because these models do not include information that cannot be quantified, these models do not provide the absolute solution to a problem. Rather, it is an efficient way of producing the optimal answer to a proposed problem.

A linear programming (LP) decision model is concerned with how to best allocate scarce resources to attain a chosen objective. LP models are designed to provide a solution to problems where the linear assumptions underlying the model are reasonable approximations. All LP models have two common features: (1) the decision to be made is subject to constraints; and (2) there is some quantity to be maximized or minimized. There are generally three steps in solving an LP problem:

1. Determine the objective function.
2. Determine the basic relationships.
3. Compute the optimal solution.

Two aspects of using LP are especially difficult to define. First, it is difficult to express the objective in a format suitable to be solved by an

LP approach. Second, reliable estimates of the information inputs used in the LP model are not always easily obtained.

LP has been used in a wide range of business problems. Transportation, resource allocation, personnel scheduling, and health planning are all settings in which LP has been used. Obviously, LP is not appropriate for all types of business problems. Hill describes four criteria for the use of LP:

1. The problem must be sufficiently complex that a simpler or even intuitive approach is unacceptable.
2. The problem's solution must be rewarding or practical enough that the added benefits of an LP analysis are worth the costs of the extra effort required.
3. It must be possible to describe the problem in quantitative terms.
4. All the mathematical relationships must be linear.

When there are only two or three variables in the objective function and a minimal number of constraints, methods that do not require the aid of computerization may be used. These methods include the spreadsheet method, the graphical solution method, and the trial-and-error method. Real situations are generally more complex and more than three variables are involved. In such cases, the "simplex method" must be used.

A spreadsheet method is useful when the user is interested in manipulating data in the model. In situations in which the user needs to find the optimal solution, software such as VINO or "What's Best!" must be utilized (Eppen, 1987).

In the *spreadsheet method,* formulas are developed that represent the objective function and the constraint functions. Parameters are computed from the formulas and the decision variables that are entered into cells in the spreadsheet. If the user is interested in a "what if" analysis, the user will enter predetermined variables into a specified cell and the formulas will be replaced with specific values. The result will be the optimal solution for the value entered. (See Example 1.)

The *graphical solution method* provides an easy way of solving LP problems with two decision variables. Using an xy graph, the optimal solution must lie on one of the corners of the "area of feasible solution," which is an area contained within the bounds created by the intersection of numerous lines representing the decision constraints. (See Example 2.)

The *trial-and-error solution method* uses coordinates of the corners of the area of feasible solutions to locate the optimal solution. (See Example 2.)

The *simplex method* utilizes standard computer software packages based on a systematic algebraic way of examining the "corners" of an LP constraint. The optimal solution is reached by solving a series of linear equations. Each corner represents a possible solution and can be represented in tabular form, known as the simplex tableau. By performing iterations on each corner or tableau, the optimal solution is reached when no further improvement can be made on a previous iteration.

EXAMPLE 1: SPREADSHEET METHOD—ASSIGNMENT OF NURSES TO DEPARTMENTS WITH VARIABLE DEMAND

The Director of Nursing at Busy Hospital is trying to determine how to staff nurses in Pediatrics. There are six shifts per day as follows:

Shift	Starting Time	Ending Time
1	Midnight	8 AM
2	4 AM	Noon
3	8 AM	4 PM
4	Noon	8 PM
5	4 PM	Midnight
6	8 PM	4 AM

The supervisor knows the minimum number of nurses required for each time slot:

Time	Minimum number of nurses required
Midnight–4 AM	8
4 AM–8 AM	12
8 AM–Noon	20
Noon–4 PM	20
4 PM–8 PM	17
8 PM–Midnight	8

The Director of Nursing, faced with the nursing shortage, would like to minimize the total number of nurses required for this department. The objective function would then be

$$\text{Min. } N1 + N2 + N3 + N4 + N5 + N6$$

where $N1$ = number of nurses working shift 1
$N2$ = number of nurses working shift 2
.
.
.
$N6$ = number of nurses working shift 6 (See Table 14–3–1).

The decision constraints would then be:

$$N1 + N6 < 8$$

$$N1 + N2 < 12$$

$$N2 + N3 < 20$$

$$N3 + N4 < 20$$

$$N4 + N5 < 17$$

$$N5 + N6 < 8$$

Nursing Staffing Symbolic Spreadsheet

I	II	III #	IV #	V #	VI
Shift	Start Time	Nurses Start	Nurses Work	Nurses Required	Extra Nurses
1	12 AM		0	8	
2	4 AM		0	12	
3	8 AM		0	20	
4	12 PM		0	20	
5	4 PM		0	17	
6	8 PM		0	8	

Table 14–3–1 Objective Function

Shift	Mid– 4 AM	4 AM– 8 AM	8 AM– Noon	Noon– 4 PM	4 PM– 8 PM	8 PM– Mid
1	N1	N1				
2		N2	N2			
3			N3	N3		
4				N4	N4	
5					N5	N5
6	N6					N6

Column VI will contain the number of nurses working less the number of nurses required to give a slack amount.

Column III will contain optimized decision values.

Two versions of the optimized spreadsheet are shown below:

Nursing Staffing Value Symbolic Spreadsheet

I	II	III #	IV #	V #	VI
Shift	Start Time	Nurses Start	Nurses Work	Nurses Required	Extra Nurses
1	12 AM	8	8	8	0
2	4 AM	4	12	12	0
3	8 AM	16	20	20	0
4	12 PM	9	25	20	5
5	4 PM	8	17	17	0
6	8 PM	0	8	8	0
TOTAL NURSES =					45

Nursing Staffing Value Symbolic Spreadsheet

I	II	III #	IV #	V #	VI
Shift	Start Time	Nurses Start	Nurses Work	Nurses Required	Extra Nurses
1	12 AM	5	8	8	0
2	4 AM	12	17	12	5
3	8 AM	8	20	20	0
4	12 PM	12	20	20	0
5	4 PM	5	17	17	0
6	8 PM	3	8	8	0
TOTAL NURSES =					45

The manager can now decide based on non-quantitative information in what shift to place the five slack nurses.

A "what if" analysis would be possible in this situation. For example, the nursing requirements might be changed due to the addition of extra beds. In this case the same spreadsheet could be used with column V altered accordingly.

EXAMPLE 2: GRAPHIC SOLUTION METHOD—PRODUCT MIX ASSESSMENT, OUTPATIENT LABORATORY

The outpatient laboratory at Busy Hospital performs two major tests—hematology and chemistry. The laboratory administrator is trying to decide which service to promote in order to achieve the maximum profits. Profits have been determined to be $5 for hematology tests and $4 on clinical chemistry tests.

The laboratory functions in the following way: Samples are collected in Department 1 and processed in Department 2. Labor requirements for the tests are as follows:

	Hematology	Chemistry
Department 1	1	1
Department 2	3	2

The supervisors of the two departments have estimated the following number of hours will be available during the next months:

Department 1	1000 hours
Department 2	2400 hours

The outpatient laboratory has taken advantage of a reagent contract available from the distributor of their hematology instruments. This places a limit on the amount of this reagent that can be purchased per month and therefore a limit on the number of tests that can be performed. It has been estimated that these constraints will limit potential services to 600 hematology tests per month.

The Linear Programming Model

Objective: Maximize Profits
In mathematical terms:

Maximize $5A + 4B$

where A = number of hematology tests
and B = number of clinical chemistry tests

so that

$A + B$	< 1000 (labor constraint, Department 1)
$3A + 2B$	< 2400 (labor constraint, Department 2)
A	< 600 (reagent constraint)

In the graph in Figure 14-3-1, Line 1 represents the Department 1 constraint, Line 2 the Department 2 constraint, and Line 3 the reagent constraint. The shaded area represents the area of "feasible solutions," which contains all the possible combinations of A and B that satisfy the constraints.

In the graphic solution, the optimal solution must lie on one of the corners of the "area of feasible solutions." In general, the optimal solution will be the point that lies on the border of the "area of feasible solutions" that is farthest from the origin, in this case (600, 400).

Therefore, in order to maximize profits, the laboratory administrator should opt to perform 600 clinical chemistry tests and 400 hematology tests in the next month.

The above example, although extremely simplistic in nature, demonstrates the value of LP. Had the laboratory administrator chosen to maximize profits on the basis of profit per test alone, the optimal solution would never have been reached since the optimal solution designates performing a greater volume of clinical chemistry tests (the choice with the lower contribution margin).

TRIAL AND ERROR METHOD

1. Using the graph, choose all corner points.
2. Determine which point gives the highest total profit.

Point M (0, 1000):	Total Profit =	$5(0) + $4(1000) =	$4000
Point N (400, 600):	Total Profit =	$5(400) + $4(600) =	$4400
Point O (600, 300):	Total Profit =	$5(600) + $4(300) =	$4200
Point P (600, 0):	Total Profit =	$5(600) + $4(0) =	$3000
Point Q (0, 0):	Total Profit =	$5(0) + $4(0) =	0

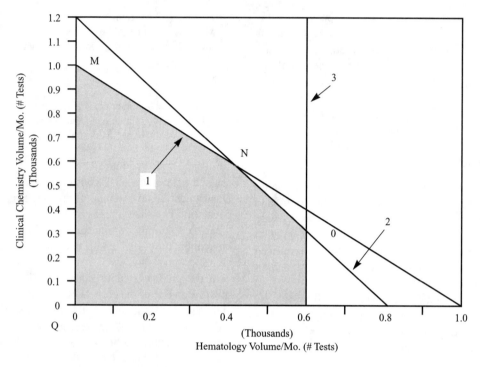

Figure 14–3–1 Linear Programming Graphic Solution

This reaffirms the conclusion that the optimal solution is 400 hematology tests and 600 clinical chemistry tests (Point N).

Obviously, LP models have limitations. As discussed above, all relationships involved in the problem must be linear. Furthermore, all variables and constraints must be described with absolute certainty. Finally, these models do not take into account variables that cannot be quantified. Therefore, users must take the "optimal" solution derived from LP as the best mathematical solution and not necessarily the best overall solution. Formal models such as LP are important, however, because they provide users with a means of eliminating inconsistencies.

Understanding how LP models work is extremely important for accountants and other management professionals. Because data from accounting are a vital input into LP, poor accounting data will affect the objective function or the area of feasible solutions, resulting in faulty decision making.

BIBLIOGRAPHY

Eppen, G.D., et al., *Introductory Management Science,* 2nd Edition. Englewood Cliffs: Prentice-Hall, Inc., 1987.

Hill, P.H. et al., *Making Decisions: A Multidisciplinary Introduction.* Reading: Addison-Wesley Publishing Company, Inc., 1979.

Horngren, C.T., and G. Foster, *Cost Accounting: A Managerial Emphasis,* 6th Edition. Englewood Cliffs: Prentice-Hall, Inc., 1987.

Turban, E., and N.P. Loomba, eds., *Cases and Readings in Management Science.* Plano: Business Publications, Inc., 1982.

15

Information Systems for Costing

Reading 15–1

Saving Money throughout the Cost Accounting Installation Cycle

Arthur J. Keegan

Almost every hospital financial information system installed in America today is obsolete and fails to properly match revenue and expenses. A hospital's laboratory used to be both a revenue center and a cost center. Today, with DRGs and capitated HMOs, the laboratory is just a cost center and the patient is the revenue center. In the good old days, the job of the hospital's financial information system was to take revenue from the patient billing system and match it to expenses in the hospital's general ledger. Now the flow reverses, and expenses must be taken from the general ledger and matched to patients' bills.

Unfortunately, the designers of the last generation of hospital information systems built the expense and revenue matching as a one-way street. Revenue can flow to expenses, but expenses can't flow to revenue.

Matching hospitalwide expenses to the patient requires some of the information processing techniques developed by cost accountants. So it is no surprise that when the Healthcare Financial Managers Association recently surveyed health care CFOs they found that the most important

Source: Reprinted from Arthur J. Keegan, "Saving Money throughout the Cost Accounting Installation Cycle," *Hospital Cost Accounting Advisor,* Vol. 2, No. 10, pp. 1–7. Copyright 1987, Aspen Publishers, Inc.

data processing (DP) systems application for the next three years will be cost accounting. Most of the hospital executives buying cost accounting services in the next three years will be first-time buyers with no experience in purchasing this type of software. The techniques laid out here will help them to select a system that offers the features they need at a reasonable price.

Always keep in mind that there are two major cost components in purchasing any software—the cost of installation and the costs of maintenance. The cost a novice buyer is most likely to overlook is the cost of maintaining the system after the software is installed. Only by minimizing the combined cost of installation and maintenance can a CFO ensure getting the best deal for the hospital.

Cost accounting systems that have low installation costs may be expensive to maintain, while a system that is more expensive to install may be much less costly to maintain over the long haul. The cost-conscious CFO must estimate maintenance costs when selecting a system.

THE COST ACCOUNTING INSTALLATION CYCLE

The cost accounting installation cycle starts with a definition of the general features of a costing system and ends with a fully installed and maintainable system. Choosing the various stages in between is an arbitrary process that no two people would ever agree on. Based on my experience as a teacher of cost accounting and as an installer of these systems, I split the installation process into the following seven steps.

- Step 1: Goal setting and general outline
- Step 2: Selecting the software
- Step 3: Finalizing the design
- Step 4: Measuring costs
- Step 5: Test drive
- Step 6: Feedback
- Step 7: Maintenance

The particular order of the steps can vary from system to system, but all steps are necessary to get a costing system in and off the ground. The costs of each step will vary according to the system chosen. Generally speaking, a greater investment in design simplifications and careful installation can lower the costs of maintenance. Designing in complexity will raise maintenance expenses.

Figure 15–1–1 shows a general curve of the work hours used during the installation cycle. The commitment normally peaks in Step 4—measuring the costs. This is the time when the most intense work is done on the system. Yet, in the long run, more hours will be devoted to maintaining the system (Step 7).

In selecting a system, it is wise to take the long view and make sure whatever is designed is not a monster to maintain—devouring resources in a time when most health care organizations have precious few hours to spare. Trading off a few more installation dollars for long-term savings in maintenance is good business.

STEP 1: GOAL SETTING

Poor planning raises the cost of installation. Abe Lincoln once said that if he had six hours to chop down an apple tree, he would spend four of the hours sharpening the ax. (He promptly forgot this advice, and sent thousands of untrained youths off to die at Bull Run.) Let's not make the same mistake. An extra hour of preparation can save a hospital staff hours of time redirecting efforts in midstream and redoing half-finished work.

The first step in planning is to learn the link between cost accounting accuracy, system timeliness, and the cost of the system. One of these factors cannot be changed without affecting at least one of the other two.

Increasing the accuracy without lengthening the time to get a report increases the cost of the system. Increasing the frequency of reports without lowering the accuracy increases the cost of the system. All cost savings eventually mean reducing accuracy or timeliness. In discussions with the controller of a major Fortune 50 corporation, which has cost accounting needs similar to those of a hospital, I learned that this corporation spends in excess of $8,000,000 per year on what its controller thinks is a reliable, timely, and accurate costing system. I know of no hospital or hospital system willing to devote even $5,000,000 annually to cost accounting, so hospitals are accepting a much lower level of accuracy than a Fortune 50 corporation.

When you have mastered the relationship between cost, accuracy, and timeliness, it will be easier to make decisions on whether increased levels of accuracy or timeliness are worth the cost.

Next, decide whether the main goal of the system is product costing or management costing (i.e., internal control). Product costing systems

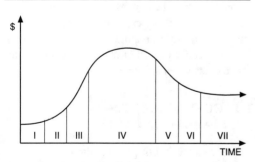

Figure 15–1–1 A Cost Profile of the Cost Accounting Installation Cycle

are designed to determine the cost of delivering the hospital's services to patients. These systems are often less elaborate than management costing systems and are less costly to install or maintain. Product costing systems do not support the flexible budgeting and management control provided by management costing systems.

Management costing systems are more elaborate, complete, and expensive than product costing systems. These systems focus mainly on properly modeling the cost behavior of service-producing departments and reporting deviations from expected levels of expenditure. Management costing systems often include standard costing features. It is easy to think of them as a very detailed, flexible budgeting system.

If internal control—management costing—is the key feature of the costing system, other managers outside the finance department must be involved in the goal-setting stage. Once the choice of the mix of product costing and management costing features is made, the following general features should be considered and reviewed for their impact on system cost.

Departmental Cost Pools

Choosing the number of departments in the hospital to cost greatly affects the cost of the system. For product costing, the choice is usually limited to patient service departments, while management costing focuses on all expense generating areas. Do not do all departments at once. Use a reasonable method to select the key departments. Later, when things are less hectic, the uncosted departments can be added to the system. Go for the big payoffs during installation.

Cost Elements

Another general design feature is how many cost elements or micro costs make up a costed item. Some sample cost elements are variable direct salary, fixed salary, variable departmental overhead, or fixed general overhead. The more cost elements, the greater the cost of maintaining the system. Many hospitals set up more cost ele-

ments than they can afford to maintain, getting little useful information for their efforts. Clear thinking and economy here can pay off.

Direct vs. Indirect Costs

The definition of direct costs, like beauty, seems to be in the eye of the beholder. It generally means costs that can be traced to an individual patient's care. Choose a definition that can be consistently applied to the departments chosen to cost. Beware of accounts like supplies that share the same account number but are a direct cost for one department and overhead for another.

Fixed and Variable Costs

Getting consensus here is difficult, and a general rule better be developed first. Remember, most managers believe "Fixed cost equals me and variable costs equals you." Hospitals, like the local firehouse, have a lot of fixed labor. Beware of thinking of labor as highly variable.

Reporting

Before looking at systems, it is wise to determine the style and frequency of reports needed. Developing pro forma reports before buying a system is a wise investment. It will save time that could otherwise be lost in dealing with suppliers who lack the reporting features needed. Frequency of reporting—timeliness—affects the cost of the system.

Once a general decision is made on system function, emphasis on management and/or product costing, and general system features, the hospital can shop for suppliers.

STEP 2: SELECTING THE SOFTWARE

The cost of cost accounting software is *not* the cost of the cost accounting system. Do not lose sight of the difference between the price of the software and the cost of the system. The cost of the system includes design, installation, and maintenance costs on top of the price for software. Relatively inexpensive software that is costly to maintain and install is no bargain.

Most hospitals require assistance in installing the software. Sometimes installation services are packaged in with a software sale, and sometimes they are sold separately. All the selection criteria below apply equally well to a full system supplier or a separate installer.

System Functionality

Determine whether the supplier sells primarily a product costing or a management costing system, and compare the system's general characteristics to the hospital's initial design.

Supplier's Experience

Obtain precise data on number of installations, years in the business, and quality of references. A supplier's reputation is a critical asset. Talk to someone who dropped the system if you can—every supplier loses some customers.

Service/Support

Find out if the supplier has regional or national service. Determine the ratio of service people to clients. What level of service is included in licensing fees and what service is charged at hourly or daily rates?

Cost Pools

All software has limits, and design decisions must be made. Make sure the vendor supports the number and types of cost pools the hospital plans for.

Cost Elements

Make sure the cost elements desired by the hospital are supported by the software. Some systems are restricted to as few as three elements of cost, while others allow an almost uncountable number. More cost elements still mean more maintenance costs, and sometimes mean slower response time.

Integration

Find out if the supplier has successfully integrated its cost accounting system with general ledger, billing, and payroll systems similar to the hospital's. Poor integration delays installation, reduces usefulness of the costing system, and raises the cost of maintenance.

Simplicity vs. Complexity

More complex software is not necessarily better. Accuracy has a higher cost of maintenance. Flexibility has more benefits than complexity.

System Speed

Inspect the costing system's response time. Determine how fast it generates test reports. Time can be money. Waiting six hours for a report may be unacceptable.

Updating Procedure

Check out how quickly and easily the system can be updated. Look at monthly processing and when reports can be run. Review the steps to changing a cost weight, changing a costing method, or adding a new procedure to cost.

License or Sale

The hospital should know if it owns or licenses the software. If the hospital merges with others, can it add other providers to its license agreement? Make sure the hospital gets all software enhancements released within six months of the installation date.

Price

Price is always important. For the same features, the lower the better. If possible, don't pay all of it until the system works.

These are the general concerns in purchasing costing software. Depending on a hospital's specific goals, other concerns may be more important. One goal may be to select a product that runs on certain hardware. Hardware restrictions significantly narrow the field of selection.

STEP 3: FINALIZING THE DESIGN

Selecting the cost accounting system software sets limits on what the system can do. Any software chosen will probably not do everything the hospital initially wanted to do. After software selection, a design should be set. This step should involve all the departments to be costed.

The big decisions in this step are how many items to cost and in how much detail they should be costed. The hospital at this stage will learn that all the knowledge needed for installing a cost accounting system does not reside in the accounting department.

Successful costing means properly describing how services are produced—the production function. The clearer the description of how a procedure is produced, the easier and cheaper it is to cost that procedure. The managers in charge of producing services can effect significant savings in installing a costing system. See Exhibit 15–1–1 for a sample production function.

One rule often used to reduce installation time is Pareto's principle (the "80/20" rule). This rule states that generally 20 percent of a department's procedures account for 80 percent of its output. Using this precept can limit precise costing to only the services most often used. Do not apply it blindly. Be on the lookout for different production methods in the same department.

Applying Pareto's principle to the radiology department will often result in overlooking angiographic procedures. Angiography uses a much different production process than routine diagnostic radiology, and is very resource-intensive.

At this stage, the number of cost components should be selected. This is very important if standard costs will be used in the system. For example, should direct labor be divided into just two components—fixed and variable—or should a la-

Exhibit 15–1–1 Sample Production Function

Procedure: Liver Scan

Labor Components

Person	Activity	Time	Cost
Technologist	Prep.	15 min.	$2.90
Aide	Prep.	2 min.	.25
Aide	Transport	14 min.	1.75
Technologist	Injection	5 min.	.97
Technologist	Treatment	15 min.	2.90
Transcriptionist	Transcription	4 min.	.60
			$9.37

Supplies

Item	Cost
8 × 10 Film	$ .89
Processing chemicals	.09
Radionuclide	11.75
Gloves	.40
Syringe	.20
	$13.33
Total	$22.70

bor component exist for each salary code or even for each job code? Critical to this decision is how many cost components the organization can afford to maintain. Don't set up a system that is detailed beyond a reasonable maintenance effort.

Overhead cost assignment to procedures is important for product costing but less critical for management costing. Spending a lot of time on overhead issues for a management costing system is a waste of time.

This step of the cycle is complete when decisions are reached on the actual procedures to cost, the description of the production functions, the number and kinds of cost elements, and exactly how overhead is to be costed. The scene now shifts to the various hospital departments where costing will take place.

STEP 4: MEASURING COSTS

After maintenance, this is usually the most costly step in the installation cycle. The hospital

CFO should make extra effort to reduce the costs of this step.

Here the hospital's cost accountants get down and dirty and measure the cost of producing services. The purpose of this step is to translate costs from the general ledger format to the individual procedures.

Before the general ledger costs can be assigned to procedures, they first have to be mapped to the cost elements. In other words, individual salary accounts have to be mapped to either fixed or variable salary or some other cost elements. Many methods exist for this mapping, and they can be broken down into four general categories, from least costly to most costly.

Declaration

This method is the least costly and requires the department manager to assign accounts directly to a cost component. Each salary account is declared either fixed or variable, likewise with nonsalary and departmental overhead. Although it seems crude, it probably is the most cost effective and should be used as often as possible.

Inspection

This method requires assigning costs to fixed and variable based on reading contracts and purchase orders. Items that are fixed charges become fixed costs, and items whose cost varies with volume purchased are variable. In this method, salaried employees' wages are assigned to fixed expenses, while hourly employees' wages are considered variable.

Observation

Observation means going in and watching the services being produced. Observational techniques include work sampling, logging work time, regression analysis, and many others. These techniques are largely used for measuring direct labor inputs.

Engineering

Engineering techniques are used when cost standards or normative costs are to be set. The engineer determines what the costs should be after modeling the production process. These are the most expensive techniques, and should be reserved for areas of highly repetitive work or for areas that have a high potential for staff reduction.

A hospital will use a combination of declaration, inspection, observation, and engineering techniques for tracing costs to products. The techniques will be chosen based on the item to be costed.

A common problem in this stage in hospitals is that hospital departments produce more than a single output, and a weighting scheme is developed to allocate departmental cost pools to outputs. This can be done simply and cheaply by using the procedure charge as the allocation statistic or a Ratio of Cost to Charges method (RCC Method).

While RCCs are relatively inexpensive, they can be unacceptably inaccurate, since most hospital charges bear no relation to costs. Therefore, labor content, nonlabor content, and overhead must be estimated for each procedure. One way to save money is to rely on published standards or the department directors' best intuition. It appears that investing in detailed studies only yields a good payback for direct labor in high revenue areas. Overhead and nonlabor are economically costed by using descriptive measures.

Because of 19 years of Medicare cost reporting, the techniques for overhead costing are highly developed in the hospital industry. Realistically, sophisticated overhead costing adds very little punch to a managerial or product costing system. For management purposes, allocated overheads are usually uncontrollable while for product purposes marginal costs without fixed overhead are much more meaningful than full costs. Be wary of investing many of a hospital's scarce accounting resources in improving overhead costing.

The way to save money in the fourth step is to limit the number of costs you measure by engineering or observational techniques. Use as much descriptive costing material as meets the hospital's accuracy goals, and don't waste a lot of time on overhead.

STEP 5: TEST DRIVE

When Step 4 is done, the hospital can address two major issues. Does the output make sense, and how often should the hospital fire this sucker up? If the output looks funny, this is the best time to fix it.

First, audit all the costs. On a test basis, the cost accountants should make sure that they can trace inputs through to outputs. Beware of accepting a system with "black boxes" where numbers go in, magic takes place, and numbers come out. Black boxes can be expensive to fix if their designers accept jobs in the fast food industry.

After correcting all the problems that are obvious to the accounting office, design standard reports and determine how often they should be distributed. Because of generally poor inventory accounting in hospitals, costing reports are best done on a quarterly basis.

Skipping Step 5 can result in tremendous credibility problems. Department managers are usually very wary and anxious about the output of the cost accounting system. Trashy output is all they need to ignite a major rejection of the system and the loss of all investment up to this point.

STEP 6: FEEDBACK

Once the hospital's cost accountants finish tuning the system, feedback should be sought from the costed departments. The next step is to ask managers to sign off on the costing work done in their departments and affirm that the work is accurate.

The benefit here is reinforcing the ownership of the data by the department managers. A lack of credibility is one of the best ways to waste a hospital's investment in cost accounting. Department managers need to be treated as intimate partners in the cost accounting cycle.

Also, involvement of departmental managers will lower the cost of maintaining the system. Managers who are well versed in the operation of the costing system will be able to alert the hospital's cost accountants to changes in the production process, emergence of new procedures, and changes in the fixed or variable nature of departmental costs. Involving the departmental managers allows the accountants to leverage off other experience and expertise and save money.

STEP 7: MAINTENANCE

This is where most of the money will be spent in a cost accounting system, because maintenance expense occurs every year the system is in operation. A small percentage savings here can mean big dollar savings over long periods of time. Therefore, an overriding concern in all decisions made during the installation should be the impact of that decision on the costs of maintaining the system.

One rule of thumb is that if a hospital cannot afford two people trained in how to run and maintain the cost accounting system, it should not go ahead with the system. Having only one "expert" in the system means when the expert goes, so goes the expertise. As Saki said, "She was a good cook, as cooks go, and as cooks go, she went." Job opportunities are expanding rapidly for trained hospital cost accountants.

Given the complexity of these products, there will always be many decisions that are not well documented except in the head of the user. A second trained user will provide a check against undocumented modifications.

Develop a schedule of periodic maintenance and revision. Using the costing system for budgeting will increase the necessity of keeping all its information up to date. Departments should be put on a schedule of review with the more significant ones being reviewed more frequently than the less important ones.

Maintenance and updating will always need to be done when a production function changes. Switching to unit dose in pharmacy or primary nursing on a nursing unit requires changing the cost accounting data. Large variances in last year's unit cost and this year's cost are a dead giveaway of changing production functions.

It can't be said often enough: The best way to save money is save money on maintenance. Do not avoid maintenance, but keep the system simple enough for easy maintenance. Having only one employee versed in the system is not a money-saving step; it is a prelude to disaster.

Common sense and proper planning are the sure way to keeping a cost accounting installation on track and under budget. Spend a little extra time sharpening your ax before cutting the costs of cost accounting.

Reading 15–2

Cost Accounting Software Design

Randall C. Stephenson

Effective October 1, 1983, when the Medicare program began paying hospitals for inpatient services under its new Prospective Payment System (PPS), hospitals began to experience a critical need for accurate cost information. Perhaps the single most important impact of prospective pricing will be to change the role that cost management plays in the overall financial management of a hospital. The achievement of positive financial results under such a system requires that management have a detailed knowledge of costs and the variables that influence them. These include

- patient case-mix and acuity
- labor productivity
- physician practice patterns
- capacity thresholds
- input-output relationships

A thorough understanding of these factors is required for management to initiate actions that will provide a positive contribution to the hospital's financial results.

Old hospital costing methodologies are based upon top-down allocation routines, in which costs are determined on an average basis for whole products or groups of services. These

Source: Reprinted from Randall C. Stephenson, "Cost Accounting Software Design," *Hospital Cost Accounting Advisor,* Vol. 1, No. 6, November 1985, pp. 1, 4–7. Copyright 1985, Aspen Publishers, Inc.

techniques do not produce cost information at a level of detail that can support marginal cost analysis, competitive pricing and bidding, performance monitoring based upon variance analysis, or product-line decision making.

The dynamics of the industry necessitate innovative decision making by hospital executives to effectively manage the delivery of health care services. Experience has shown that accurate and detailed cost information has a wide variety of management applications in hospitals, including the following areas:

- product-line profitability analysis (case mix)
- flexible budgeting and control
- strategic planning
- department cost variance analysis
- decision support/modeling
- trend analysis

To address the need of hospitals to access timely and accurate cost accounting information, Management Science America (MSA) has developed software that enables hospitals to make use of proven "bottom-up" cost accounting techniques. The MSA Health Care System consists of three primary modules that are organized and integrated to fully support a hospital's varied uses of cost information. The three modules are Health Care Costing, Health Care Accounting, and Case-Mix Management. Their functions are summarized in Exhibit 15–2–1.

In developing a health care cost system, a number of distinct, yet interrelated requirements for a cost accounting system must be recognized. Hospital managers at all levels of the organization will require concise, meaningful, and timely cost information to understand and control the costs for which they are responsible. Cost information must be organized to support management decision making throughout the organization. The cost accounting system must have the flexibility and adaptive structure to meet the specific and varying needs of strategic analysis and planning. Patient services must be appropriately and consistently costed on a timely basis by DRG or other appropriate product-line classification. To the extent possible, the hospital cost accounting system should be integrated with existing financial systems to ensure cost-effective operation.

The general design of the MSA system is derived from job costing systems that have evolved over the years in industry. (See *Hospital Cost Accounting Advisor*, Vol. 1, No. 5 for a discussion of job costing.) The job costing model is appropriate for a hospital because it can recognize the following factors that are inherent in providing patient care services:

1. Each patient's treatment is uniquely defined and modified to meet the patient's specific needs and the varying conditions of that patient.
2. Patient treatment and care can be defined as a number of service units, which are similar to component parts. The total treatment of a patient can be defined as a list of service units provided, that is, a bill of services.
3. The individual service units provided are fairly uniform in nature and for the purpose of costing can be defined in terms of standard cost units.

HEALTH CARE COSTING

The Health Care Costing Module identifies the cost of procedures and services performed

Exhibit 15–2–1 Features of the MSA Health Care System

Health Care Costing Module

- defines products and product structure relationships at the procedure, subprocedure, or service unit levels
- establishes and maintains rates for labor, material, and overhead categories
- defines and maintains up to 16 cost elements for each product or service
- simulates the impact of changes in cost variables at any level
- provides extensive where-used reporting and same-as-except-for capabilities to reduce the clerical effort required to define and maintain cost standards
- supports engineering (microcosted), relative value unit, and average costing techniques

Health Care Accounting Module

- measures departmental performance in up to 16 cost categories
- calculates major operational variances based on volume changes and efficiencies
- provides statistical and cost information
- integrates with general ledger systems for management reporting

Case-Mix Management Module

- provides standard reporting on the basis of diagnosis-related groups (DRGs) or other user-defined product groupings
- provides utilities for ad hoc reporting online
- provides extensive outlier, net income, profitability, physician, and patient demographic reporting capabilities
- supports marginal cost analysis using standard cost profiles and detailed cost elements from the Health Care Costing Module

throughout the hospital. Standard cost information is maintained at a detailed level in this module, and this information can be readily accessed and used by the other system modules.

The objective of the module is to develop a standard cost profile for each of the procedures or services performed throughout a hospital. These standard cost profiles can be developed for both charge items (e.g., discrete items or services typically detailed on the charge description master file or your hospital's patient accounting system) and service unit items (e.g., patient-oriented services that are not typically part of the patient billing process, but can be used as a means of assigning and transferring costs to patients as services are provided). An example of a service unit item might be a medical records chart workup or an admissions workup.

The module develops procedure-level or service-unit-level standard cost profiles using a mix of engineered (microcosted), relative value unit (RVU), and average costing techniques. This feature of the system facilitates the use of the 80/20 rule as it applies to cost accounting for hospitals. Experience has shown that in most hospital departments, a relatively small percentage of services performed will typically account for a majority of the department's costs.

For such high-volume, high-contribution procedures, a hospital may deem it appropriate to use microcosting (engineered costing) techniques to ensure data accuracy and reliability. The module enables hospitals to develop and maintain itemized procedure-level schedules of material costs, or *bills of material*. It also keeps track of where and by whom labor effort is expended as products, procedures, and services are delivered to patients. This information is referred to as a *routing*, which is the series of tasks done in a specific sequence by different people at different work centers. Through the use of these bills of material and standard routing concepts, a hospital can engineer (microcost) standard cost profiles for those items for which a high degree of costing accuracy is required.

Other services or products may make only a small contribution to a department's overall operation, and hence may be less critical from an accuracy standpoint. Microcosting techniques can be combined with RVU and average costing techniques to arrive at an overall costing solution that is both accurate and cost-effective.

The module enables hospitals to define and maintain up to 16 cost elements for each item to be costed. Cost elements in this case refer to components of the total standard cost of an item, identifying details such as direct labor, materi-

als, fixed and variable overhead, and so on. These cost elements are user controlled and can be tailored to meet your hospital's specific needs. For example, you may need to define a unique cost element for depreciation or fringe benefits. Or you may wish to track indirect materials or indirect labor as separate cost elements. One key design feature is that costs are always tied to their origins in the general ledger. For example, a fixed cost element remains a fixed cost whether it is viewed as part of a DRG's total cost or part of a product line's total cost: Fixed or variable costs are clearly identifiable as such at any product level. This gives you a tremendous advantage in marginal cost analysis and competitive pricing.

In today's environment, modeling and cost simulation capabilities are more critical than ever. This system keeps track of the quantity and unit cost of inputs by using a bill of material. Six months later if the quantity consumed or unit cost of one of these inputs changes, the hospital doesn't have to recalculate the entire cost. It just changes one number on the bill of material for that product, and the system does the rest.

You can also input *new* cost factors (e.g., change the basis for cost allocation) and perform a cost rollup to see the impact on the overall cost. The ability to perform cost simulations enables administrators to determine the impact of changes in a wide range of cost factors. You can see the impact of anticipated changes for factors as simple as a payroll rate change or as complex as volume and method changes. If a factor has an impact on the cost of a procedure, material, patient, DRG, or service, the impact of that change can be modeled to aid in analyzing the results.

Users can develop, store, and maintain standard cost profiles using full absorption costing techniques. These fully absorbed cost standards can be used in the process of measuring and analyzing product-line profitability. Simultaneously, standard cost profiles can also be developed and stored from direct costing efforts for the purpose of support marginal cost analyses. Thus, one cost database can be used to support the varied requirements of profitability analysis, competitive bidding and pricing analyses, and managerial decision support. The ability to use one common database maximizes user flexibility and minimizes user maintenance requirements.

HEALTH CARE ACCOUNTING

With the Health Care Accounting Module, you can accurately and fairly measure performance in each department. Using procedural-level standards and statistical information about actual services provided, variances are calculated. Since costs are developed by element in the Health Care Costing Module (e.g., direct labor, direct supplies, depreciation, and variable overhead), the information sent to General Ledger can produce variances such as the following:

- volume variance
- patient mix (case-mix) variance
- labor rate variance
- labor efficiency variance
- material price variance
- material usage variance
- overhead spending variance
- overhead utilization variance

The ability to calculate and report variances at this level of detail can assist you in your effort to increase managers' understanding of their role in the cost management process. When cost variances are analyzed in terms of the components listed above, your managers can understand the cause and effect relationship that exists between their day-to-day decision-making efforts and the bottom line financial performance of the hospital. In addition, you can hold managers accountable only for those items that they control or influence. In short, the Health Care Accounting

Module can be used to enhance your hospital's overall management control effort.

CASE-MIX MANAGEMENT

Today, case-mix management systems are recognized as invaluable tools in analyzing clinical, marketing, and financial trends in the health care environment. The Case-Mix Management Module provides you with the tools to analyze patient and product-line trends. This module will handle such tasks as identifying patient demographics in each DRG or the resource consumption profiles by DRG and by physician.

The Case-Mix Management Module is built around a matrix concept, as shown in Exhibit 15–2–2, which relates service programs of a hospital to its operational units. Service programs are defined using diagnostic groups of patients, medical organizations, or even specific physician groups. Operational units are groups of revenue centers as defined by aggregations of specific charge codes. Each cell in the matrix could contain information such as revenue or cost, or a service statistic such as patient days or number of procedures.

The Case-Mix Management Module is directly interfaced to the Health Care Costing Module, and can use the cost element data from the costing module. Because of this interface, the case-mix reports reflect standard cost data as opposed to cost data calculated by cost-to-charge ratio methods. This design feature is a significant advancement over older case-mix systems, where costs are based entirely on ratio of cost to charges or other top-down methodologies. The ability to utilize detailed procedure-level standard cost data in the Case-Mix Management Module means you can now engage in marginal cost analyses by program or product line, for the purpose of competitive bidding and pricing analyses.

Exhibit 15–2–2 Example of the Matrix Concept

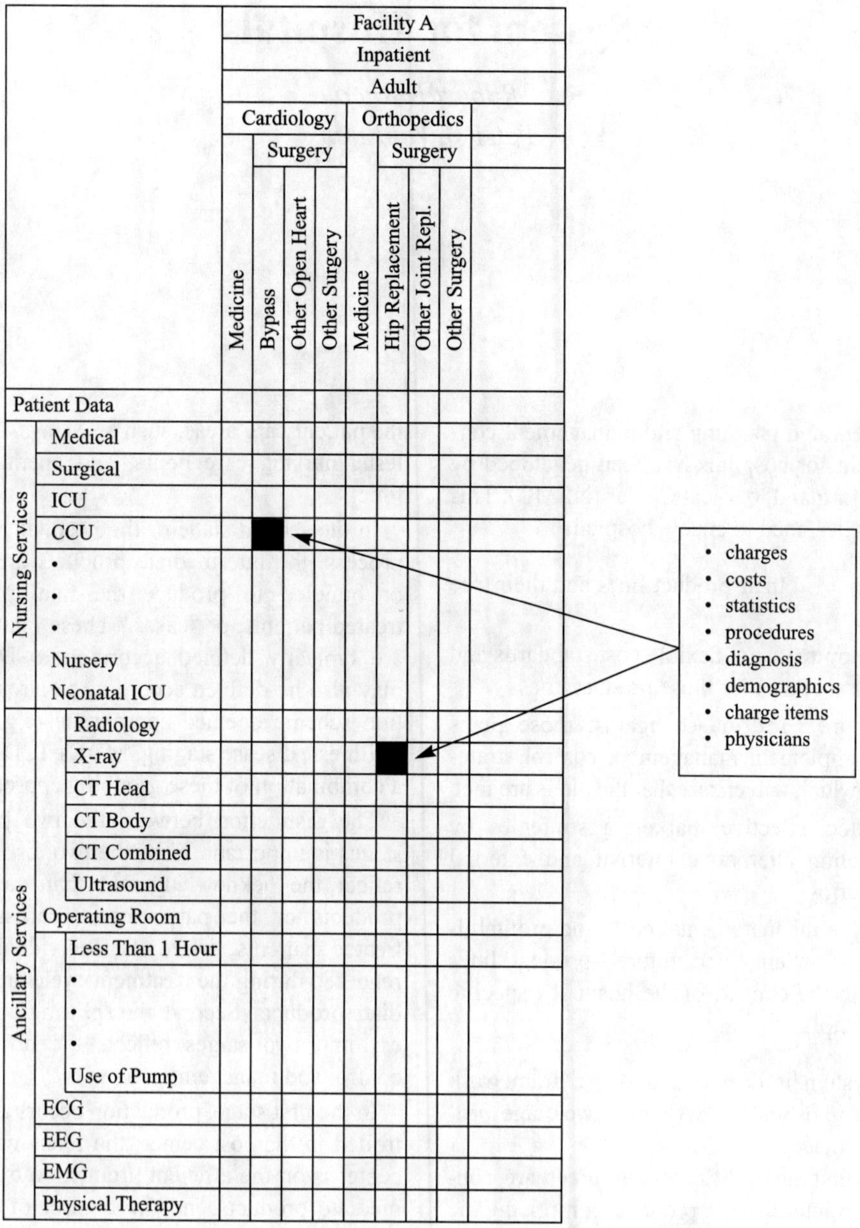

		Medicine	Bypass	Other Open Heart	Other Surgery	Medicine	Hip Replacement	Other Joint Repl.	Other Surgery	

(Facility A — Inpatient — Adult; Cardiology Surgery; Orthopedics Surgery)

- charges
- costs
- statistics
- procedures
- diagnosis
- demographics
- charge items
- physicians

Nursing Services rows: Patient Data, Medical, Surgical, ICU, CCU, •, •, •, Nursery, Neonatal ICU

Ancillary Services rows: Radiology, X-ray, CT Head, CT Body, CT Combined, Ultrasound, Operating Room, Less Than 1 Hour, •, •, •, Use of Pump, ECG, EEG, EMG, Physical Therapy

Source: Reprinted from *Hospital Cost Accounting Advisor,* Vol. 1, No. 6, p. 7, Aspen Publishers, Inc., © 1985.

Reading 15–3

An Integrated Planning and Management Control System for Hospitals

Robert F. Raco
Peter W. VanEtten

An integrated planning and management control system for hospitals has been developed by the New England Medical Center (NEMC). This system is designed to enable hospitals to

- understand their product lines and their true costs
- develop realistic, flexible cost standards and financial plans for those product lines
- measure performance against those plans and implement management control strategies which will ensure that the plans are met
- develop effective marketing strategies by modeling alternative internal and external scenarios
- analyze the incremental costs and profitability of current—and future—product lines within the context of the hospital's specific marketplace

The system is designed within a framework that views hospital activity as a two-stage production process.

In the first stage, hospital resources are converted into intermediate products comprising the individual procedures and services provided in

Source: Reprinted from Robert F. Raco and Peter W. VanEtten, "An Integrated Planning and Management Control System for Hospitals," *Hospital Cost Accounting Advisor,* Vol. 1, No. 7, pp. 4–7. Copyright 1985, Aspen Publishers, Inc.

the patient care areas, such as X-rays, laboratory tests, nursing care hours, and operating room time.

In the second stage of the hospital production process, the intermediate products are grouped or bundled to produce the final products—treated patients, or "cases." These final products are typically defined according to DRGs, but may also be defined according to any classification scheme deemed appropriate (e.g., severity of illness, disease staging, MDCs, ICD-9-CM, or a combination of these grouping approaches).

The distinction between the two production stages is important. First, the two distinct stages reflect the acknowledgment that the ultimate products of the patient-care process are the treated patients, while the individual services rendered during the treatment cycle are intermediate products. Second, the splitting of the process into two stages reflects the difference in control and management focus.

In the first stage, production occurs and is controlled in the cost center; the focus within each center is on the efficient production of the intermediate products and the control of unit cost. The second stage, however, is generally controlled by the physician. Thus, the focus of the second stage is on the number and mix of intermediate products "bundled" to produce final products.

NEMC's system consists of three integrated systems that provide software to support the management of the two production stages: Department Cost Manager (DCM), Clinical Cost Manager (CCM), and Clinical Financial Planner (CFP).

Department Cost Manager

DCM focuses on the control and management of costs associated with intermediate products. DCM enables hospital managers to identify intermediate products, develop standard costs, perform variance analysis and marginal cost analysis, and simulate changes in department costs.

Clinical Cost Manager

CCM is a planning, control, and intervention system that focuses on costs associated with the hospital's end product, or patient case. CCM enables managers and physicians to define the hospital's end products (using any of several case classifications), develop standard treatments and protocols for those classifications, cost out hospital case-mix, and perform variance analysis for cost, revenue, and profitability.

Clinical Financial Planner

CFP is a financial modeling system that enables managers to perform a broad range of budgeting, planning, and simulation functions.

As a decision-support tool, it can be used to model a variety of user-defined activity, cost, and revenue scenarios to determine their profitability. CFP is also used to develop the hospital budget, establish new standards for intermediate product costs and treatment protocols, and project the effect of different marketing strategies.

Information to support these systems is fed from the hospital's existing operational and financial databases through interfaces. Interfaces have been designed to transmit data to these three systems with minimal or no changes to a hospital's current systems and/or operations.

Figure 15–3–1 presents an overview of the flow of information among these three systems and the base information systems. Note that the only required hospital feeder systems are General Ledger, Medical Records, and Billing. Optional feeder systems include Payroll and Materials Management as well as department-specific systems (e.g., Nursing Acuity, or Operating Room Information System).

DEPARTMENT COST MANAGER

DCM is a management control system for use primarily by direct (ancillary and routine) hospi-

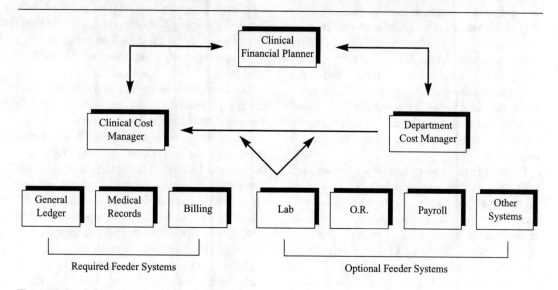

Figure 15–3–1 Information Flow among the Three Management Systems

tal departments. DCM's methodology views departments as cost centers rather than revenue centers (since end products, not intermediate products, generate revenue—particularly under a prospective payment system).

DCM focuses on the control and management of costs associated with intermediate products—procedures and services—that make up the end product or patient case. As a management tool, DCM performs the following functions:

- identifies intermediate products
- builds a standard cost for each intermediate product
- simulates changes in standard unit costs, department budgets, and staffing
- reports cost variances by product and department
- performs marginal cost analysis

In the DCM *product identification* process, the user selects and groups procedures and services into definable intermediate products. DCM's approach is based on the assumption that a relatively small number of procedures and services make up a high percentage of volume and cost. DCM interfaces directly with the hospital's database, which allows the user to complete this grouping and selection process on-line.

DCM's *product costing* process builds standard costs for each intermediate product. Within this framework, DCM identifies each department's direct costs by labor, supplies, and direct overhead components, distinguishing between fixed and variable costs. Because DCM is based on true cost accounting methodology, it can be applied to all hospital ancillary and routine departments.

DCM offers *department cost simulation* within the standards building process. By changing relative value units (RVUs) associated with each cost type, or changing labor productivity goals, overtime rates, wage rates, and so on, the user can model standard costs, department budgets, and staffing.

Variance analysis is a powerful DCM function and an effective mechanism for management control. Through variance analysis, DCM explains the difference between budgeted and actual costs by subdividing the variance into its component parts. By identifying these component causes of variance (volume and mix, utilization, and direct overhead variances), DCM provides clear definitions of cost accountability. Managers can thus be held responsible for costs they truly control.

DCM also provides information for *marginal cost analysis.* Because DCM distinguishes between variable and fixed costs, a hospital can estimate the effect of a projected change in volume on department costs. Such marginal cost data are also useful for determining the costs of additional cases or new programs. Other uses of DCM's marginal cost information include profitability analysis and more accurate pricing.

The DCM system includes these modules:

- Product Identifier
- Interface
- Standards Builder
- Reports

Product Identifier Module

Users define intermediate products by selecting and grouping hospital procedures and services in an on-line process. The end result is a defined, manageable number of intermediate products.

Assuming that, in general, a relatively small number of procedures and services make up a high percentage of volume and cost, Product Identifier allows users to select the exact volume percentage that will account for that small number of specific, individual intermediate products. The remaining low volume procedures and services can be grouped into one or more "other" intermediate product(s). Subsequent standard cost development and cost analysis then focuses on the specific intermediate products.

The product identification process is based on data that are fed directly from hospital volume and cost-related systems through the DCM interface table. This interface function minimizes the need for user input and allows the user to perform product identification on-line.

Interface Module

This module represents the interface between DCM and the hospital's database for volume, cost, and variable labor statistics.

An essential byproduct of the product identification process is the volume conversion factors that map the hospital's procedures (e.g., billing data) to the newly established intermediate products. The user can enter a multiplication or division factor for each procedure code to spread that procedure's volume to the products. These conversion factors become part of the interface table.

The user provides cost information to the interface table by specifying the unique feeder systems and account codes to be used for obtaining each department's costs and variable labor hours. As in procedure volume conversion, the user specifies any conversion arithmetic required for these cost and variable labor feeder keys.

All of this information becomes part of an interface table that is used to map hospital feeder data to intermediate products and departments. This key interface table is repeatedly used in building standard costs, generating cost variance reports, and so on.

If the user does not want to use volume and cost data provided through the Interface Module, DCM offers an override capability. This function allows the user to enter alternate data for standards development. The override capability has two primary purposes: to account for unforeseen changes in volume and cost after standard costs have been developed, or to enter information that cannot be accessed through feeder system interfaces (e.g., new procedures or departments).

Standards Builder Module

This module develops detailed cost standards by intermediate product. The key to this process is DCM's ability to associate intermediate products and their respective volumes with budgets

and user-defined RVUs. Cost standards are built by cost type and cost category.

DCM defines nine specific cost types:

1. Variable Labor
2. Variable Supplies
3. Variable Other
4. Fixed Direct Labor
5. Fixed Direct Equipment
6. Fixed Direct Facilities
7. Fixed Direct Other
8. Variable Indirect
9. Fixed Indirect

DCM allows the user to establish a virtually unlimited number of categories within each cost type. Categories are subclassifications of cost types. For example, the variable labor cost type for nursing could be subdivided among RN, LPN, and Nurse Technician categories. Unit cost standards would subsequently be developed separately for those and any other defined categories.

RVUs by cost type/category form the foundation for building cost standards. In an on-line process, the user defines RVUs for each product. RVUs represent minutes for variable labor but can represent *any* weighting scheme for all other cost types. Product volumes, combined with RVUs, yield a weighted volume for each intermediate product. The total budget for each product's cost type (or category, if applicable) is then spread back to the intermediate products according to the weighted volumes.

The Standards Builder Module provides additional functional information for variable labor costs. Standards Builder not only distinguishes among the various types of variable labor hours (e.g., worked hours, overtime hours, and vacation/sick/holiday hours) but also generates productivity measures in the form of standard ratios based on these different types of hours. The standard ratios can then be compared to actual ratios to monitor productivity.

The Standards Builder Module is designed to allow both "build-up" and "back-in" methods for establishing budgets and staffing levels for variable labor costs. Calculations for both methods are based on the given number of "specified work hours" to produce the products (as established by the weighted volume data described above—minutes × volume).

The *build-up method* determines the required variable labor staffing and budget given user-defined labor productivity goals and wage rates. The user establishes how many full-time equivalents (FTEs) and dollars are needed by projecting certain labor ratios and salary rates against the given number of specified hours.

The *back-in method* develops labor standards and productivity measures based on an already set amount of FTEs and labor budget. The user "backs in" to labor productivity standards given certain parameters for overtime salary rates, vacation/sick/holiday percentage of regular paid hours, and so on.

Reports Module

DCM's cost variance and statistical reports can be generated at multiple levels, ranging from the whole hospital to a group of departments or to a specific cost category within a specific cost type of one department.

A user can obtain both single entity reports (which report one department or a group of departments combined into one total) and multiple entity reports (which report two or more departments separately on the same report). Single entity reports are most useful to a department manager. Multiple entity reports are more likely to be used by a higher level manager or administrator responsible for more than one department.

DCM variance reports explain cost variances from budget and thus provide direction for a hospital concerned with cost control. While a hospital cost center manager in the past has had access to the center's total variance (total budgeted cost less total actual costs), DCM can provide a variance analysis explaining changes in

- product volume
- product mix
- labor efficiency and price
- supplies utilization
- direct overhead utilization

The real power of this variance breakdown is that it allows for better cost control through identification of costs in categories linked with specific responsibility levels. Activity (volume and mix) variances are primarily the responsibility of physicians or case managers. Variances related to cost per unit (labor, supplies utilization, and direct overhead) are the responsibility of the cost center manager. Thus, DCM variance analysis allows for clearly defined accountability for both favorable and unfavorable variances from budget and will significantly aid the cost control process.

16

Performance Evaluation and Incentive Compensation

Reading 16–1

Measuring Segment Performance: New Ventures of Today's Innovative Hospital Systems Pose Evaluation Challenges

Steven A. Finkler

As hospitals have become more innovative in recent years, their performance evaluation systems have not always kept pace. How does one evaluate the performance of a new rehab center and its manager? How about a new home care service? Many of the traditional hospital approaches to performance evaluation are not adequate for consideration of the various new ventures hospitals are undertaking.

Hospital management has traditionally measured organizational performance based on profitability of revenue centers and adherence to budgeted expenses for cost centers. About a decade ago, prospective payment systems forced hospitals to place a greater focus on adherence to expense budgets for all departments. It hardly pays to reward radiology for doing more X-rays and making a profit on each one when they are done on an inpatient with a fixed overall DRG reimbursement. That provides an incentive to do

Source: Reprinted from S.A. Finkler, "Measuring Segment Performance: New Ventures of Today's Innovative Hospital Systems Pose Evaluation Challenges," *Hospital Cost Management and Accounting,* Vol. 8, No. 9, pp. 1–7. Copyright December 1996, Aspen Publishers, Inc.

more X-rays, even though revenues would not increase.

In such a situation, the profit is an accounting artifact with no substance. The motivation system rewards incurring costs that generate no added revenue. One of the major purposes of a performance measurement system is to establish a system that gives managers incentives to act in a cost-effective manner.

Most hospitals have been successful in developing approaches to rein in the use of clearly unnecessary testing and other procedures. They have reacted appropriately to the prospective systems in place. However, most hospitals have had a not-for-profit orientation. As such, they lack some of the performance measurement approaches in place in for-profit organizations.

As hospitals enter more and more new ventures, whether those ventures are established on a for-profit or not-for-profit basis, a major motivation to generate profits for the hospital system remains. These profits can subsidize the central inpatient acute care mission, which may not be able to sustain itself on its own. Approaches to evaluating new venture performance and an evaluation of their effectiveness in providing managers with appropriate incentives follow.

PROFIT CENTER EVALUATION

As hospitals enter new ventures, often their first approach to evaluation is to establish profit centers. A profit center is responsible for both its expenses and its revenues. Therefore, it is evaluated based on how much profit it makes. This approach has both advantages and disadvantages.

In a profit center, managers can be evaluated based simply on how much profit they make. However, some profit centers are inherently likely to be more profitable than others. Reimbursement rules may favor one venture over another. While the total profit of each center is important for decisions related to the continued existence of the center, performance evaluation is better done using comparisons to a budget.

Thus, using a profit center approach, each profit center should have a budgeted profit. Performance can then be judged by comparing the actual results to that budget.

While this is a clear step forward, it may still put a manager in a position of being held accountable for things the manager cannot control. For example, central administrative costs may be allocated to the segment of the integrated system. While this has benefits for external reporting, it makes sense to recast the income statement for performance evaluation.

The income statement presented in Exhibit 16–1–1, for example, starts with revenues and then splits costs into variable and fixed components. This is based on the belief that managers have the most control over revenues and variable costs, at least in the short-run. Thus, the *contribution margin* shown in the exhibit represents the element that the manager should be held most accountable for. In comparing the budgeted and actual contribution margins, managers should be most rewarded for favorable contribution margin variances, and vice versa for unfavorable ones.

The next section of Exhibit 16–1–1 highlights the fixed costs of the venture itself. This new venture has some control over the fixed costs directly assignable to it. On the other hand, fixed costs are not very responsive to short term volume varia-

tions. Therefore, the *venture margin* is a better measure of whether or not the venture is financially viable than it is of managerial performance.

Lastly, central overhead costs are subtracted to arrive at *net income*. These are generally joint costs that for the most part do not change as ventures are added or removed. If the net income is negative, but the venture margin is positive, then the segment is still adding financial benefit to the overall system.

Thus, each measure is valuable. The last measure, net income, provides useful information for external reporting. All divisions of the organization can have their net incomes added together to arrive at the overall net income of the system. The middle measure, venture margin, provides useful information because it tells whether the segment or venture adds to profits of the system. The first measure, contribution margin, focuses on the actual performance of the manager.

Care should be exercised in making decisions about ceasing operations of a division. The fixed costs in Exhibit 16–1–1 may in fact contain some joint costs. It is essential that one determine whether such costs could actually be avoided before deciding that it would be better to close down a specific hospital subsidiary.

Another problem that the profit center approach to evaluation does not adequately address

---

Exhibit 16–1–1 Recast Income Statement for Performance Evaluation

Revenues	$5,000,000
– Variable Operating Costs	2,000,000
– Variable Segment Administrative Costs	500,000
Contribution Margin	$2,500,000
– Fixed Operating Costs	1,000,000
– Fixed Segment Administrative Costs	600,000
Venture Margin	$ 900,000
– Allocated Costs	400,000
Net Income	$ 500,000

relates to the investment made in the venture. Does the profit have to be as great if we only invest $50,000 as it would have to be if we risk $5 million in the new venture? Probably not. Therefore, when substantial investments are required, an investment center approach may provide a better basis for performance evaluation.

INVESTMENT CENTERS

Investment centers are often evaluated based on the return on investment (ROI). Suppose, for example, that Exhibit 16–1–1 represented the profit on a proposed outpatient facility that cost the hospital $10 million to acquire and start up. The net income from Exhibit 16–1–1, divided by the $10 million investment, shows an ROI of only 5 percent.

$$ROI = \frac{\text{Net Income}}{\text{Investment}}$$

$$ROI = \frac{\$500,000}{\$10,000,000}$$

$$ROI = 5\%$$

The hospital might have two other alternative projects that have projected profits of only $400,000 and $300,000, respectively. If profits are the primary focus, we might select the first project with the $500,000 profit.

However, what if the required investment for the second and third projects were $4 million and $2 million, respectively. Their ROIs would be as follows:

$$ROI = \frac{\$400,000}{\$4,000,000}$$

$$ROI = 10\%$$

$$ROI = \frac{\$300,000}{\$2,000,000}$$

$$ROI = 15\%$$

If the hospital has only $10 million available to invest, looking for the most profitable project is clearly incorrect. It can earn $500,000 on the first project, which requires investment of the full $10 million. Or else it can earn $700,000 in total on the two latter projects, which require an aggregate investment of $6 million, and still have $4 million left over for additional investments.

Thus, ROI may be a much better indicator than profits when investment decisions have to be made.

UNINTENDED CONSEQUENCES OF RETURN ON INVESTMENT EVALUATION

Although the ROI measure is generally better for evaluating investments than a simple profit measure, it is not without its problems.

For one thing, different projects tend to have different levels of risk. An 8 percent ROI on a very safe venture may be considered superior to a 10 percent expected ROI on a very risky project.

A second problem arises if we are considering two mutually exclusive projects that have very different sizes. For example, suppose that the hospital has a piece of land available for use. One proposal has been made to build a multideck parking garage on the land. The cost of the garage is estimated to be $5 million. Parking space is in great demand, and the expected ROI for the project is 35 percent. This is well in excess of any other projects available to the hospital. Some planning committee members want to get started on the garage as soon as possible.

The next best alternative is to build an outpatient testing facility on the site. This would include a variety of diagnostic testing capabilities. The area of the city where this would be built is currently underserved, and there would be a strong demand for the services offered. However, the facility would earn only a 20 percent ROI, substantially less than the parking garage.

While some members of the planning committee argue that the testing center is more in line with the hospital's mission, others argue that it cannot afford the financial sacrifice. (For this example, assume that the testing center would not generate any additional admissions or other revenues for the hospital. This is probably not true, but we want to put the parking garage in the best possible financial light for the moment. Also assume that no other land suitable for the testing center is available. We can do only one or the other of the projects. We cannot do both.)

The testing center would cost $40 million to build and equip. At a 20 percent ROI, it would generate an annual profit of $8 million. The garage, at 35 percent, is generating an annual profit of only $1.75 million ($5 million × 35% ROI). The testing center will generate a substantially higher profit. In general, we try to avoid simply looking at profit because it fails to reflect the amount of our investment, as discussed earlier. That is why ROI is often a better measure.

On the other hand, it is not just the ROI on one project, but rather on our entire range of investments that is critical. One must consider what the hospital will do with the money that it could invest in the testing center if it chooses to build the parking garage. If, for example, the hospital could invest the remaining $35 million at a 25 percent ROI, the garage would make sense. We would make 35 percent on the garage and 25 percent on the rest of the money. This is much better than investing the entire $40 million at an ROI of 20 percent.

But what if the next best alternative, aside from the garage and the testing center, earns an ROI of only 15 percent? Which is better? Thirty-five percent and 15 percent on the garage and another project, respectively, or 20 percent on the testing center? We must take a weighted average to find out.

$$\frac{\$\ 5,000,000}{\$40,000,000} \times 35\% = 4.375\%$$

$$\frac{\$35,000,000}{\$40,000,000} \times 15\% = +13.125\%$$

$$17.50\%$$

The garage and the 15 percent project will give an average ROI of 17.5 percent. This is lower than the 20 percent that could be earned on the testing center. It turns out that, overall, the hospital will have a higher ROI on its investment of the $40,000,000 if it bypasses the high-yielding, smaller garage project.

The key to this conclusion is the fact that the two projects are mutually exclusive. Ideally, we would do both the garage and earn 35 percent, and the testing center and earn 20 percent. That total $45 million investment would then have an average ROI of 21.67 percent, as follows:

$$\frac{\$\ 5,000,000}{\$45,000,000} \times 35\% = 3.889\%$$

$$\frac{\$40,000,000}{\$45,000,000} \times 20\% = +17.778\%$$

$$21.67\%$$

If the projects cannot both be done, however, then the testing center is more attractive. The hospital's evaluation approach should clearly reflect that fact.

RESIDUAL INCOME

There is one other problem created by the ROI approach to evaluation. The problem is created when managers are evaluated based on their ROI. The higher their department or division's ROI, the bigger their bonus. The incentive created by such a system is to reject any new venture that would lower the division's ROI, even if the venture would be financially attractive to the hospital organization.

For example, suppose that we have an outpatient testing facility that currently earns a 25 percent ROI. Assume that the hospital is willing to take the risk of new projects if they can be expected to earn at least a 15 percent ROI. What if the testing center becomes faced with the possibility of adding additional equipment that will earn a 20 percent ROI?

From the hospital's perspective, this will add to profits, and at 20 percent, it is an attractive investment. From the manager's perspective, however, the weighted average ROI of the division will be lower if a 20 percent investment is averaged in with the current investments, which are earning 25 percent, than if it is not.

This problem may be solved by using the residual income approach. This approach attempts to combine the benefits of using both net income and ROI. Using this method, any project is required to earn a specific minimum ROI. For example, the hospital might require that all investments earn at least 15 percent to be acceptable, as noted above.

The division is then credited with all net income in excess of that desired ROI. This amount is called the *residual income.* The higher the residual income, the better the manager has performed.

Suppose that in the above case, the testing center currently had $40 million invested and was earning an annual profit of $10 million. The ROI is 25 percent. The proposed new equipment would cost $5 million and has an expected ROI of 20 percent. That means that it is expected to yield an annual profit of $1 million. Under an ROI approach, it is rejected by the manager because the new total $11 million profit on a total investment of $45 million brings down the ROI from 25 percent to 24.4 percent.

With a residual income approach, however, the manager starts out with a residual income of $4 million. This is calculated as follows: The initial investment is $40 million, and the hospital requires a base return of 15 percent. Fifteen percent of $40 million is $6 million. The profit of $10 million provides the required $6 million, and also leaves over an additional or residual income of $4 million above the requirement.

The new project has a profit of $1 million. At an investment of $5 million, the 15 percent base requirement is $750,000. There is a residual income from the project of $250,000. Under the residual income approach to performance evaluation, rather than decreasing the performance from an ROI of 25 percent to 24.4 percent, the new investment increases the residual income from $4 million to $4.25 million.

The goal of performance measures is always to generate a system that gives individuals an incentive to do what is in the best interest of the organization. The benefit of residual income is that it now pays for the manager to do the thing that is good for the organization.

HOW DO YOU MEASURE THE INVESTMENT?

It is required for both the ROI and residual income methods that you know how much investment is involved. However, there is some ambiguity as to what is meant by "investment."

Stockholders' Equity vs. Total Assets

We could simply think of the investment as the amount of money spent initially to acquire the project. However, that is a simplistic approach. There are several possible ways to consider the investment.

For-profit corporations generally focus on their *stockholders' equity* as a measure of investment. For not-for-profit organizations, this is equivalent to net assets. Consider a hospital that borrows $30 million and puts up $10 million of its own cash to build a $40 million testing center. How much is the investment?

Clearly, the testing center cost $40 million. That is the hospital's asset. However, the hospital has really invested only $10 million of its own money. The asset is $40 million, the liability is $30 million, and the net assets are $10 million. Ten million dollars is the stockholders' equity measure of investment. Note that given this approach, a profit of $2.5 million is needed for a 25 percent ROI ($2.5 million net income divided by a $10 million investment = 25%).

If the hospital had put up the full $40 million itself, it would need a profit of $10 million for the same ROI. That effect is referred to as *leverage.* You can earn a higher ROI if you borrow money than if you supply all of the money yourself. Note, however, that the hospital will have to pay interest on any amount it borrows.

Suppose, for example, that the interest rate is 10 percent. Also suppose that the profit before interest payments is $5 million. If you do not borrow any money, your profit is $5 million and you have invested $40 million (that is both the assets and the net assets, since there are no liabilities). The ROI is 12.5 percent ($5 million net income divided by $40 million investment = 12.5%).

If you borrowed $30 million at 10 percent interest, there will be a $3 million interest expense. The net profit after paying interest will be only $2 million rather than $5 million. However, you have reduced the hospital's own investment from $40 million to $10 million. On that $10 million investment, the $2 million profit after paying interest results in a 20 percent ROI.

The ROI is higher because of the loan. However, so is the risk. If things go badly, the bank will still want to receive its interest payments. Borrowing can enhance returns, but it increases risk.

Suppose that profit before interest falls to $2 million because of changes in government payments for Medicaid. For the hospital that does not borrow, it earns an ROI of 5 percent ($2 million profit divided by a $40 million investment). If we borrowed $30 million, the $3 million interest payment would drive us into a loss position. Rather than earning a modest 5 percent ROI, we would have a negative 10 percent ROI (based on a $1 million loss after paying interest, divided by our $10 million investment). "He who lives by the sword dies by the sword."

Who decides whether or not to borrow? That is a critical question in performance evaluation. If the manager of the testing center makes that investment decision, then the manager should be held accountable for the ROI, good or bad. In other words, if the manager decides to borrow money to gain the leveraged ROI, the manager should be held accountable if things turn out poorly.

In many cases, however, top organizational management decides how to finance the project. The venture's manager is simply responsible for running the venture effectively. In that case, the impact of interest should not swing ROI up and down, affecting the manager's performance evaluation.

We can deal with this by holding the manager accountable for elements that are controllable. For example, rather than using stockholders' equity or net assets, we can measure investment as stockholders' equity plus long-term debt. In such an instance, the investment in our example would be $40 million, whether the money was borrowed or not.

This will tend to reduce the level of ROI in situations in which there actually is borrowing. However, as long as the approach is consistent and the manager is not expected to produce a "leveraged" level of ROI from an "unleveraged" measurement, it should not create any disincentives.

Similarly, we can use net income or income before interest in the ROI and residual income calculations. Which is appropriate? Using income before interest shows that the manager is not responsible for interest because the manager doesn't make the borrowing decision. Therefore, the manager is not held accountable for the impact of interest.

However, many would argue that since interest is a real cost, we should not give the manager the impression that it does not impact the hospital's income, because it does. Therefore, there is strong support for using net income in the calculations, even though it is not fully controllable by the manager.

The measure of stockholders' equity plus long-term debt seems a bit cumbersome. In our example, this is the same as total assets. Why not just measure the investment as being the organization's total assets?

That is another alternative approach. The choice should depend on who manages and controls current liabilities. If the manager can control short-term debt, using net assets plus long-term debt is appropriate. As the manager uses more or less short-term debt, the ROI will be affected. If the manager does not have the ability to control short-term debt, but rather working capital is done on a centralized basis, then the evaluation should be based on total assets as a measure of investment.

ACQUISITION VS. DEPRECIATED COST

The next problem in investment measurement concerns the decision as to whether to use asset acquisition cost or depreciated value in measuring investment. Unfortunately, both approaches are somewhat flawed.

The problem with *acquisition cost* is that over time, equipment and buildings decline in productive capability. Since managers are "charged" for their full initial cost year after year, there is a temptation to replace them too soon with newer, more productive facilities.

The problem with using *depreciated cost* is just the reverse. If we only count the depreciated cost as an investment, there is a tendency to keep buildings and equipment too long. Since they have a low valuation in the ROI measurement, old facilities tend to boost ROI. But over time, the equipment and buildings become so old that we may lose a competitive edge due to the declining productivity of the facilities.

An additional problem with this approach is that managers that are rewarded based on either ROI or residual income will receive increased rewards for static performance. Each year, as the equipment and buildings depreciate, the investment base is lower. A constant level of net income will increase both ROI and residual income.

For example, suppose that income were $1 million on a $10 million investment base that is being depreciated over 20 years on average. Assume that the hospital has a required rate of return of 8 percent. Therefore, there is a residual income of $200,000 ($10 million × 8% = $800,000 required return; $1 million net income – $800,000 required = $200,000 residual income). The ROI is 10 percent.

The next year, the investment has been depreciated down to $9.5 million. If net income is exactly the same, the ROI rises to 10.5 percent ($1 million net income divided by the lower investment of $9.5 million). The residual income rises to $240,000 ($9.5 million × 8% = $760,000 required return; $1 million net income – $760,000 required = $240,000 residual income).

Since the division's performance hasn't really improved, the manager's evaluation should not imply that it has. The ideal solution to this problem is to use the *market value* of facilities for investment measurement. Unfortunately, market value is a number that is not generally available.

However, we should not be discouraged. Perfect solutions often do not exist. But we can give better incentives and we can better evaluate performance by shifting to ROI and/or residual income approaches when we are evaluating separable divisions, segments, or ventures the hospital has undertaken, or is planning to undertake.

Reading 16–2

The Impact of Motivation and Incentive Programs on Financial Budgets

Janice Alger

In today's economy, many organizations are taking a harder look at their financial plans and strategies to determine their past effectiveness and efficacy for the future. One of the key tools used in this evaluation is a financial budget. Budgets are an integral part of an organization's managerial functions in that they provide a financial outline of its goals. In order for the organization to meet its goals, it is important that the objectives expressed in the budget are adhered to. However, achieving this is not always easy.

Many organizations have designed programs to provide incentives to managers and/or employees to meet budget objectives. Such programs can enhance the financial position of an organization as well as improve morale and job satisfaction among employees. The purpose of this article is to describe various motivation and incentive techniques and discuss how these techniques can be used to assist a department or organization in attaining its financial objectives.

BACKGROUND

Budgets

A budget "is a plan...formalized (written down) and quantified (e.g., stated in dollar

terms). It represents management's intentions or expectations."[1] Simply put, a budget is a plan. Preparing a comprehensive budget requires extensive planning at all levels. In this process, specific objectives and activities are put into place in a combined effort to meet the goals of the organization.[2] Since budgets are prospectively oriented, managers are forced to focus on potential opportunities and pitfalls and can therefore develop appropriate courses of action to address them. Failure to comply with the budget means the objectives are not met and the organization's goals are not being achieved.[3] It is easy to see the importance of developing a budget and sticking to it. In order for this to happen, budget objectives must be realistically established; that is, managers (or budget planners) must consider all factors that influence results. For example, there may be obstacles out of the manager's control that adversely affect his/her budget. These factors must be considered in the budget development process. It is futile to set budgets that are unattainable. Such practice results in frustration for managers and employees and they may become discouraged and view the budget process as a waste of time.

In addition to planning, budgets are an effective tool to improve communication among departments and employees. Some organizations state their goals and subsequently convert them into departmental budgets. This enables employees within these departments to become familiar with management's plans and foster better understanding of their individual roles. Employees

Source: Reprinted from Janice Alger, "The Impact of Motivation and Incentive Programs on Financial Budgets," *Hospital Cost Management and Accounting,* Vol. 5, No. 8, November 1993, pp. 1–7. Copyright 1993, Aspen Publishers, Inc.

who feel they are involved in the overall plan tend to be more satisfied with their jobs and may work harder to help the organization meet its goals.

The budget process must also consider the structure of the organization as well as its management style. Some employers seek input from middle and lower level managers when preparing a budget, while others restrict its development to top management or the controller. The term "participative budgeting" is the practice of permitting individuals to participate in the development of the budget. There are two primary advantages associated with participative budgeting:

- It provides a sense of challenge and responsibility among employees.
- It increases the probability that the goals of the budget will be "internalized" by the managers involved. That is, they accept the organization's goals as their own.

Some budgeting situations may lend themselves to more participation by managers and employees whereas others may not. Greater participation in the budget process is often associated with better quality budgets and a higher level of employee acceptance.[4] One of the consequences of participative budgeting is that the process may require more time and effort if more individuals are involved. In addition, some executives argue that managerial involvement may result in "organizational slack" where managers underestimate revenues and overestimate costs to ensure their departments will meet the established budget parameters. Each organization is different and should therefore seek a level of participation in the budgeting process that meets its specific needs and is acceptable to the managers who will be responsible for the budget.

Incentives

In recent years, there has been a dramatic increase in the number of organizations that have implemented incentive and reward systems. This change has occurred in all types of industries— from manufacturing to service. The purposes of these systems are to:

- link pay to performance, productivity, and quality
- reduce compensation costs by improving efficiency
- improve employee commitment and involvement
- increase teamwork[5]

By and large, most managers are dedicated to their employers and assist in the organization's success. However, the employee's personal goals may not fully converge with those of the organization. That is, managers may work to help the organization reach its mission, but may have personal or professional goals that are not shared by the organization. This concept is termed "goal divergence." Clearly, the organization should take steps to blend its interests with those of employees, enabling the two to work together toward mutual goals or "goal congruence."[6] Once apprised of the organization's goals, a manager can be more efficient in striving toward a specific end. Further, managers may be even more motivated to adhere to a budget if rewards are available for reaching them; hence, the development of incentive programs for attaining budget goals.

Generally, most incentive plans focus on individuals rather than groups, although a few offer incentives for departments or units. Money is the most common and most popular type of incentive; however, nonmonetary rewards such as praise, participation in the planning process, and recognition are also successful motivators. The following sections describe some incentive plans and how to design them, along with some positive and negative aspects of these programs.

TYPES OF INCENTIVE PLANS

There are a host of programs organizations can adopt to motivate managers and employees to comply with budget objectives. Many, however, are modifications of similar, more commonly used programs. The following is an explanation of some incentive programs that may be used to assist managers in meeting departmental or organizational budgets.

Bonus—This approach provides an incentive for managers or employees to use resources more efficiently. An individual employee or a complete department can be rewarded for keeping expenses below budget or by generating revenues above budgeted figures. For example, if a department's expenses are lower than the budgeted amount, the department would be permitted to retain a fixed percentage or dollar amount of the savings.[7] This system is effective because it can reduce expenses; however, opponents of these programs argue that quality may decline if employees cut corners to reduce expenses. Also, jealousy and competition may become more prominent if rewards are distributed on an individual basis and all employees or managers do not receive them.

Suggestion System—Suggestion systems are designed to reward employees for money saving or revenue generating suggestions. This type of program has been widely used in industry for some time. In fact, in 1969 General Motors paid out nearly $17 million in monetary awards to employees for their valuable suggestions.[8]

Suggestion programs are popular because they involve all levels of employees and afford everyone an opportunity to receive a reward. Many employers incorporate "suggestion boxes" into their programs that provide employees, who may be intimidated to express ideas or concerns publicly, an opportunity to make themselves heard. Negative aspects of this system include the fact that participants are not always informed of the results of their suggestions and that the financial rewards are small, particularly in instances when savings or additional revenue to the organization is significant. Finally, from a production standpoint, some manufacturing organizations have found that suggestion systems increase good ideas but do not have a direct impact on output.[9]

Group Level Incentive Plans—In some departments or organizations, it is difficult to measure individual performance. In these instances, individual incentives may not be appropriate because they do not provide a good indication of teamwork and cooperation within a department that may be essential to its success. Group level incentive plans were developed to address these situations.

To design a group level plan, objective performance levels are set by management with employee input. The objectives should be challenging; however, it is also important that employees feel the objectives are realistic and attainable. One of the potential problems with group incentives is that some group members often do more work than other group members, which can lead to hostility and possibly sabotage. Some industries use group incentives in conjunction with individual level or plant level incentives to help offset frustration for employees who do not "pull their weight."

Profit Sharing Plans—Profit sharing plans give employees the opportunity to participate in a program that shares in the profits of the organization. These plans typically include a predetermined, defined formula for allocation of profit shares among employees and management. One drawback with these schemes is that they do not always reward employee efforts. For example, if profits decline for reasons that are out of the employee's control, employees may become frustrated. Another approach is to reward employees for something they can control—labor costs. The next item is an example of such a program.

Scanlon Plan—This plan was developed in the 1930s by Joseph N. Scanlon, the president of a steel and tin plate company in Ohio. The plan emphasizes employer-employee participation and sharing in the operations and profitability of a company. The centerpiece of this plan is the theory that "efficiency of operations depends on company-wide cooperation and that bonus incentives encourage cooperation."[10] The bonus is determined on reductions in overall labor costs, such as reducing overtime. The difference between expected and actual costs is shared with employees.

Today, the Scanlon plan is recognized as a system built around assumptions of human behavior. Quality suggestions and employees sharing shortcuts and cooperating with each other are vital to its success. Studies show that this plan has resulted in better quality of output, and a better acceptance of technological change.[11] This plan may be used for not-for-profit or profit organizations.

Management by Objectives—This type of incentive is actually a management style where a manager and employee work together to develop a set of objectives from which a performance evaluation for the employee is developed. Employees who are more involved in the setting of objectives may be more likely to work harder to achieve them.[12]

Special Achievement Awards—This program is self-explanatory. It provides rewards for outstanding employee contributions within a department or the overall organization. The awards are typically cash payments ranging from $500 to $100,000. Other noncompensation rewards include better office space or furniture, increased technical or clerical assistance, or more influence over budget decisions. The federal government offers a program similar to this model to its employees.[13]

Contests—A number of organizations hold contests, games, or promotions to foster effort among employees. Contests focus on many topics, including productivity and quality improvement, development of safety techniques, or methods to reduce costs, absenteeism, or tardiness. The premise behind contests is to focus on individual efforts and emphasize the spirit of competition. Winners receive recognition and "bragging rights" over their peers. Prizes include items such as cash, merchandise, special trips, and time off. The negative impact of contests can be the competition it stirs within the organization. Hostility and other unanticipated results can undermine the contest idea. Thus, prior to implementing a contest program, organizations should evaluate its potential impact on the overall organization.

The Memorial Employees Retirement Incentives Trust (MERIT) program—This program was designed exclusively for not-for-profit organizations. In this plan the size of the reward is based upon savings in overall budgeted expenses. The incentives are placed in a trust that employees may withdraw from after retirement. There are five key steps to the plan:

- Standard efficiency testing is conducted to establish controllable expenses as a percent of the total operating revenue for the base period.
- Current year efficiency percent is deducted from the performance base. This is typically limited to a 5 percent deviation from performance base and cannot be negative.
- Employers' contribution is developed by applying the efficiency percentage obtained by payroll. Limit on the maximum and minimum adjustment is usually set.
- Final contribution amount is calculated.
- Employees' contributions are determined by the ratio of their earnings to the total earnings of all participants.

INCENTIVE DESIGN

Once the organization has determined what incentive programs will be offered, it must determine how they will be funded. According to a recent compensation study by KMPG Peat Marwick, there are four primary funding mechanisms for distribution of the incentives. They are:

- Goal attainment, where achievement of planned financial results is rewarded
- Fixed formula, which rewards performance that exceeds a predetermined threshold
- Peer comparison, where rewards are calculated based on data from comparable companies

- Discretionary rewards, which are provided at the discretion of the board, compensation committee, or the chief financial officer[14]

Further, the study also indicates a strong preference among organizations for option one, Goal attainment. Recommended guidelines for implementing goal attainment incentives include the use of a top down and bottom up process where the top down provides direction for attaining goals by establishing objectives and linking them to performance measures. The bottom up approach encourages commitment from employees at all levels and builds support for goals and objectives. Participants must be able to influence the objectives over time, although they may need instruction of how to effect the measures; keep it simple. The incentive plan should be simple and easy to understand. Otherwise it will not reach its objectives.

From the employer's standpoint, the advent of budget incentives in an organization helps meet budget objectives. They also provide other advantages to the organization, such as improved job satisfaction and motivation among employees. As indicated earlier, if employees realize they are helping the organization meet its goals and are receiving added benefits for it, they are likely to be more satisfied with their job. Thus, the organization may see reductions in turnover and absenteeism, which tend to be associated with job satisfaction.[15]

Conversely, there are a few drawbacks of budget incentives worth noting. Depending upon the organization, some employees believe incentives imply a lack of trust of workers by management. That is, management is not convinced employees are working at their best levels. In this instance, these programs may do more harm than good. Also, employees may view the incentives as "too good to be true" and conclude they probably don't work the way they are presented. This problem can be overcome with time as word gets around that rewards are being distributed. Similar to this, some employees fear the incentives will be cut if too much money is paid out. Finally, managers may also experience problems

when incentive programs are not available at all levels of management—employees may not want to be promoted if the higher level does not offer incentives.

Although some of these issues present problems for organizations, a good relationship between management and employees can work these issues out and reverse negative feedback on these programs.

SIMPLE INCENTIVE PLANS

I.

The following incentive plan was implemented for site managers of a local company in the service industry. The plan provides financial incentives to site managers based on profit performance of his/her site as well as area. Profit objectives are paid as a percent of base salary based on the following scale:

Profit Performance Objective

Achievement of YTD Site Profit Plan	% of Base for Site Performance	% of Base for Area Performance	Total Potential
Less than 90% of Budget	0%	0%	0%
91% to 95% of Budget	3%	3%	6%
96% to 99% of Budget	4%	4%	8%
100%+ of Budget	5%	5%	10%

In addition to these incentives, the company provides quarterly incentives of up to 10 percent based on performance objectives set by the district manager and reviewed by the general manager and site manager. These objectives include a variety of issues, including goals to contain expenses such as absenteeism, expenses, turnover, productivity, etc. Exhibit 16–2–1 provides a worksheet that lists the profit objectives as well as performance objectives.

Exhibit 16–2–1 Departmental Performance Objectives

Department: _____

Department Head: _____

Profit/Revenue Objectives

YTD Achievement	Incentive for Dept. Performance	Incentive for Organization Performance
90% or Less	0%	0%
91%–95%	2%	2%
96%–99%	3%	3%
100+%	5%	5%

A. Dept. Revenue Objective _____ %

B. Achieved Year to Date _____ %

Performance Objectives

Objective	Description	Target	Actual
Absenteeism			
Expenses			
Chargeback %			
Employee Productivity			
Turnover			
Department Inspection			
Turnaround Time			
Growth			

_____ % Earned from Profit Objectives

_____ % Earned from Performance Objectives

_____ % Total Incentive Earned

Prepared by: _____

Approved by: _____

Date: _____

In order to ensure that quality or reputation is not sacrificed in attaining these objectives, the company has added qualifiers that must be met prior to any incentive payout. These qualifiers are:

- Loss of an existing account eliminated the profit incentive for the quarter in which the account is lost. Site managers, however, are still eligible for the performance incentive for that quarter.
- Budgets cannot be adjusted during the year unless approved by regional director and corporate controller.
- In order to be eligible, managers must conduct themselves and fulfill their duties in a manner consistent with company policies and procedures.

II.

The above example is an incentive program designed to promote revenue growth. The following examples are select programs directed toward expense management in an insurance company. The concepts are readily applicable to the hospital industry.

Expense Management Bonus Program

Persistency—The purpose of the persistency bonus is to provide a direct incentive for retention of existing business. Each local office is allotted a "lapse maximum," which they must meet to receive this bonus. When a customer terminates, the premium loss counts against the lapse maximum. The bonus is calculated based on the amount the lapsed revenue beats (is less than) the lapse maximum and is paid based on a schedule. This program is designed so employees focus on existing business and not only on commissions paid for new business.

Deficit Recovery—Under this program a "bonusable" event is deemed to have occurred if a customer (active or lapsed) pays a portion (or all) of a deficit resulting from the group's experience. In an insured plan, customers are not legally required to pay deficits; however, some groups do so to reduce premium increases. Payable bonus is 1 percent of the amount recovered up to a maximum of $5,000.

Stop Waste Campaign—This program is the newest incentive designed to keep expenses down in the local marketing offices and the home office. Individuals are asked to submit ideas to eliminate waste in any area of the company. Rewards paid out are twofold. The employee submitting the idea receives free lunch with the chief financial officer and the departments implementing the idea receive thank you gifts at the close of the year. (In this organization, the latter reward is more popular than the former.)

CONCLUSION

With increased competition and increases in job mobility, I believe employee incentive programs of all types will continue to increase in popularity. From a personal point of view, I am very happy with the incentives my organization provides. Previously, I have held jobs where bonuses and incentives have been paid for increasing revenues. In my current position, I am afforded the opportunity to receive bonuses for keeping expenses low and helping my department stay within its budget. I think the presence of these programs leads me to "go the extra mile" to keep expenses low and keep customers happy. I also believe that by adopting these programs organizations are emphasizing to employees how important it is to stay within budget and work efficiently. Employees will then begin to think, "if the organization is paying me extra for this effort, it must be important."

One caveat I have with regard to these programs in the hospital industry in particular is that employees may act in their own best interests to obtain a bonus rather than in the best interests of the patient. I would suggest that qualifiers be added to incentive plans to alleviate this problem.

At this point it seems to me that the issue of incentives is no longer controversial. The issue that is now controversial is the type of program offered and to whom it should be offered—management or employees or both.

NOTES

1. Steven A. Finkler, *Budgeting Concepts for Nurse Managers,* 2nd ed., W.B. Saunders Company, Philadelphia, 1992, p. 1.

2. Paul J. Wendell, CPA, *Corporate Controller's Manual,* 2nd ed., Warren Gorham & LaMont, Inc., Boston, 1992, p. D3–4.

3. Paul J. Wendell, p. D3–4.

4. Robert Moncur and Robert Swieringa, *Some Effects of Participative Budgeting on Managerial Behavior,* National Association of Accountants, New York, 1975, pp. 2–3.

5. Keith Davis and William Werther, Jr., *Human Resources and Personnel Management,* McGraw-Hill, Inc., New York, 1989, p. 363.

6. Steven A. Finkler, *Budgeting Concepts for Nurse Managers,* 2nd ed., W.B. Saunders Company, Philadelphia, 1992, p. 44.

7. Steven A. Finkler, p. 45.

8. Randall S. Schuler, *Personnel and Human Resources Management,* West Publishing Company, St. Paul, 1981, pp. 294–295.

9. Ibid.

10. Randall S. Schuler, p. 296.

11. Richard Henderson, *Compensation Management: Rewarding Performance,* 5th ed., Prentice Hall, Englewood Cliffs, pp. 338–339.

12. Steven A. Finkler, pp. 44–45.

13. Richard Henderson, p. 339.

14. John Bloedorn, Partner KMPG, "The Compensation Model: A Contemporary Design," *Compensation Briefs,* August 1992, pp. 5–7.

15. Randall S. Schuler, p. 298.

Part IV

Cost Accounting for the Year 2000 and Beyond

For the last decade there has been a growing literature critical of current cost accounting practices throughout all United States industries. The concern is that costing has evolved primarily into a tool for external reporting of financial results, rather than for the management of the organization. The concern has led to a movement to drastically revise cost accounting practices to make them more relevant. The criticisms of cost accounting, along with a number of suggested approaches for improvement are discussed in the first chapter in this part of the companion text, *Essentials of Cost Accounting for Health Care Organizations, Second Edition.*[1]

One technique which has received great attention in recent years is activity based costing (ABC). The underlying focus of activity based costing is that overhead has become a major component of costs, and that it is possible to drastically improve the accuracy of product costing by more closely considering the activitieswhich cause overhead to be incurred. This

technique is explained, discussed, and applied to health care in the three readings in this chapter, "Activity-Based Costing in the Operating Room at Valley View Hospital," "Activity-Based Costing for Hospitals," and "ABC Estimation of Unit Costs for Emergency Department Services."

The second chapter in this section, Chapter 18, looks at Total Quality Management (TQM). Toward the end of the 1980s businesses in this country, based on their observations of international industry, found that better quality does not necessarily mean higher costs. In fact, doing things right the first time, every time, might not only lead to a better product, but might also save costs in the long run. One popular application of TQM in cost accounting is to show how the additional costs of appraising quality and preventing failures can be offset by the savings from reductions in internal and external failure costs. Reading 18–1 lays a foundation in this area by providing a discussion of measuring the costs of quality. Then Reading 18–2 explains the Total Cost Management technique which merges cost accounting and total quality management. That article gives an application of the technique in a laboratory setting.

---

[1]Steven A. Finkler and David M. Ward, *Essentials of Cost Accounting for Health Care Organizations, Second Edition*, Aspen Publishers, Inc., Gaithersburg, MD, 1999.

17

New Approaches to Cost Accounting

Reading 17–1

Activity-Based Costing in the Operating Room at Valley View Hospital

Judith J. Baker

Georgia F. Boyd

In today's health care environment, the hospital cost accounting system should accomplish three aims. The cost accounting system should accomplish cost efficiency without a negative impact on the quality of service delivery. The system should provide information for management to maximize resources. In addition, the system should assist in continuous quality improvement (CQI).

This article presents an example of how one hospital reports the results of activity-based costing (ABC). It examines the composition and supporting assumptions of an ABC report for a particular procedure in the operating room (OR). It describes management uses of the information generated. It also comments on how the CQI initiative at Valley View Hospital is synchronized with the ABC reporting.

ABC CONCEPT

ABC measures the cost and performance of activities, resources, and cost objects. Resources are assigned to activities, and then activities are assigned to cost objects based on their use. ABC recognizes the causal relationships of cost drivers to activities.

The treatment of allocated costs differs from traditional systems in that overhead is allocated first by tracing actual cost, by activity, where possible. The balance of overhead is allocated through a cause-and-effect relationship with activities. Another advantage for managers is that non–value-added activities can be readily isolated and identified.

Expenses are separated and matched to the level of activity that consumes the resources. Specifically, the expenses needed to produce individual units of a particular service or product are separated from the expenses incurred to produce different products or services or to serve different payers. This separation is independent of how many units are produced or sold; it is not volume driven.

In other words, costs are traced by activities across departments or cost centers. ABC produces data that are more accurate and give a clearer view of costs.

Source: Reprinted from J.J. Baker and G.F. Boyd, "Activity-Based Costing in the Operating Room at Valley View Hospital," *Journal of Health Care Finance*, Vol. 24, No. 1, pp. 1–9. Copyright Fall 1997, Aspen Publishers, Inc.

BACKGROUND

Valley View Hospital is a nonprofit community hospital. It is located in Glenwood Springs, in north-central Colorado. Valley View Hospital serves a three-county area. It also operates a clinic in the town of Eagle, 30 miles to the east.

ABC AT VALLEY VIEW HOSPITAL

Valley View's ABC was commenced about 2 years ago. The costing has been set up on a parallel system and is not integrated into the general ledger system. ABC can successfully function as a supplemental, or parallel, system. This is a great advantage, as the information system in place does not have to be disturbed.[1] ABC has been implemented internally department by department at Valley View. The ABC components of a management report, the detail of a Bill of Activity, and the ways certain Capital Equipment Costs are handled in this ABC application are examined here.

ABC IN THE OR

Consider the application of ABC to a single OR procedure. The overall cost of any OR procedure incorporates direct labor and direct supplies used along with equipment cost for the specialty equipment utilized in the procedure. In addition, total procedure cost would include the particular procedure's portion of allocated costs for items such as administrative personnel. Finally, total procedure cost would include the institutional overhead attributable to the particular OR procedure.

The Valley View OR was converted to ABC within the last one third of the hospital's departmental conversion process. OR costing is by type of procedure. Highest volume procedures were converted first. Three reports are most commonly used at Valley View to document costing in the OR:

1. The Gross Margin Analysis (GMA) Activity-Based Costing Report
2. The Bill of Activities (BOA)
3. Specialty Capital Equipment (Technology) Costs

The three reports represent three levels of costing documentation. The GMA represents a decision-making level of reporting. It utilizes the costing figures in conjunction with other decision-making information. The BOA assembles the costing components that are utilized in the GMA. The Specialty Capital Equipment (Technology) Costs report presents the supporting line-item detail for each item of specialty capital equipment directly associated with the procedure that is accounted for on a per-patient basis.

The GMA ABC Report

The OR cost information appears in the form of a GMA ABC report. The GMA for knee arthroscopy is presented as Table 17–1–1. Recall that ABC measures both cost and performance. This report format functions as a measure of both elements.

There are eight individual costing elements listed within the report:

1. Acuity 3 surgery per minute
2. arthroscope
3. general closure suture/A
4. IV [intravenous] set-up
5. Phase II recovery
6. Surgical preparation
7. Tourniquet equipment
8. Video equipment

Activities include surgical preparation, IV set-up, the surgery itself, and Phase II recovery. Technology directly related to the activities for this procedure includes the arthroscope, the video equipment, and the tourniquet equipment. Each activity classification (surgical preparation, IV set-up, the surgery itself, and Phase II recovery) includes labor, supplies, equipment, and overhead costs.

The GMA report contains an average count column for each line item. The average count is multiplied by the relevant cost per unit column to arrive at the extended cost column. Thus, "Acuity 3 surgery per minute" is listed at a cost of $9.27 per minute. The average count of 55.9 minutes for a knee arthroscopy is multiplied times the $9.27 cost per minute to arrive at the extended cost amount of $518.19.

In a similar manner, the average count is multiplied by the relevant Charge per Unit column to arrive at the Extended Charge column. Thus, "Acuity 3 surgery per minute" is listed at a charge of $18.00 per minute. The average count of 55.9 minutes for a knee arthroscopy is multiplied times the $18.00 charge per minute to arrive at the extended charge amount of $1,006.20.

The difference between the extended charge amount of $1,006.20 and the extended cost amount of $518.19 accounts for the reported gross margin amount of $488.01 for this particular line item. Note that there can be both positive and negative amounts in the gross margin column. Further note that the overall gross margin calculated for this procedure is 36.5 percent ($1,483.11 less $941.79 equals $541.32; $541.32 divided by $1,483.11 equals 36.5 percent).

BOA Costing Components

The BOA for "Acuity 3 surgery per minute" is presented as Table 17–1–2. A bill of activities is a list. In this case, it is a list of the activities required and the associated costs of the resources consumed by a procedure.

Table 17–1–1 Knee Arthroscope GMA: DRG 22; Primary Procedures 80.26, 80.6, 81.47; Knee Arthroscopy; N = 47 Patients

Procedure Name	Procedure	Category	Average Count	Unit Charge	Standard Cost	Extended Charge	Extended Cost	Gross Margin ($)	% of Total Charge
Acuity 3 surgery/min	36003176	360OR	55.9	18.00	9.27	1,006.20	518.19	488.01	
Arthroscope	36004042	360OR	1.0	188.50	3.40	188.50	3.40	185.10	
General closure suture/A	36006502	360OR	1.4	19.40	0.42	27.16	0.59	26.57	
IV set-up	36001303	360OR	1.0	20.30	2.52	20.30	2.52	17.78	
Phase II recovery	36001162	360OR	161.1	0.50	2.35	80.55	378.59	(298.04)	
Surgical preparation	36003200	360OR	1.0	64.00	15.08	64.00	15.08	48.92	
Tourniquet equipment	36006734	360OR	1.0	18.40	0.01	18.40	0.01	18.39	
Video equipment	36006752	360OR	1.0	78.00	23.41	78.00	23.41	54.59	
OR						1,483.11	941.79	541.32	53.3
Gross margin %								36.5%	

Source: Copyright © Georgia F. Boyd, Glenwood Springs, Colorado.
Note: Avg ct = average count; chg = change; Std = standard; Extd = extended.

Table 17–1–2 BOA Cost Components: OR Acuity 3, Standard Unit Cost of $9.27

Cost Group	Resource	Usage	Direct Quantity	Allocated Usage	Computed Std Cost
Direct variable labor	RN	Hr.	1 min.		0.37
Direct variable labor	RN, circulation nurse	Hr.		0.01	1.09
Direct variable labor	Scrub nurse	Hr.	1 min.		0.32
Indirect fixed labor	Director			0.01	0.30
Equipment direct		Usage	1		0.21
Equipment allocated				1.00	0.30
Direct variable materials				1.00	0.33
Indirect fixed materials				1.00	0.56
Variable overhead				1.00	3.19
Fixed overhead				1.00	2.60
			Acuity std cost		$9.27 per min.

Source: Copyright © Georgia F. Boyd, Glenwood Springs, Colorado.
Note: Std = standard.

This type of BOA is termed *a Service Cost Bill of Activities.* A Service Cost BOA represents all the activities necessary to provide a service.[2] Thus, for a hospital setting out the cost of an already developed service, the major costs to be found in a Service Cost BOA would include direct labor, supplies, technology (including depreciation), along with associated support costs. That is true in the case of Valley View Hospital.

The terminology for this BOA-Acuity 3 surgery per minute-reflects the OR acuity formula. The formula takes nurse skill level, skill mix, and quantity of staffing into account. In this case, "Acuity 3 surgery" requires two registered nurses (RNs) and a circulation nurse.

There are 10 cost groups in the Table 17–1–2 BOA:

1. direct variable labor—RN
2. direct variable labor—RN, circulation nurse
3. direct variable labor—scrub nurse
4. indirect fixed labor—director
5. equipment—direct
6. equipment—allocated
7. direct variable materials
8. indirect fixed materials
9. variable overhead
10. fixed overhead

Assumptions regarding OR Acuity 3 BOA are summarized as follows:

- Direct variable labor categories (1, 2, 3) represent the appropriate skill level, skill mix, and quantity to meet the criteria for OR Acuity 3 for this procedure.
- Indirect fixed labor (4) represents the Director's time.
- Equipment—direct (5) requires a bit more explanation. All specialty equipment utilized in a procedure is directly charged to the patient as a separate line item. Thus, the arthroscope appears as a separate line item. However, there is also "nonchargeable" specialty equipment, such as the surgical table, OR lights, central warming cabinets, and

sterilizer. This equipment is charged within the BOA as "Equipment—Direct."

- Equipment—allocated (6) represents all other items, such as instruments that are spread under an equipment allocation rather than being charged direct as specialty equipment.
- Direct materials (7) are computed as a unit cost based on department supply expense levels. The actual supplies utilized are charged along with built-in overheads coming out of central supply, thus resulting in a "loaded" direct charge.
- Indirect materials (8) are computed as an allocated cost based on department supply expense levels.
- Variable and fixed overhead (9 and 10) are computed as unit costs based on overhead allocations. This article is not the forum for dissecting the computations for fixed and variable overhead. Suffice it to say there are 33 elements of OR overhead, each with its own driver and its own allocated unit cost.

The 10 elements within the Table 17–1–2 BOA result in a $9.27 acuity standard cost per minute. This figure is carried forward to the GMA report. On the GMA, the $9.27 per minute for OR Acuity 3 is multiplied by the 55.9 minutes utilized for the knee arthroscope procedure.

In an ABC system, the allocation bases utilized for applying costs to services or procedures are called *cost drivers.* Cost drivers include any causal factor that increases the total costs of an activity. Both volume-related allocations bases and other volume-unrelated allocation bases can be used as cost drivers in an ABC system.[3] (The use of a multitude of allocation bases that can be either volume-related or non-volume-related is a major distinction of the ABC system.) In this case, direct labor is the primary cost driver.

Specialty Capital Equipment (Technology) Costs

The second line item in the Knee Arthroscope GMA (Table 17–1–1) is listed as "Arthroscope."

This entry indicates the arthroscope equipment utilized in the OR for the procedure.

All specialty equipment utilized in a procedure that is directly charged to a patient is a separate line item. An illustration of the direct charge for specialty capital equipment is composed of five line items as illustrated in Table 17–1–3.

Table 17–1–3 shows the asset acquired value and the annual depreciation on cost for each of the five equipment line items. The annual usage for the past 2 years is set out, then the annualized usage for the current year is set out. The final column calculates the current year cost per use. This figure is obtained by dividing the annual depreciation by the current year's annualized usage figure: $930.60 annual depreciation divided by 274 annualized usage equals $3.3964 cost per use.

The knee arthroscope GMA charges one unit for a single usage of the arthroscope. That is, one procedure performed equates to one unit.

Note that Valley View's OR cost is at an advantage here. The arthroscopy camera—the most expensive item on the direct-charge OR capital equipment charges (see Table 17–1–3)—is fully depreciated. Thus, the annualized cost per use for this year is one half or less of what it would be if depreciation was still being charged for the arthroscopy camera.

Management Uses for the ABC Reports

Within ABC, the cost object drives the composition of the final cost reporting. A cost object is anything for which a separate measurement of costs is desired.[4] Brimson calls the cost object a "cost objective" and says the cost objective depends on the management decision to be made.[5] Thus, the cost objective influences the reporting objective, and the reporting objective influences the cost objective.

Valley View management's primary use for the ABC reports is in four areas:

1. performance measurement/evaluation
2. strategic planning
3. managed care contract negotiations
4. managed care contract management

Valley View management's secondary use for the ABC reports is in two areas: (1) resource allocation and (2) cost control. Valley View management's future use for the ABC reports is in two additional areas: (1) departmental budgeting and (2) staffing decisions.

Management reports are at the procedure level in this OR example. The decision-making viewpoint is primarily from the service line, or product line, analysis. That is, the individual procedure reported upon in this example is part of a service line. The management information presented in these reports fits into an overall service line analysis. It should be emphasized that there is no one right way for choice of cost objectives or reporting objectives. Each organization will respond according to its own situation.

Table 17–1–3 Capital Equipment Charges: OR 01.660 Arthroscope

Asset No.	Description	Service Unit No.	Asset Acquired Value	Annual Depreciation Cost	Annual Usage			1996 Cost per Use
					1994	1995	1996 Annualized	
	Arthroscope	36004042			229	266	274	
	Avg chg per product				$177.54	$181.20	$188.39	
(O) 000372	Arthroscopy camera (fully deprec)		9,761.20	0.00				
(O) 000373	Telescope and lenses		6,361.36	636.12				
(N) 000073	Duckbill Upbiter and basket punch		1,531.25	153.12				
(N) 000106	Forceps 3.4 mm backbiter/Arthrotek		905.45	90.60				
(N) 000289	Isometric ligament positioner		507.06	50.76				
			19,066.32	930.60			274	$3.3964

Source: Copyright © Georgia F. Boyd, Glenwood Springs, Colorado.
Note: Avg chg = Average charge.

Synchronizing ABC and CQI

Valley View Hospital is committed to CQI. CQI allows a never-ending search for higher levels of performance within the organization; "if you're not going forward, you're going backwards."[6]

Deming's philosophy is taught to Valley View staff. W. Edwards Deming was a pioneer in the development of process improvement. His process improvement concept is summarized in "Deming's wheel," which involves repeated application of the steps of planning, doing, checking, and acting.[7] As the wheel revolves, the cycle is repeated over and over, illustrating the concept of continuous, or never-ending, improvement. The commitment of Valley View to CQI is best illustrated by this fact: there is a "quality management" line item within the array of general overhead expenses. This line item includes a budgeted amount available for CQI training.

Synchronizing ABC and CQI is logical. ABC's activity analysis and cost-driver analysis allow the exploration of process. This exploration of process from both the performance measurement and the costing aspects of ABC flow directly into the process improvement elements of CQI. Thus, the highest and best use for ABC

and for CQI occur when the two initiatives are synchronized.

The Valley View OR ABC reporting example demonstrates compliance with the three aims of a hospital cost accounting system. The underlying reporting objective is fulfilled in that the information provided can accomplish cost efficiency, provide information for management to maximize resources, and assist in CQI.

NOTES

1. Baker, J.J. "Activity-Based Costing for Integrated Delivery Systems." *Journal of Health Care Finance 22,* no. 2 (1995): 59.

2. Brimson, J., Antos, J. *Activity-Based Management for Service Industries, Government Entities, and Nonprofit Organizations.* New York: John Wiley & Sons, 1994, 240.

3. Chan, Y. "Improving Hospital Cost Accounting with Activity-Based Costing." *Health Care Management Review 18,* no. 1 (1993): 72.

4. Horngren, C., et al. *Cost Accounting: A Managerial Emphasis,* 8th ed. Englewood Cliffs, NJ: Prentice Hall, 1994, 248.

5. Brimson, J. *Activity Accounting: An Activity-Based Costing Approach.* New York: John Wiley & Sons, 1991, 161.

6. Horngren, C., et al. *Cost Accounting,* 7.

7. Cryer, J., Miller, R. *Statistics for Business: Data Analysis and Modelling.* Boston: PWS-Kent Publishing Co., 1991, 12.

Reading 17–2

Activity-Based Costing for Hospitals

Suneel Udpa

The challenges posed by managed care, capitated payments, and other restrictive hospital reimbursement mechanisms such as diagnosis-related groups (DRGs) provide an ideal setting for the implementation of activity-based costing (ABC) in hospitals. Current health care practices and procedures such as DRGs, patient-acuity systems, case management, critical path analysis, utilization review, and others can be used in the implementation of the ABC system.

ABC in the manufacturing sector has remained a focal point of interest for practitioners and academics for a number of years. Studies applying the basic principles of ABC used in manufacturing firms to health care organizations have appeared in health care journals only recently. However, a majority of the studies of ABC in health care settings focus on a narrow application of ABC to a department within the health care organization. For instance, Chan[1] examines the application of ABC to the costing of laboratory tests, Ramsey[2] examines the application of ABC to the hospital's radiology department and a nursing station, and finally, Canby[3] applies ABC to the X-ray department of the hospital. In this article, I provide a framework for the implementation of ABC for a health care organization's total operations and its specialized services.

The study described in this article examines the application of ABC to the hospital's inpatient services. Application of ABC to a hospital's outpatient care service requires additional considerations. Outpatient care generally involves a much larger number of units of service with relatively small cost per unit. Also, databases on outpatient services and related costs are often poorly developed and bills are often generated at multiple sites. ABC can nonetheless still be applied to a few selected high-volume and high-cost–low-profit margin outpatient services using the principles and techniques described in this article.

NEED FOR A NEW COST SYSTEM

In conventional cost accounting systems, direct costs such as costs of specific services (e.g., use of the operating room, diagnostic procedures, laboratory tests, pharmacy, and physical therapy) are billed directly to patients. However, indirect costs or overhead for the entire hospital operation (including individual departments) are typically accumulated and divided by the total number of patient days to determine the per diem cost. In this system, hospitals assume overhead cost per patient day is the same irrespective of the patient type, level of care, procedure being performed, or length of stay (LOS).

However, not all overhead costs vary on a patient-day basis. For instance, overhead costs relating to admissions and registration do not vary

Source: Reprinted from S. Udpa, "Activity-Based Costing for Hospitals," *Health Care Management Review,* Vol. 21, No. 3, pp. 83–96. Copyright Summer 1996, Aspen Publishers, Inc.

with the number of patient days but vary with the number of patients admitted, that is, the cost associated with admitting patients is independent of LOS. Also, the cost per patient day is not the same across all patients. Patients with short stays but who require extensive nursing support have a higher cost per patient day compared to patients who require long stays with minimal nursing attention. Therefore, conventional hospital cost systems can report seriously distorted cost per patient when patient care is diverse in terms of either level of care (acuity) or amount of care (patient days).

Pricing, which historically has not been a key factor in hospital marketing, is now an important criterion through which hospitals compete for business from large organizational buyers such as managed care organizations (e.g., health maintenance organizations [HMOs] and preferred provider organizations [PPOs]), third party insurers, and employers. This price competition and the resulting importance of accurate cost information make the need for a new cost system urgent in most hospitals.

ACTIVITY-BASED COSTING

ABC is an information system that maintains and processes data on a firm's activities and products/services. It identifies the activities performed, traces costs to these activities, and then uses various cost drivers to trace the cost of activities to the final products/services. Cost drivers are factors that create or influence cost and reflect the consumption of activities by the products/services. An ABC system can be used by management for a variety of purposes relating to both activities and products/services.[4]

ABC involves a two-stage allocation process. In the first stage, we assign hospital costs to activity pools such as "admit patients," "cardiac catheterization," "administer ECG tests," and so on. In the second stage, costs are assigned from these activity pools to individual patients, or units of episodic care, using appropriate cost drivers that measure the patients' consumption of these "activity resources."

DEVELOPING THE ABC MODEL

This section details the development and implementation of ABC on a hospitalwide basis, weaving together the principles and techniques of ABC with current health care practices such as case management, critical path analysis, acuity levels, and total quality management (TQM). The steps in developing and implementing the ABC model are outlined below.

Step 1: Form a Cross-Functional Steering Committee

In order to establish a process for implementing ABC, first form a committee that will ultimately be responsible for the implementation and evaluation of the ABC system. A cross-functional steering committee could consist of the following members:

1. RN case coordinators/case management specialists
2. physicians
3. accountant
4. information systems manager
5. medical records personnel
6. outside consultant (if necessary).

The committee and its members should meet regularly with physicians, hospital staff, and management to identify issues that could affect the implementation of the ABC system, such as utilization of resources, quality patient care, communication between the nursing staff and physicians, information systems, and process improvements. It is very important to gain staff and physician support for the ABC system. Personnel will more readily accept the new system if they are educated about the nature of the system and are concurrently involved in the development and implementation phases.

Step 2: Identify Case Types/DRGs for Analysis

Case types for analysis are typically selected based on case volume (high volume), financial impact (high cost, low profitability), variance measure (high variance from DRG estimate), quality assurance issues (high risk), or special interest (new service). Also, for initial analysis, case types with predictable hospital delivery paths are selected. When a high-volume or high-cost case type is selected, a decrease in LOS of even 1 day has a very significant impact on costs.

Figure 17–2–1 shows a sample graph based on case volume and contribution margin (Price – Variable Cost) per case for each DRG. DRGs in the top left quadrant have the highest case volume and low margin. The hospital is likely to gain the greatest benefit from activity analysis and ABC analyzes these DRGs.

DRGs should not be the only classification system used to develop and implement critical paths and the ABC system. Cost distortions can result when DRGs are broad based and include case types that are non-homogeneous. In some cases, it might be more accurate to use the *International Classification of Diseases—Ninth Edition—Clinical Modifications* (ICD-9-CM di-

agnosis codes) instead of DRGs to analyze particular case types.

Step 3: Profile the Health Care Delivery System

Using case management and critical path analysis, perform activity analysis across all operations and processes that are required to move the patient from preadmission to discharge.

Case management is both a model and a technology for restructuring the clinical production process to ensure that a patient receives needed services in a supportive, efficient, and cost-effective manner. When integrating case management with the hospital cost accounting system, two perspectives of case management should be considered: the hospitalwide systems/processes and the direct patient care delivery system or critical path. Analyzing the hospitalwide processes involves examining in detail the activities involved in the preadmission process, the hospital stay process, and the patient discharge process. For instance, in performing an activity analysis of

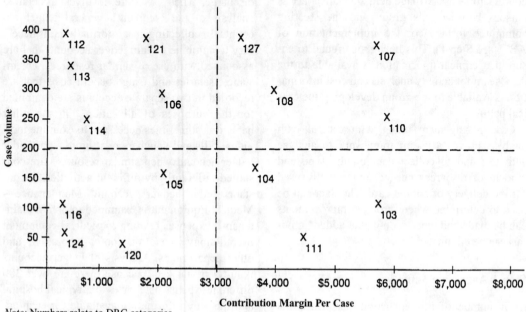

Note: Numbers relate to DRG categories.

Figure 17–2–1 Sample DRG Volume–Profitability Matrix

the hospital stay process, the hospital should review the following activities: ordering and receiving drugs from the pharmacy, ordering and providing therapeutic and diagnostic services, utilizing specialty services, and using all the auxiliary services such as laundry, dietary, administrative, and janitorial.

The direct patient care delivery system or critical path analysis is an abbreviated report that shows the critical or key incidents that must occur in a predictable and timely order to achieve the hospital's medical and financial goals. Critical paths are tools that, once individualized by the primary nurse and physician for a particular patient within the first 24 hours of admission, are used on every shift on each consecutive unit to plan and monitor the flow of care.[5] Table 17–2–1 presents a sample critical pathway for acute myocardial infarction for days 0–6.

Case management and critical path analysis are developed and implemented typically by a multidisciplinary group of staff consisting of physicians, nurses, physical therapists, diagnostic specialists, quality and utilization review specialists, and other support personnel. RN case coordinators/case management specialists act as liaisons between this group and the steering committee formed for the implementation of ABC (see Step 1). This linkage is crucial to ensure that clinical information is available to the ABC team for activity analysis and cost information is available to the group developing the critical path.

Case management along with critical path analysis proves a useful framework to analyze activities and to collect data on the type and amount of resources needed and actually used for the delivery of patient care. The data can be used to determine where process improvements can be made and where non–value-added activities can be eliminated.

Step 4: Aggregate Activities

The number of different actions performed in a typical hospital facility is so large that it is economically unfeasible to create an activity pool for each separate action. Therefore, many individual actions have to be aggregated to form a few separate distinct activity pools. A single cost driver is then used to trace the cost of these activities to different procedures/patients. For instance, the different actions associated with the admissions / registration process such as reservations/scheduling, inpatient registration, admissions testing, and patient placement are aggregated into one activity pool—"admit patients." One must note that as more and more actions are aggregated into an activity, the ability of a cost driver to accurately trace the resources consumed by patients decreases. On the other hand, creating separate activity centers for actions that are either similar or inseparable just adds complexity to the ABC system without providing any new insights into how resources are consumed.

Step 5: Analyze Cost Flow Using Cost Drivers

The hospital cost management system is used to develop cost information on different activities along the critical path from preadmission to discharge. The procedure involves a detailed analysis of the company's general ledger accounts. In collecting cost information it is necessary to combine certain ledger accounts that are associated with use of similar resources. For instance, salaries and fringe benefit costs that are recorded in two separate accounts are combined for the purposes of allocation. On the other hand, it is sometimes necessary to examine individual bills and vouchers relating to a particular ledger account when similar resources are consumed differently by different activities. For instance, the ledger account Maintenance—Medical Equipment is examined to obtain maintenance expenses relating to medical equipment in radiology, operating room, laboratory, and other departments. Analysis of ledger accounts is not a trivial task because there are over 300 different expense categories at a typical hospital and the only information available for each account is the account name and concise explanations of different transactions.

Table 17–2–1 Critical Pathway: Acute Myocardial Infarction

Activities	Day 0 (Preadmission)	Day 1	Day 2	Day 3	Day 4	Day 5	Day 6
Admit patients	Patient reservation Insurance verification Routine admission testing						
Provide nursing care		Complete blood chemistry	Complete blood chemistry	Complete blood chemistry	Complete blood chemistry	Complete blood chemistry	Complete blood chemistry
Perform diagnostics		CBC with differential Cardiac isoenzymes q 8 hr PT, PTT, ACT initially and PTT q 6 hr Beta hCG 12-lead ECG daily Chest X-ray	CBC PTT (if on heparin) Cardiac isoenzymes if not at baseline 12-lead ECG daily and per protocol MUGA scan or echocardiogram, if indicated	CBC PTT (if on heparin) Cardiac isoenzymes if not at baseline 12-lead ECG daily and per protocol	CBC PTT (if on heparin) Cardiac isoenzymes if not at baseline 12-lead ECG daily and per protocol	CBC 12-lead ECG daily and per protocol	CBC 12-lead ECG
Provide nursing care		ECG monitoring	ECG monitoring	ECG monitoring	ECG monitoring	ECG monitoring	ECG monitoring
Administer ECG & other tests		HR, RR, BP q 1 hr Rhythm strip q shift and p.r.n. Continuous oximetry Heart sounds, breath sounds q 1–2 hr	HR, RR, BP q 2 hr Rhythm strip q shift and p.r.n. Continuous oximetry Heart sounds, breath sounds q 2 hr	HH, RR, BP q 2 hr Rhythm strip q shift and p.r.n. D/C oximetry Assess other body systems as needed	HR, RR, BP q 4 hr Rhythm strip q shift and p.r.n.	HR, RR, BP q 4 hr Rhythm strip q shift and p.r.n. Assess other body systems as needed	HR, RR, BP q 4 hr Assess other body systems as needed
Provide nursing care **Cardiac catheterization** **Dispense medications**		Heparin IV NTG continuous IV infusion Beta blocker Calcium channel blocker ACE inhibitor ASA Morphine IV, analgesics Stool softener Sedative Antiemetic	Heparin IV Titrate and D/C NTG infusion NTG SL, transdermal Beta blocker Calcium channel blocker ACE inhibitor ASA Analgesics Stool softener Sedative	Heparin IV NTG SL, transdermal or spray Beta blocker Calcium channel blocker ACE inhibitor ASA Analgesics Stool softener Sedative	D/C heparin NTG SL, transdermal or spray Beta blocker Calcium channel blocker ACE inhibitor ASA Analgesics Stool softener Sedative	NTG SL, transdermal or spray Beta blocker Calcium channel blocker ACE inhibitor ASA Analgesics Stool softener Sedative	NTG SL, transdermal or spray Beta blocker Calcium channel blocker ACE inhibitor ASA Analgesics Stool softener

Table 17-2-1 continued

Activities	Day 0 (Preadmission)	Day 1	Day 2	Day 3	Day 4	Day 5	Day 6
Provide meals		Low-salt, low-fat, low-cholesterol, or ADA diet	Low-salt, low-fat, low-cholesterol, or ADA diet	Low-salt, low-fat, low-cholesterol, or ADA diet	Low-salt, low-fat, low-cholesterol, or ADA diet	Low-salt, low-fat, low-cholesterol, or ADA diet NPO after 2400 for stress test	Low-salt, low-fat, low-cholesterol, or ADA diet
Provide nursing care		Bed rest (semi-Fowler's) assistance with ADLs	OOB to chair Assistance with ADLs	OOB to chair Assistance with ADLs	Ambulation, ADLs with assistance	Ambulation with supervision	Ambulation with supervision
Provide therapy		IV access Antiembolism stockings Intake and output Oxygen 2 liters/min	IV access Antiembolism stockings Intake and output Oxygen 2 liters/min	IV access Antiembolism stockings Intake and output Possibly D/C O_2	IV access Transfer to telemetry unit Antiembolism stockings D/C intake and output	IV access Antiembolism stockings	Stress test D/C IV access after
Provide nursing services—teaching		Orientation to CCU and hospital routines Review of C.P. Cardiac teaching begins	Instruction on diet Cardiac teaching	Orientation to the difference between CCU and telemetry unit Cardiac teaching	Cardiac teaching	Explanation of stress test Complete cardiac teaching	Written instructions: medications, what to report, activity limits, and next appointment
Discharge planning		Social services Discharge teaching	Dietary and cardiac rehabilitation Plan for family teaching	Discharge teaching	Discharge teaching	Discharge teaching Plan discharge	Discharge to home

First-stage cost drivers are used to trace the cost of inputs into cost pools for each activity center (see Figure 17–2–2). Direct costs are directly assigned to activity centers. For instance, salaries of employees working entirely within an activity center (department) can be directly assigned to that activity center. Common and indirect costs are assigned to different activity centers using different first-stage cost drivers. Table 17–2–2 lists different first-stage cost drivers (allocation bases) used to allocate hospital overhead costs to activity centers.

Second-stage cost drivers are used to measure the amount of activity resources consumed by different procedures (DRGs) or patients (see Figure 17–2–2). Table 17–2–3 lists second-stage cost drivers used for the different activity centers.

Step 6: Educate Hospital Staff about the ABC System

On-site training seminars are held throughout the design and implementation stage to introduce and educate hospital administrators, nurses, and physicians to the concepts and benefits of ABC, case management, and critical path analysis. Hospital staff meetings are used to report progress and to discuss any problems that the steering committee has encountered. These seminars and periodic meetings have two main objectives: to ensure that the design and implementation are appropriate and to build commitment to the ABC and case management system among the hospital staff.

Step 7: Evaluate and Analyze Data and Results

ABC systems in combination with case management and critical path analysis provide crucial financial and clinical measures to conduct variance analysis and evaluate the efficiency of the health care delivery system in terms of achieving expected patient outcomes, timely discharge of patients, appropriate utilization of resources, and cost control.

Table 17–2–2 First-Stage Cost Drivers

	Hospital Overhead Costs	First-Stage Cost Drivers
Labor-related	Supervision	Number of employees/payroll dollars
	Personnel services	
Equipment-related	Insurance on equipment	Value of equipment
	Taxes on equipment	Value of equipment
	Medical equipment depreciation	Value of equipment/equipment hours used
	Medical equipment maintenance	Number of maintenance hours
Space-related	Building rental	Space occupied
	Building insurance	Space occupied
	Power costs	Space occupied, volume occupied
	Building maintenance	Space occupied
Service-related	Central administration[*]	Number of employees/patient volume
	Central service[†]	Quantity/value of supplies
	Medical records, and billing/accounting	Number of documents generated/patient volume
	Cafeteria	Number of meals/number of employees
	Information system	Value of computer equipment/number of programming hours
	Laundry	Weight of laundry washed
	Marketing	Patient volume

[*]Central administration costs include salaries of the president, vice president, and other central administrative staff.
[†]Central service costs include supplying, reclaiming, and sterilizing supplies such as gloves, needles, glassware, syringes, linens, surgical packs, and instruments.

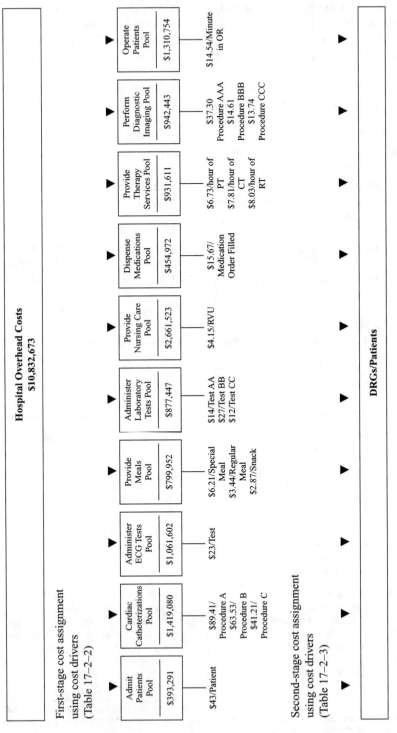

Figure17–2–2 Graphic Example of Activity-Based Costing

Table 17–2–3 Second-Stage Cost Drivers

Activity Center	Activities	Cost Drivers
1. Admit patients	Reservation/scheduling, inpatient registration, billing and insurance verification, admission testing, room/bed/medical assignment	Number of patients admitted
2. Cardiac catheterization	Scheduling, prepare patient, administer medication, cardiac catheterization, film processing, interpret results, patient education	Number of procedures by type[*]
3. Administer ECG tests	Scheduling, prepare patient, perform ECG procedure, interpret results	Number of tests
4. Provide meals/nutritional service	Plan meals, purchase supplies, prepare food, deliver food, clean and sanitize	Number of meals by type[†]
5. Administer laboratory tests	Obtain specimens, perform tests, report results	Number of tests by type[‡]
6. Provide nursing care	Transport patients, update medical records, provide patient care, patient education, discharge planning, inservice training	Number of Relative Value Units
7. Dispense medications	Purchase drugs and medical supplies, maintain records, fill medication orders, maintain inventory	Number of medication orders filled
8. Provide therapy	Schedule patients, evaluate patients, provide treatment, educate patients, maintain records	Number of hours by type
9. Perform diagnostic imaging	Schedule patients, perform procedures, develop film, interpret results, transport patient	Number of procedures by type[§]
10. Operate patient	Schedule patients, order supplies, maintain supplies, instruments & equipment, provide nursing care, transport patient	Number of hours of surgery by surgical suite type

[*]Cardiac catheterization procedures include therapeutic procedures such as angioplasty, thrombolysis, and diagnostic procedures such as left heart catheterizations, ventriculography, and coronary angiograms.
[†]Different meal types include special meals, regular meals, and snacks.
[‡]Laboratory tests include pathological tests, chemical tests, blood tests, immunological tests, and nuclear medicine.
[§]Diagnostic imaging procedures include radiographs of spine, neck, chest, and extremities; mammography; and fluoroscopic procedures such as gastrointestinal series, barium enema, and gallbladder examinations.

Variances can be categorized into the following:

1. *Patient variances:* These are due to complications or changes in the patient's health, for instance, conditions such as allergic reactions, infections, diarrhea, and hemorrhages that affect LOS and costs.

2. *Caregiver variances:* These can be due to physician variances or nursing variances.

Examples include inappropriate use of equipment, untimely tests, insufficient protection, inadequate discharge planning, failure to promptly notify appropriate personnel, and inadequate patient education.

3. *Environmental variances:* Causes for these variances include equipment breakdown, unavailable beds, scheduling problems, lab delays, and power outages.

4. *Price variances:* These are variances caused by paying higher than budgeted prices for supplies, drugs, instruments, and labor.

5. *Efficiency variances:* These usually include duplicated tests or labwork due to faulty procedures, wastage, patient delay, inadequate credit and insurance screening, staffing schedules, inefficient records location and retrieval systems, absenteeism, and medication dispensing errors.

A variance analysis report for each activity center is completed during a patient's stay at the hospital. The report, in addition to providing patient identification and medical information, lists the different categories of variances, possible reasons for the variances, and resources lost or consumed as a result of the negative variances. Resources consumed are measured in units of cost drivers used specific to each activity center, for instance, for nursing care activity pool, resources consumed are measured in number of relative value units (RVUs).

Figure 17–2–3 illustrates the application of variance analysis under an ABC system using a hypothetical example based on costs associated with the nursing care activity pool. Although

---

Assume the following information for the nursing activity center of St. Joseph Hospital for the month of September.

Nursing Activity Center
Cost Driver = Number of Relative Value Units (RVUs)

Budget	**Actual**
Activity Level = 600,000 RVUs	Activity Level = 641,331 RVUs
Overhead Costs = $2,700,000	Overhead Costs = $2,661,523
Budgeted Cost per RVU = $4.50	Actual Cost per RVU = $4.15

Information obtained from the Variance Analysis Reports of all patients for the month of September.

Patient Variance = 8,231 RVUs
Caregiver Variance = 11,624 RVUs
Environmental Variance = 14,275 RVUs
Efficiency Variance = 7,201 RVUs

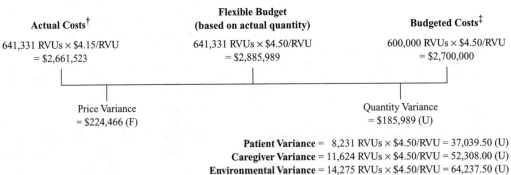

Summary Variance Report for Nursing Activity Center[*]

Actual Costs[†]	**Flexible Budget (based on actual quantity)**	**Budgeted Costs**[‡]
641,331 RVUs × $4.15/RVU = $2,661,523	641,331 RVUs × $4.50/RVU = $2,885,989	600,000 RVUs × $4.50/RVU = $2,700,000

Price Variance = $224,466 (F)

Quantity Variance = $185,989 (U)

Patient Variance = 8,231 RVUs × $4.50/RVU = 37,039.50 (U)
Caregiver Variance = 11,624 RVUs × $4.50/RVU = 52,308.00 (U)
Environmental Variance = 14,275 RVUs × $4.50/RVU = 64,237.50 (U)
Efficiency Variance = 7,201 RVUs × $4.50/RVU = 32,404.50 (U)

[*]It is recommended that individual cost drivers be used for different activity pools in analyzing price and quantity variances. In this example, it is assumed that a single cost driver—number of RVUs—adequately captures the consumption of resources in this activity center.
[†]Here overhead costs for the Nursing Care Activity Center are assumed to be essentially variable in relation to the cost driver used (number of RVUs). For fixed costs, variances can be further divided into strategic and operational capacity variances.
[‡]For simplicity, budgeted activity level is assumed to equal standard activity level.

Figure 17–2–3 Illustrative Example of Variance Analysis under an ABC System

the variance analysis proposed under the ABC system is similar in structure to a traditional variance analysis, there are two significant differences. First, since under the ABC system variance analysis is applied to each activity pool rather than the entire hospital's operation, more homogeneous cost pools and more causal cost drivers are used in the analysis. Second, with the use of a detailed variance analysis report and the emphasis on "activity analysis" under the ABC system, hospital administrators are better able to pinpoint weaknesses in the health care delivery system and focus their improvement efforts.

NUMERICAL EXAMPLE OF ABC IN HOSPITALS

To provide a numerical example of ABC in hospitals, assume the following information:

St. Joseph Hospital offers two services/procedures, DRG 1X1 and DRG 1X2. DRG 1X1 is a procedure requiring high-acuity care with a 5-day stay (LOS = 5 days) in the hospital, after which the patient is moved to a nursing home. DRG 1X2 is a procedure requiring low-acuity care with a LOS in the hospital also of 5 days.

Conventional Cost System

The cost of the two procedures under the conventional cost accounting system is computed in Table 17–2–4. Note that direct costs are all costs that can be directly assigned to the patient or DRG including physician fees, direct nursing costs, room costs, medications, laboratory tests, and therapy services. Hospital overhead allocated includes hospital and departmental overhead that is not directly assigned to the patient or DRG. In a conventional cost accounting system, overhead is allocated on a patient-day basis, as follows:

$$\text{Hospital overhead allocated/patient-day} =$$
$$\text{Hospital overhead costs /Number of patient days} =$$
$$\$10,832,673/54,838 \text{ patient days} =$$
$$\$197.54/\text{patient day}$$

Activity-Based Cost System

Let us next assume that St. Joseph Hospital has analyzed its operations using case management and critical path analysis and has identified 10 activity centers (Figure 17–2–2) and its first- and second-stage cost drivers (Tables 17–2–2 and 17–2–3, respectively). It has also analyzed the activities involved within each of the activity centers. Figure 17–2–4 presents the analysis of 1 of the 10 activity centers, Perform Diagnostic Imaging Pool, as an illustration.

As shown in Figures 17–2–2 and 17–2–4, the hospital has determined the amount of overhead cost traceable to each of the 10 activity centers and has computed the overhead rate for each activity center using first- and second-stage cost drivers respectively. In Table 17–2–5, these rates have in turn been used to assign the hospital overhead costs to the individual patients/DRGs based on the actual number of activity transactions. Note from Table 17–2–5 that the use of ABC has resulted in $3,079.78 in overhead cost being assigned to DRG 1X1 and $835.11 in overhead cost being assigned to DRG 1X2. These amounts are used in Table 17–2–6 to determine the total cost of DRG 1X1 and 1X2 under ABC. For comparison purposes, we also

Table 17–2–4 Cost under Conventional Cost Accounting System

	DRG 1X1	DRG 1X2
Patient days	5	5
Direct cost	$8,451.00	$2,421.00
Hospital cost allocated (5 patient days × 197.54)	987.70	987.70
Total Costs	$9,438.70	$3,408.70

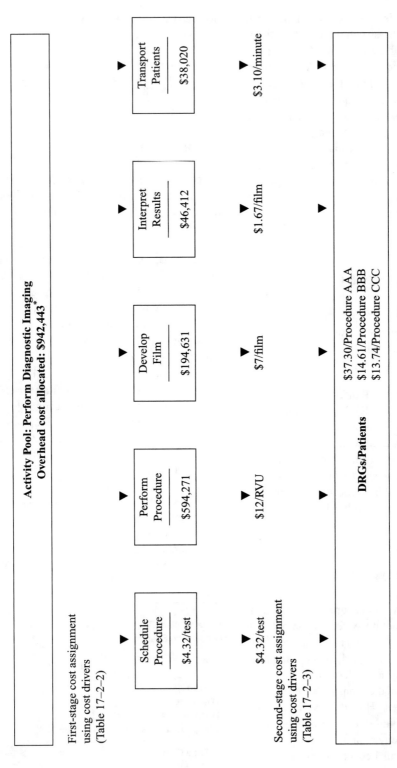

Figure 17–2–4 Graphic Example of Activity Center: Perform Diagnostic Imaging Pool

*These are overhead costs relating to the activity center. Direct costs such as salaries of the radiologists, technologists, technicians, and staff, cost of supplies, and depreciation and maintenance of screening equipment etc. are directly assigned to the activity pools.

Table 17-2-5 Overhead Cost per DRG

Activity Center	DRG 1X1			DRG 1X2		
	Number of Transactions	Rate per Transaction	Overhead Cost	Number of Transactions	Rate per Transaction	Overhead Cost
Admit patients pool	1 patient	$43/patient	$43.00	1 patient	$43/patient	$43.00
Cardiac catheterizations pool	2 Procedure A	$89.41/Procedure A	178.82	1 Procedure C	$41.21/Procedure C	41.21
Administer ECG tests pool	7 tests	$23/test	161.00	4 tests	$23/test	92.00
Provide meals pool	9 special meals	$6.21/special meal	55.89	9 regular meals	$3.44/regular meal	30.96
	6 snacks	$2.87/snack	17.22	6 snacks	$2.87/snack	17.22
Administer laboratory tests pool	4 tests BB	$27/test BB	108.00	3 tests AA	$14/test AA	42.00
Provide nursing care pool	312 RVUs	$4.15/RVU	1,294.80	104 RVUs	$4.15/RVU	431.60
Dispense medications pool	14 medication orders	$15.67/medication order filled	219.38	6 medication orders	$15.67/medication order filled	94.02
Provide therapy sessions pool	7 hrs CT	$7.81/hour of CT	54.67	2 hrs CT	$7.81/hour of CT	15.62
Perform diagnostic imaging pool	2 procedures AAA	$37.30/procedure AAA	74.60	2 procedures CCC	$13.74/procedure CCC	27.48
Operate patients pool	1 hr in OR	$14.54/minute in OR	872.40			
			$3,079.78			$835.11

Table 17-2-6 Cost per DRG under ABC and Conventional Cost System

	Activity-Based Costing		Conventional Cost System	
	DRG 1X1	DRG 1X2	DRG 1X1	DRG 1X2
Direct costs	8,451.00	2,421.00	8,451.00	2,421.00
Hospital overhead allocated	3,079.78	835.11	987.70	987.70
Total costs	11,530.78	3,256.11	9,438.70	3,408.70
			Undercosted by 22.16%	Overcosted by 4.47%

present costs for DRG 1X1 and 1X2 under the conventional cost system (see Table 17–2–4). Under the conventional cost system, DRG 1X1 is undercosted by over 22 percent and DRG 1X2 is overcosted by almost 5 percent. Using ABC, we have been able to identify the overhead costs that are traceable to each DRG/patient based on consumption of activity resources and thus obtain more accurate cost data.

Accurate costs reported by the ABC systems reduce the risk that poor case-mix decisions, faulty pricing decisions, and suboptimal capital budgeting decisions will be made because of inaccurate costs. This risk can be particularly high when competitor hospitals can take advantage of a hospital's poor decisions that can occur as a result of inaccurate costs.

• • •

ABC is a relatively new concept for hospitals. Integrating ABC with case management, critical path analysis, and other hospital control processes represents an exciting new development. It provides a structured approach to analyzing activities, costing services, reducing costs, and improving quality. In addition, it brings to bear the skills of employers from different functional areas of the hospital and helps generate ideas and innovative solutions to the problems at hand.

There are numerous challenges in implementing an ABC system in hospitals. First, collecting the data needed to establish an ABC system is time consuming and expensive. An ABC system is much more complex and detailed than a traditional cost system because costs are allocated to different activity pools and each of these pools is further broken down into several separate activities. This requires detailed analysis of financial accounting records as well as inquiries and interviews to identify and gather costs and other information on specific activities. In some cases, information required for an ABC system is almost impossible to obtain. Also, the statistical analysis required to allocate costs is much more complex for an ABC system. Another barrier to successfully implementing the ABC system is that many organizations view it as a quick fix and purely an exercise in accounting concerned only with developing better cost data. A successful implementation of an ABC system requires a comprehensive paradigm shift in management—a move from a functional departmental view of the hospital management structure to a more cross-functional view of hospital activities and processes. This requires reeducation of the entire organization from physicians to nurses to administrative staff. For this to happen, the initiative and impetus for change should come from senior management. Very often, changing management's perspective is far more complex and challenging than designing the system.

This article introduces the application of ABC to the management of hospitals. As more and more hospitals gain experience with ABC, their shared experiences will provide further insights into the integration and implementation of ABC in hospitals.

REFERENCES

1. Y.C. Chan, "Improving Hospital Cost Accounting with Activity-Based Costing." *Health Care Management Review 18,* no. 1 (1993): 71–77.

2. R. Ramsey IV, "Activity-Based Costing for Hospitals." *Hospital and Health Services Administration 39,* no. 3 (1994): 385–396.

3. J. Canby IV, "Applying Activity-Based Costing to Healthcare Settings." *Healthcare Financial Management 49,* no. 2 (1995): 50–56.

4. P.B.B. Turney, "What is the Scope of Activity-Based Costing?" *Journal of Cost Management 3,* no. 4 (1990): 40–42.

5. K. Zander, "Nursing Case Management: Strategic Management of Cost and Quality Outcomes." *Journal of Nursing Administration 18,* no. 5 (1988): 23–30.

ABC Estimation of Unit Costs for Emergency Department Services

Richard L. Holmes

Richard E. Schroeder

Traditional costing methods used in health care determine the "full costs" for services provided—critical information when payers are willing to compensate the hospital based on either changes or actual costs. Such payers are a vanishing breed, as Medicare, Medicaid, major insurers, and managed care companies all turn to prospective payments or fee schedules to determine provider compensation. In such an environment, the so-called full cost of any individual service may have little bearing on its profitability or management (Finkler, 1994). Although the business is not financially viable unless its total revenues meet the aggregated full costs of all products and services, this relationship of costs and revenues is misleading at the individual service level. The presence of numerous payers who will not pay full charges invalidates full costs as a charge-setting mechanism because some of the costs must be shifted to other payers. In addition, the full cost of any one output includes substantial fixed cost that is usually allocated arbitrarily. Such a full cost might have been helpful in setting prices in an era when any prices would be paid, but it is not helpful today in pricing competitive bids or resolving make-or-buy dilemmas.

Instead, decisions should be based on the relevant costs for the situation at hand. Often, the relevant cost is the incremental cost of an additional unit of service, or the avoidable cost if one unit less is provided (Garrison, 1991). This type of information applies to decisions to seek increases in volume or market share, or to curtail existing volume. Armed with incremental cost information, the manager may ensure that services targeted for marketing are profitable, that services discontinued are "losers," and that prices bid to managed care companies are advantageous.

The concept of incremental cost is neither new nor novel, but decades of cost accounting tradition have limited its measurement to easily traceable costs and allocated the remaining costs based on arbitrary or "equitable" bases (Belkaoui, 1983). For the last 15 years, a growing literature has decried such techniques as misleading because the true causes of costs are not discerned or assigned by such bases. Led by industrial firms (especially manufacturers), management accountants have embraced new techniques that tie costs to their true causes, termed activity-based costing (ABC) (Borden, 1990). However, there are very few success sto-

Source: Reprinted from R.L. Holmes and R.E. Schroeder, "ABC Estimation of Unit Costs for Emergency Department Services," *Journal of Ambulatory Care Management,* Vol. 19, No. 2, pp. 22–31. Copyright April 1996, Aspen Publishers, Inc.

Note: The opinions expressed herein are strictly those of the authors and do not reflect the official policy or position of the Department of the Army, the Department of Defense, or the U.S. government.

ries for the implementation of ABC in health care settings.

A SIMPLE APPROXIMATION OF ACTIVITY-BASED COSTING

There are a variety of reasons why ABC is more difficult for the health care industry (Rotch, 1990). First, products are more difficult to define and measure. Second, processes and their costs are more complex and less readily tied to easily counted "triggers" or activities. Third, intermediate products are rampant in many settings, adding another layer of analysis for each product and adding to the time and cost of implementation. Finally, the historical cost-based reimbursement payment methods of health care have insulated it from the competitive marketplace, postponing the recognition of the need for accurate unit cost information and control (Orloff, Littell, Clune, Klingman, & Preston, 1990).

Not only is each of these difficulties applicable to the emergency department (ED), but the heterogeneity of patients and services of emergent medicine magnifies their impact. Nevertheless, better decisions can result by accepting feasible imperfect information on incremental activity-based costs in lieu of traditional full cost data. To learn these costs requires:

1. Identification of all relevant costs.
2. Sorting of costs in support of ED functions, discarding those that are not relevant or not affected by volume or availability of services.
3. Clustering into groups for counting and costing (such as Ambulatory Patient Groups [APG] or Physicians' Current Procedural Terminology [CPT] groups) those services that create similar demands for ED functions.
4. Identifying and counting the activities or cost drivers for each service group. (Such activities or drivers are the characteristics of the service that trigger the performance of an ED function.)

5. Estimating the costliness of each ED function, permitting quantification of the relationship between costs and the triggering characteristics.
6. Aggregating the "functional costliness" (individual activity costs) for all ED functions of a service to determine the incremental cost of one unit.

After completion of these six steps, a rough unit incremental cost has been calculated.

IMPLEMENTING INCREMENTAL COSTING WITH LIMITED DATA

Hospital settings may be not-for-profit, governmental, or for-profit. Only in the for-profit setting is there a history of charge capturing systems designed to maximize revenues. In the not-for-profit and governmental hospitals there has often been less emphasis placed on billings, and the charge-capture systems vary from good to nonexistent. Estimating incremental costs for such a governmental or nonprofit setting is more difficult and less accurate than where resource use has been captured as it is in the for-profit sector. Nevertheless, the estimated incremental costs are far more useful for many decisions than having no information at all. Incremental costing for a fictitious ED is used here to illustrate the approach, but if better data were available more accurate unit costs could be found through the same method.

Step 1: Identification of All Relevant Costs

Relevant costs may be incurred at three levels of traceability to a service. The least traceable groups of costs are incurred in other cost centers of the facility, such as administration or laboratory. Much more measurable are the costs incurred by the service-producing department, even if these are not readily tied to a specific patient or service. The most traceable costs are those resources whose use by an individual service is captured directly. In this discussion, we will term the outside costs *external,* those within the producing center will be called *departmental,* and those captured directly will be termed *direct* cost.

Even hospitals with no charge-capturing system tend to have at least a traditional step-down cost-finding system, because the annual cost reporting required for Medicare details this method (Health Care Financing Administration [HCFA], continuous). Such systems assign to any organizational department two kinds of costs: *external* and *departmental.* The *external* costs were allocated to the department from other cost centers, while the *departmental* costs were traceable directly to the cost center of the department. The first two columns of Tables 17–3–1 and 17–3–2 illustrate the entry of *external* and *departmental* costs into a spreadsheet. These

and all subsequent tables are actual excerpts of the spreadsheets described. While the displayed tables include only two columns for types of services, the actual spreadsheets have additional columns to the right so that all types of services may be costed.

If any costs are captured directly for specific department services, the estimation of unit costs can be improved. Such costs are termed *direct* costs of the individual services offered by a department. Table 17–3–3 illustrates the entry of such *direct* costs into a spreadsheet. Because the *departmental* costs of the existing step-down system are likely to include these costs within its totals, note that the third column of Table 17–3–2 subtracts these *direct* costs out of the *departmental* costs so that they will not be double-counted.

Table 17–3–1 External Costs Charged to the Emergency Department (ED) by the Traditional Cost Accounting System[*]

Cost Center	*Amount*	*Relevance*	*% Variable*	*Driver*	*DRG[†] 193 (Biliary Tract)*	*DRG 209 (Major Joint/Limb)*
Pharmaceuticals	$2,544	1	70%	Wtd procs	$312	$534
Clinical pathology	$1,648	1	60%	RVUs	$271	$415
Anatomical pathology	$433	1	10%	DRG-wts	$7	$12
Blood bank	$654	1	90%	BUs	$133	$233
Diagnostic radiology	$3,781	1	30%	Radfilms	$123	$246
Electrocardiography	$476	1	80%	EKGs	$73	$73
Pulmonary	$537	1	40%	RTs	$72	$0
Central sterile	$2,358	1	90%	DRG-wts	$335	$564
Anesthesiology	$3,561	1	70%	ORmins	$580	$1,035
Operating room	$6,443	1	45%	ORmins	$675	$1,203
Recovery room	$2,766	1	55%	ORmins	$354	$631
Depreciation	$43,577	0				
Corporate office	$12,433	0				
Clinical spt division	$1,542	1	5%	DRG-wts	$12	$20
Special staff	$2,677	0				
Nursing	$4,877	1	70%	NAcuity	$636	$773
Preventive med	$3,778	0				
Immunizations	$745	1	80%	Shots	$0000	$0000
Total	$143,039				$3,670	$5,886

[*]Some rows have been omitted from the display, as have all columns for other types of services to the right of those shown. The abbreviated cost drivers in the fifth column are described in Table 17–3–4.
[†]Diagnosis-related group.

Table 17–3–2 Costs Recorded Specifically against the Emergency Department (ED) Cost Center

| Indirect Costs of Services Traced to the ED | | | | | | | June 1995 | | |
Cost Type	Gross $	– Direct $	= Indirect $	Relevance	% Variable	Cost Driver	DRG[*] 193	DRG 209
Number services							8	16
Clinician labor	$62,355	$31,250	$31,105	1	90%	Protocol-C	$4,923	$9,300
Nursing labor	$61,056		$61,056	1	95%	Protocol-N	$7,975	$12,722
Paraprofessional	$8,576		$8,576	1	100%	Protocol-T	$892	$1,903
Admin/clerk	$3,615		$3,615	1	60%	Protocol-A	$317	$605
Supplies	$201,356	$163,246	$38,110	1	90%	DRG-wts	$5,414	$9,118
Equipment	$22,334		$22,334	0		DRG-wts	$0	$0
Contracts	$15,015		$15,015	1	95%	Protocol-C	$2,509	$4,738

[*]Diagnosis-related group.

Table 17–3–3 Direct Traceable Costs Recorded against Each Type of Service[*]

| Direct Costs of Each Type of Service | | June 1995 | |
Cost Type	Department Total	DRG[†] 193	DRG 209
Clinical labor	$31,250	$ 2,300	$ 7,200
Nursing labor			
Paraprofessional			
Admin/clerk			
Supplies	$163,246	$49,988	$93,254
Equipment			
Contracts			

[*]Blank rows have no direct costs recorded in this ED.
[†]Diagnosis-related group.

Step 2: Sorting of Costs

An incorrect decision can result from including in the analysis any costs that are not affected by the decision. Such inappropriate costs include *sunk* costs that were spent in the past and cannot be recovered, as well as those *fixed* costs that do not vary with the production of a service and would not be avoided in its absence (Garrison, 1991). Such irrelevant costs may exist at *external* or *departmental* levels (but normally would not be included in *direct* resource capture). Some costs are viewed as irrelevant in their entirety, and are indicated by a "0" entry in the Relevance column in Tables 17–3–1 and 17–3–2. Some costs are relevant but for only a portion of their total amount; so the relevant (or *variable)* percentage is entered in the % Variable column.

The proper percentages might be measured empirically, or might only reflect the opinion of a skilled administrator when the cost of more accurate measurement did not appear to be justified. In this example, the standard cost pools (names of accumulated costs in the hospital's step-down cost reporting system) were accepted.

Step 3: Clustering and Counting of Services

A unit cost cannot be found for a type of service unless the service exists (that is, has been defined). Only after the service is well defined can it be counted unambiguously. Systems that sort services into countable defined clusters are called classification systems.

There are many classification systems applicable to and that have been tested in EDs, but the three most likely candidates are:

- Common Procedural Terminology, 4th Edition (CPT-4) codes, which are currently used by HCFA to reimburse clinicians for ED services (using the derivative HCFA common procedure codes) (Gapenski, 1993).
- APGs, which have been proposed to Congress by HCFA for all future reimbursement of hospitals for ED services (Howland, 1994).
- Broader local classifications.

Since there are over 7,000 CPT-4 codes and 297 APGs (HCFA, 1994), implementing these classifications in a new setting requires a substantial learning curve. Any local classification system presents an alternative that can be implemented more quickly. However, make-or-buy decisions will be complicated if the internal service to be costed is not the same service by which an outside source would receive payment. The two right-most column headings in Tables 17–3–1 through 17–3–7 are the names of some of the services identified in this hypothetical ED.

Step 4: Identifying Activity Measures or Cost Drivers

The estimate of the share of costs caused by a particular service, whether the cost is *external* or *departmental,* depends on the degree to which that service caused the cost to be incurred. For different costs, there are different service characteristics that may be driving the cost. For example, clinician labor cost may be the result of the average number of clinician minutes required to provide an average patient with the individual service. Table 17–3–4 shows the cost driver factor for an average patient for each of the services identified in the ED. The same names of factors are shown in Tables 17–3–1 and 17–3–2 beside the types of costs to which they apply. Like the variability, these factors may be measured or may reflect expert opinion (protocols or clinical pathways) or published norms, depending on the accuracy desired.

Step 5: Estimating the Costliness of the Factors

This can be viewed as an estimate of how much new cost is created when one of the factors increases by one unit for a particular cost. (For example, how much more nursing labor cost is incurred for one additional minute of nursing time?) Mathematically, this can be expressed as the quotient of the total variable cost of that type, divided by the total recorded quantity of the factor for all services and patients (for example, total variable nursing labor dollars divided by the total quantity of nursing minutes). A spreadsheet performs such calculations instantly and results in the costs associated with each type of service in the right-most columns of Tables 17–3–1 and 17–3–2.

Step 6: Aggregating the Functional Costliness of a Unit of Service

The concept is to add every cost caused by an additional unit of any one service, which in turn is the sum of the costliness of each of its factors times the number of that factor it uses. For example, the cost of one more service adds the costliness of its nursing minutes to the costliness of its clinic in minutes, unit supply costs, clerical costs, and so forth. In the illustration, the cost of external, departmental, and direct costs is shown for each type of cost for each service in Tables 17–3–1, 17–3–2, and 17–3–3, respectively. In Table 17–3–5, all of these costs are aggregated automatically into two tables. One table shows the aggregate cost of treating all of the patients who received each individual service; the table below it shows the incremental cost of treating a single (average) patient who received each individual service.

Refinements

The accuracy of this estimate can be improved by incurring additional costs for better informa-

Table 17–3–4 Cost Drivers and Allocation Bases Used To Assign Costs to Services

Cost Driver Statistics per Procedure			June 1995	
Cost Driver	**Brief Description**	**Total Basis**	**DRG[*] 193**	**DRG 209**
BUs	Expected units of blood	141.5	4	3.5
DRG-wts	DRG weights from Medicare	96.3	1.9	1.6
EKGs	Standard electrocardiographs	84	2	1
NAcuity	Nursing acuity hours	2190	51	31
ORmins	OR minutes	11063	322	287
Protocol-A	Protocol minutes/admin or clerk	1148	21	20
Protocol-C	Protocol minutes/clinician	81.88	1.8	1.7
Protocol-N	Protocol minutes/nurse	34796	598.0	477.0
Protocol-T	Protocol minutes/technician	3461	45	48
RTs	Standard respiratory therapies	24	1	0
RVUs	Laboratory tests in relative value	991	34	26
Radfilms	Radiology films	369	5	5
Shots	Standard immunizations (tetanus)	7	0	0
Wtd procs	Pharmaceuticals in weighted amount	20	7	6

[*]Diagnosis-related group.

Table 17–3–5 Total Incremental Costs, and Incremental Unit Costs, for Each Service

Emergency Department Summary June 1995		
Product list (by DRG[*] or APG[†])	**DRG 193**	**DRG 209**
Brief description of service:	biliary tract	major joint/limb
Quantity provided during the period:	8	16
Aggregate costs for type of service		
External costs	$3,669.96	$5,886.12
Indirect costs	$22,029.83	$38,385.77
Direct costs	$52,288.00	$100,454.00
Total	$77,987.79	$144,725.89
Incremental unit costs		
External costs	$458.74	$367.88
Indirect costs	$2,753.73	$2,399.11
Direct costs	$6,536.00	$6,278.38
Total:	$9,748.47	$9,045.37

[*]Diagnosis-related group.
[†]Ambulatory patient group.

tion. For example, a mechanism to capture actual costs as they are caused by a type of service would improve accuracy over the extrapolation from a cost driver described in step 5. Whether such accuracy warrants the added cost is a managerial decision. Cooper (1988) suggests such information cost should be accepted only when it is outweighed by the costs to be saved from the improved decision.

Another refinement would be to track unit costs not just to individual services, but to the individual clinicians responsible for the services. This would improve the economic profiling of clinicians (current practice in 52% of hospitals [Prospective Payment Assessment Commission, 1994]) and permit the alerting of those whose common care practices are more costly than those of their peers. Tables 17–3–6 and 17–3–7

Table 17–3–6 Quantity of Services Provided by Each Clinician[*]

Physician Case Workload		June 1995	
Product	Total	DRG[†] 193	DRG 209
Quantity for all providers	48	8	16
Abrams, Dr. William		2	7
Jones, Dr. Sherry		6	9
Smith, Dr. John L.		0	0
Thomas, Dr. Enid		0	0
Cases unaccounted by provider		0	0

[*]This portion of the spreadsheet is optional. However, if any clinician profiling is to be calculated, this table must also be present.
[†]Diagnosis-related group.

show how the approach presented here could be expanded to clinician levels, where economic profiling is desired. If this added information cost is accepted, the corresponding rows in Table 17–3–4 can be replaced with "links" to these other pages of the spreadsheet instead of being entered directly.

Approaching True ABC Costs

The system proposed here retains much of traditional cost accounting and cost capture systems in order to approximate costs as ABC might derive them. The system can be refined to accommodate ABC when and if they become available. For example, ABC might identify "patient scheduling" or "patient registration" as an ED function to be costed (Brimson & Antos, 1994). Study of this function might discover both direct and external labor costs to accomplish it, as well as computer or supply costs. The study might find, for example, that patient registration was twice as intensive for admissions as for patients treated and released. (ABC would then determine the registration cost for each service by dividing up the total registration costs in proportion to the number of services performed, weighting those services causing admissions by two.) To integrate the new ABC study information into this system, all ABC-determined registration costs are removed from the *external, departmental,* and *direct* portions of the model. Without them, the model calculates the unit in-

Table 17–3–7 Laboratory Testing Ordered by Each Clinician, for Each Type of Service[*]

Physician Laboratory Testing		June 1995	
	Total Basis	DRG[†] 193	DRG 209
Aggregate	991	274	414
Abrams, Dr. William		65	161
Jones, Dr. Sherry		209	253
Smith, Dr. John L.		0	0
Thomas, Dr. Enid		0	0
Unaccounted		0	0
Per case average:		34	26
Comparison to mean			
Abrams, Dr. William	–0.8811	32.5	23
Jones, Dr. Sherry	1.05819	34.83	28.11
Smith, Dr. John L.	0.97701	0	0
Thomas, Dr. Enid	1.11538	0	0
Unaccounted	1.25	0	0

[*]This table illustrates clinician use of one resource—laboratory testing. Additional tables could be created for other resources, such as pharmaceuticals, supplies, radiography, etc.
[†]Diagnosis-related group.

cremental cost *except* for patient registration. To get the full incremental cost, all that is required is to add back in the ABC-determined unit cost of patient registration for the service, and the new answer has been improved by the added ABC accuracy.

If the hospital adopts a broader implementation of ABC, other numbers provided the model will also improve. For example, *external* costs previously allocated from the laboratory and radiology might be re-sorted into external functions like "diagnose disease," "monitor recovery," and "verify normal health." These new types of costs would need their own "cost driver" factors to be entered in the model. (For example, the cost driver for "monitor recovery" might be the expected number of postsurgical days for a service.) However, the approach presented here never requires ABC to be implemented anywhere—it only permits improving the estimates by using the best cost information already available.

INTEGRATING COSTS AND QUALITY

The joint consideration of quality and cost is as important in the ED as for inpatient care. Outcome measures (whether by CPT, APG, or local classification) are essential to assess the quality and effectiveness of the ED. Frequently, clinicians and administrative staff work together to derive and implement a system of protocols and measures assessing quality. Since the same protocols can provide valuable allocation bases for many indirect costs, the accounting staff should be included in quality circles or process action teams that are charged with the responsibility for measuring resource usage and outcomes. Only when quality and cost management are integrated into a total quality management effort can the data illustrated in Tables 17–3–6 and 17–3–7 provide meaningful insight into efficient and quality care.

The combination of awareness of unit costs and clinician economic profiles permits more

timely and cost-effective decisions about adding or curtailing services. It also provides a ready monitor of performance to permit continuous improvement approaches for the cost or variance reductions typical of total quality management. Good decision making cannot be accomplished solely by sound motivation and ethics—timely and adequate information is also required. This methodology provides the ED clinician or manager with a technique to face impending decisions without waiting for a massive overhaul to the accounting system.

REFERENCES

Belkaoui, A. (1983). *Cost accounting: A multidimensional emphasis.* New York. NY: Dryden.

Borden, J.P. (1990, Spring). Review of literature on activity-based costing. *Journal of* Cost *Management,* 5–12.

Brimson. J.A., & Antos, J. (1994). Activity-based management: For service industries, government entities, and non-profit organizations. New York, NY: Wiley.

Cooper, R. (1988). The rise of activity-based costing—Part 2: When do I need an activity-based cost system? *Journal of Cost Management, 1*(3), 41–48.

Finkler, S.A. (1994). *Essentials of cost accounting for health care organizations.* Gaithersburg, MD: Aspen Publishers.

Gapenski, L.C. (1993). *Understanding health care financial management.* Ann Arbor, MI: Association of University Programs in Health Administration.

Garrison, R.H. (1991). *Managerial accounting.* (6th ed.). Homewood, IL: Irwin.

Health Care Financing Administration (1994, July). Report to Congress, draft. Washington, DC: Author.

Health Care Financing Administration (continuous updates). Provider reimbursement manual. (Part 1). Washington, DC: Government Printing Office.

Howland, D. (1994). PPS for Medicare outpatients proposed. *American Hospital Association News, 30*(21), 3.

Orloff, T.M., Littell, C.L, Clune, C., Klingman, D., & Preston, B. (1990). Hospital cost accounting: Who's doing what and why? *Health Care Management Review, 15*(4), 73.

Prospective Payment Assessment Commission (1994). *Medicare and the American health care system: Report to the Congress.* Washington, DC: Government Printing Office.

Rotch, W. (1990). Activity-based costing in service industries. *Journal of Cost Management, 4*(2), 8.

18

Total Cost Management: Measuring the Costs of Quality

Reading 18–1

Measuring the Costs of Quality

Steven A. Finkler

The increasing pressure on hospitals to control costs has resulted in cutbacks that threaten quality. At the same time, the total quality management (TQM) movement has shown that in many instances costs can be saved by improving quality. The key strategy that is coming to the forefront is to use high quality as a device to generate increased volume, while at the same time using those quality improvements to reduce the costs of providing patient care. To maximize the results of efforts in this area, hospital managers need to focus to an ever greater extent on measuring the costs of quality.

QUALITY COSTS

The confounding issue in quality cost measurement is the problem of defining and measuring quality. This task often falls on hospital accounting departments. As Hansen and Mowen note, "While the quality department may initially track the cost of poor quality, the accounting department must integrate the quality cost management system with other cost management systems. A fundamental prerequisite for this reporting is measuring costs of quality. But to

measure these costs, an operational definition of quality itself is needed.[1]

In industry, there is a growing philosophy of viewing quality from the customer perspective. Manufactured products that meet customer expectations are considered to be quality products. Customers, however, may have different expectations. Therefore, a product or service does not have to be the best product or service to be of high quality. It simply needs to be good value for the money. Health care has not yet fully focused on this issue. Historically, everyone has wanted the "best" health care possible.

To start to think about quality costs, product quality can be segmented into design quality and conformance quality.[2] To understand design quality, imagine a person buying a thermostat to regulate the heat in a room. For $50 that person can get a model that will regulate the temperature within a 6° range. Therefore, if the thermostat is set for 70°, the temperature in the room should always be between 67 and 73°. For $250 the person can get a thermostat with a 2° range, keeping the room between 69 and 71°. Which thermostat is better quality? The first reaction of most people is that the latter thermostat is higher quality. That higher quality requires higher manufacturing costs. TQM does not argue that the more accurate $250 thermostat will be cheaper to make than the less accurate $50 thermostat because it is higher quality. Different design

Source: Reprinted from S.A. Finkler, "Measuring the Costs of Quality," *Hospital Cost Management and Accounting,* Vol. 7, No. 11, pp. 1–6. Copyright February 1996, Aspen Publishers, Inc.

quality has different costs, and a product with a higher quality design may well be more costly than another with lower design quality, no matter how efficiently it is produced.

For each of the two thermostats, however, there is a question of how well their manufacture conforms to their design. This is considered to be *conformance quality*. The less expensive thermostat may be viewed as a desirable product, even with its lower quality design specifications, if people feel that the ±3° range is acceptable, given the lower price. If the actual temperature swings are ±10°, then the product is not conforming to its specifications and customers are likely to be unhappy with its quality.

When each of the two types of thermostats is set to 70°, the goal is to be as close to 70° as possible. Suppose the cheaper thermostat actually conforms to its stated 6° range (±3°). If the thermostat is set for 70°, the room temperature never drops below 67° or goes above 73°. However, suppose that the more expensive thermostat really works with a 4° range. It keeps the room between 68° and 72°. Which thermostat is better quality?

Because the goal is to keep the room as close to 70° as possible, the more expensive thermostat comes closer to that goal. However, it may still be viewed as being of lower quality than the other one. The less expensive thermostat is conforming within its design specifications, whereas the more expensive one is not. Customers often view quality based on price and expectations rather than absolute performance.

Quality experts focus on meeting design standards rather than on maximizing those standards. Measuring the costs of quality relates not to the costs of the two different thermostats but rather to the costs of conforming to the quality design standards for any one type of thermostat.

SERVICE QUALITY

Hospitals and other health care providers have the added problem of providing a service rather than a product. Nevertheless, they are still subject to the same basic constraints of design quality and conformance quality. This problem is complicated by the fact that it is difficult to make an objective measurement of quality. Is quality limited to outcomes? Bedside manner of a physician may be an overlooked element of the quality of service. Does that mean that good bedside manner is essential? Not necessarily. One could market a "no frills" health care service by advertising good outcomes, but limited bedside manner, at a low cost.

What elements go into the basic design quality for health care services? Berry and Parasuraman[3] list five dimensions of service quality: (1) reliability, (2) tangibles, (3) responsiveness, (4) assurance, and (5) empathy. To understand the costs of quality in providing a service, managers must confront first the design specifications for each of these dimensions and then ensure conformance with those specifications.

The five dimensions go beyond the qualities of the thermostat discussed earlier. Reliability is a measure of the ability to deliver the promised service, similar to a thermostat keeping the promised temperature range. Tangibles relate to things such as the physical appearance of the organization. What kind of a visual impression is made on the patient? Responsiveness represents the degree to which the organization promptly responds to patient wants. Assurance relates to the intangible of providing the patient with the feeling that the service is being provided correctly. That is, does the patient feel that staff members know what they're doing? Empathy is the degree to which the care is provided with the individualized attention patients desire.

Providing service along all these dimensions costs money. Therefore it is essential to explicitly, rather than implicitly, design the specifications for the quality of the service to be provided along each dimension. Then the employees can work to find the lowest cost way to generate service that meets those design specifications.

MEETING THE DESIGN SPECIFICATIONS

One can define the costs of quality as being the costs that the organization must incur in order to provide its services in conformance with its specifications. If it does the job well, the organization can minimize these costs. However, one must clearly consider the fact that quality costs include both the costs to ensure quality and the costs of failing to provide quality.

This means that quality costs include the costs to prevent failure to conform with specifications as well as the costs of finding and correcting failures. It also includes the costs the hospital incurs because of its failure to identify and correct poor quality (for example, lawsuits or lost customers).

The costs of quality, therefore, have frequently been broken down into the categories of prevention costs, appraisal costs, internal failure costs, and external failure costs. Because it costs money when things go wrong and it costs money to prevent things from going wrong, quality costs should never be expected to be zero. Rather, organizations should try to minimize the total costs related to quality.

Prevention is viewed as the ideal if its costs are not excessively high. A dollar spent on prevention is more beneficial than a dollar spent on correction, because poor quality, even if later corrected, leaves a bad taste in a patient's mouth. The long-term negative ramifications of the general impact on reputation are hard to quantify. It took Detroit auto manufacturers many years of work to try to overcome the general reputation that Japanese cars were of superior quality.

Appraisal costs represent the money spent to uncover failure to conform with quality design specifications. The goal of such appraisal is to prevent failures to conform from going undetected. A special concern for hospitals is that the patient often receives service on a real-time basis. A product is not manufactured, inspected, and then shipped to the customer only if it passes inspection. Hospitals' customers get the product (service) as it is being produced. For this reason, control of quality costs in health care must place a higher emphasis on prevention than many other industries.

Internal and external failure costs are the costs that result from failure to conform to design specifications. Examples of this include the cost of redoing an X-ray or laboratory test, the cost of longer patient lengths of stay, or the cost of lawsuits for malpractice.

REPORTING SYSTEMS FOR QUALITY COSTS

Although many hospitals have worked on TQM initiatives, it is not clear where these initiatives are going. Reporting systems have been woefully inadequate. A recent report in *Medicine and Health* indicated that:[4]

> A new study questions the impact on quality of work restructuring strategies like total quality management.... The Economic Policy Institute report, funded by the Joyce Foundation and the Office of Technology Assessment, finds that patient satisfaction is enhanced. But hospitals and HMOs that implement such strategies cannot demonstrate that clinical quality is maintained, let alone enhanced. And in most cases they can't show where and how much cost savings are achieved.

Although patient satisfaction is clearly one element of quality, this report indicates that other aspects of quality and quality cost are not being adequately monitored.

To some extent, this is understandable. In health care there is great difficulty measuring outcomes. How much has a patient's health improved? If outcomes cannot be measured, then how can quality be measured? If quality cannot be measured, how can the costs of quality be measured?

Industry, however, has started to adopt formalized quality cost reporting. Such reporting is possible if one views quality costs from the perspective of design quality and conformance quality. Such a report would include the four quality cost categories discussed earlier: (1) prevention, (2) appraisal, (3) internal failure costs, and (4) external failure costs. Exhibit 18–1–1 provides an example of a quality cost report.

Consider the elements of this report. The first item listed under prevention is work redesign. If the current operations structure is not capable of achieving the specified quality design, then re-engineering of operations may be necessary. Such redesign will require staff time and perhaps consulting costs. These are tangible, measurable costs of preventing failure costs.

Sometimes work redesign will call for a change in staffing. Perhaps lower qualified staff will be replaced with more qualified, more expensive staff. In Exhibit 18–1–1 this is shown as position upgrades. The higher staff cost is a prevention cost. It is money being spent to reduce the quality costs of failures.

The last item listed under prevention in the example is training. Suppose a hospital carefully considers its design specifications for its services and decides that to achieve those specifications it will need to provide its employees with additional training. If the training is not provided, the chances are higher that failures will occur. There will not be conformance with the quality design. There will be costs related to those failures. However, it will cost money to provide that training.

The cost of providing training can be explicitly measured and included in a quality cost report.

Similarly, appraisal costs can be measured and included in reports. In Exhibit 18–1–1, appraisal costs are incurred for inspections and tests. For instance, X-rays have to be inspected to see whether they provide the appropriate information. If they do not, they will have to be redone. The hospital can make cost estimates for the elements of its operations that are inspections searching for conformance failures. Similarly, many laboratory tests and other clinical tests are undertaken to verify that procedures and therapeutic treatments have had their desired affect. Again, the costs of such tests can be quantified.

Measuring the costs of failures represents a more difficult challenge. If a test or procedure is not done well the first time and must be done a second time (do-over costs), those costs can be measured. To generate a quality cost report, however, there must be a decision to identify those do-over instances, determine the cost of the instances, and gather the information into the report. Is the cost of this data collection and cost analysis worth the effort?

If the effort is not made, then one must question the level of commitment to a TQM effort at the hospital. Is it adequate to assume that all TQM efforts have a positive financial result? Or must the hospital also make a commitment to reporting? That reporting provides a basis for evaluating the results of the hospital's efforts in this area. Bear in mind that a commitment to generating a report does not commit the hospital to spending inordinate amounts on collecting data. Sampling can be done; estimates can be made.

Similarly, the costs of downtime that occurs before a test can be done over (shown as an internal failure cost in Exhibit 18–1–1) or the cost of delays that occur before a patient can be discharged (shown as an external failure cost in Exhibit 18–1–1) are extremely difficult to accurately determine. Nevertheless, the hospital may find it worthwhile to at least try to estimate how frequently discharge delays occur because of conformance failures, how long they last, and the average cost per delay.

Exhibit 18–1–1 HCMA Hospital Quality Cost Report for the Year Ended December 31, 1995

Prevention costs	
Work redesign	$ 100,000
Position upgrades	280,000
Training	150,000
Appraisal costs	
Inspections	290,000
Tests	550,000
Internal failure costs	
Do-over costs	130,000
Downtime	120,000
External failure costs	
Discharge delay	410,000
Bounce-back costs	140,000
Malpractice	1,650,000
Poor reputation	???
Total quality costs	$3,820,000

Even harder to deal with are malpractice costs and the impact of poor reputation. Improved conformity to quality standards should lead to reduced malpractice costs and improved reputation (and financial benefits arising from that improved reputation). Often, however, it is necessary to compare all other costs and then qualitatively and judgmentally consider the impact of such factors.

On the other hand, bounce-back costs are more likely to be measurable. These would be costs of providing care to patients rehospitalized after discharge because of hospital failures.

QUALITY COST CHANGES OVER TIME

One of the primary reasons for quality cost reports is to be able to report comparisons before and after changes. In a TQM environment, one would expect changes to be made that generally show shifts toward higher prevention and appraisal costs and lower failure costs. Reports can be used to show *pro forma* expectations of the impact of changes. They can also be used after the implementation of changes to assess the actual or estimated impact of the changes.

Reports similar to Exhibit 18–1–1 can and should be prepared giving a comparison column and a variance column to show budgeted quality costs, actual quality costs, and any differences. This will allow managers to focus on whether their TQM efforts are having the desired impacts.

Similar reports should also be compiled showing quality costs trending from year to year. Figure 18–1–1 shows how quality costs can be tracked to show progress, or lack thereof, over a period of several years.

It has been argued that in some cases it is possible for TQM-type initiatives to actually decrease costs in all categories![5] For example, it is conceivable that a work redesign effort will not only reduce failures but also reduce the need to incur appraisal costs, and will replace other existing prevention efforts that are more costly and not needed after the work redesign. Determining whether this is the case, however, requires attention to quality cost measurement and reporting.

QUALITY CERTIFICATION

A relatively new certification process, called ISO 9000, exists to attest to an organization's

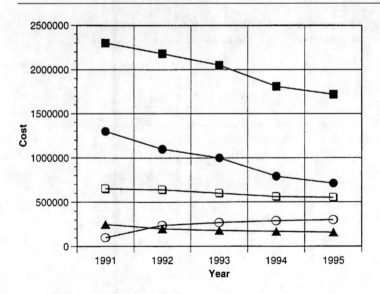

Figure 18–1–1 Quality Costs over Time

quality processes. Developed by the International Organization for Standardization in Switzerland, ISO 9000 is a set of standards for evaluation of quality.[6(p. 910)]

> These standards center around the concept of documentation and control of nonconformance and change.... Companies that attain ISO 9000 certification have been audited by an independent test company that certifies that the company meets quality standards. These standards do not apply to the production of a particular product or service. Instead, they apply to the way in which a company ensures quality, by, for example, testing products, training employees, keeping records, and fixing defects.

Major purchasers sometimes require ISO 9000 certification for their suppliers. For example, Motorola might require manufacturers of components for its products to have such certification. This certification provides some assurance about the likelihood of acceptable quality in the supplies acquired.

The process of preparing for certification and the actual certification process itself have been found to be both time consuming and expensive. On the other hand, as with any accreditation process, the time spent on preparation often results in valuable insights and ultimately valuable system improvements.

ISO 9000 does not have wide use in hospitals currently. One could conceive of a time when HMOs, however, might encourage hospitals to obtain such certification.

Regardless of whether this particular certification process becomes widespread in health care, it is clear that the issue of quality costs is here to stay. The dramatic changes occurring in the provision of health care services require all providers to seek ways to provide quality care at the lowest possible cost. Addressing this issue and developing a quality cost reporting system are activities that all hospitals should seriously consider.

NOTES

1. D.R. Hansen and M.M. Mowen, *Cost Management: Accounting and Control.* (Cincinnati, OH: South-Western College Publishing, 1995), 895.
2. Hansen and Mowen, *Cost Management.*
3. L.L. Berry and A. Parasuraman, Marketing services: Competing through quality, *The Free Press.* (New York: Macmillan, 1991).
4. P. Cotton (Ed.). *Medicine and Health, 49*, no. 31(1995): 3.
5. Hansen and Mowen, *Cost Management.*
6. Hansen and Mowen, *Cost Management,* 910.

Reading 18–2

Total Quality Management: An Application in a Biomedical Laboratory

David B. Latzer

Over the past several years, the penetration of managed care and its concomitant focus on cost savings have had a profound effect on the health care industry. A subsequent debate has erupted over the issue of whether or not decreasing the level of spending on health care also decreases the quality of services provided. In light of this, total quality management (TQM) has been purported as a way to maintain or improve the quality of care despite reductions in cost. TQM attempts to continually improve the quality of services rendered by preventing costly errors and problems before they arise.

One of the largest obstacles to TQM implementation is the inverse relationship between costs and quality.[1] High quality is associated with high costs, and low costs are associated with low quality. Fewer resources (e.g., personnel) prohibit engaging in activities that ensure high quality (e.g., double-checking orders before administering medication.) On the other hand, to raise standards, more resources are required. A consumer is willing to pay $2,000 for a set of fine china, but only $500 for everyday place-settings. Health care is an area where consumers want the highest quality of care available, and although some people are willing to pay top dollar,

the current trend is to reduce costs. This is the essence of TQM—continuously improve services, but only at a cost-effective level.

To make effective decisions regarding costs and quality, we can apply TQM to the cost accounting process. In order to visualize the costs associated with a procedure, Cleverley modeled a standard treatment protocol.[2] The standard treatment protocol details all the necessary intermediate products used to produce the desired output. These intermediate products, or service units, are accompanied by a standard cost profile—the actual cost of providing each service unit.

Compiling all the service units and the sum of standard cost profiles provides the standard treatment protocol. Based on this information, a health care provider is better able to make decisions regarding expanding or shrinking the service or negotiating with managed care companies.

Using the example of a broken leg, a full standard treatment protocol can be formed. The service units (intermediate products) provided to treat the patient include triage, X-rays, tetanus shot, patient prep, casting, and setting the leg. Also, room operating charges could be included. Each of these service units has its own individual standard cost profile comprised of the direct labor and supplies used in the procedure as well as fixed and variable overhead costs and allocations from other departments. The sum of the service units and standard cost profiles equals the standard treatment protocol and the cost of treating a broken leg. When negotiating payer rates, it is

Source: Reprinted from D.B. Latzer, "Total Quality Management: An Application in a Biomedical Laboratory," *Hospital Cost Management and Accounting,* Vol. 9, No. 2, pp. 1–6. Copyright May 1997, Aspen Publishers, Inc.

helpful to know how payment relates to both marginal and average costs.

Another part of the health care industry that also works under a form of capitated payments is biomedical research. Awarded a grant for a year or several years, labs must work under the preset budget. Knowing the costs entailed in carrying out the necessary experiments is crucial in delineating the scope of the project. Cleverley's standard treatment protocol can be extrapolated into the laboratory: a standard experiment protocol. A diagnostic tool to test for recombinant genes is the polymerase chain reaction (PCR). However, many steps are necessary to perform the experiment in addition to just the PCR. The PCR standard experiment protocol's service units include blood collection, mRNA isolation, PCR, and gel visualization. The costs associated with each of these steps can be delineated in standard cost profiles and summed into the total cost for the PCR standard experiment protocol.

Having established a standard experiment protocol and cost profile, the laboratory can improve the quality of services provided by applying the principles of TQM. This requires applying a monetary value to its notions of quality.[3] Reducing errors such as having to repeat gels because of inadequate information on the first one requires extra time, labor, and supplies, and may cause delays in the final diagnosis. The additional supervisory time required to properly train the laboratory technician can also be quantified. The important point is to identify the costs associated with providing quality services.

In an attempt to categorize and quantify the costs associated with quality, Simpson and Muthler have identified four areas: external failure costs, internal failure costs, appraisal costs, and prevention costs.[4] Although Simpson and Muthler's model was theorized for the manufacturing industry, it can be adapted for use in the biomedical research laboratory. External and internal failure costs rise in inverse proportion to the level of quality produced; increased errors (failures) have a negative impact on the test diagnosis. Appraisal and prevention costs and quality

are directly proportional. As these costs rise, so does the level of quality.

According to Simpson and Muthler, external costs in the manufacturing industry are related to the need for repairs, shipping and handling, warranty repairs and replacements, and the associated administrative costs. The company's goodwill is also included. Biomedical laboratories endure similar external failure costs. Since research labs usually work under a capitated form of payment, there is pressure to perform experiments quickly and at low cost. However, publishing inaccurate results can have a profound effect on both the institute's goodwill and the principal investigator's reputation (a significant factor in awarding grants).

To apply TQM to the need to rerun a genetic screening experiment, the total costs associated with the rerun must be calculated. Additional runs of an experiment may be warranted if paper peer reviewers deny the paper for publishing because the results were unclear. The need to redraw blood samples could also be considered an external failure. The technologist needs to revisit the animal colony to gather another blood sample. All the costs incurred drawing the second sample should be included in calculating the external failure costs, and are summarized in Exhibit 18–2–1. Often, a visit to the animal facility will be necessary to draw samples from more than one animal; therefore the number of visits, 250, is less than the 847 blood samples drawn.

The TQM cost worksheet identifies six areas where costs are incurred in having to draw another blood sample. These include labor, supply, and other costs such as machine maintenance. The amount of time it takes for the technician to travel between the lab and the animal facility constitutes a significant amount of added costs ($546). The time and supplies necessary for maintaining sterile environment in the animal facility and drawing the sample add another $896 and $2,981, respectively, to the total costs. The line centrifuge and prepare samples is the most costly activity in the retest, at $5,050. The amount of time required is significant, as is the supply cost.

Exhibit 18–2–1 TQM Cost Worksheet: External Failure Costs

Subject of TQM Analysis: Recombinant Gene Diagnostic Retests

Part A: External Failure Costs
Volume of Failures <u>250</u> instances per annum; <u>847</u> blood samples

Type of Cost	Labor Hours	× Average Rate	= Labor Costs	+ Supply Costs	+ Other Costs	= Total Costs
Travel to animal facility	42	13	$ 546			$ 546
Sterile precautions	21	13	271	$ 625		896
Draw blood	34	13	440	2,541		2,981
Centrifuge & prepare samples	200	13	2,600	1,875	$575	5,050
Extra animals				375		375
System delays						
Total			$3,857	$5,416	$575	$9,848

Cost per failure instance: Total failure cost/instances = $9,848/250 = $39.39

Source: Adapted from *Essentials of Cost Accounting for Health Care Organizations,* Aspen Publishers, Inc.

Unlike other industries where personnel accounts for the overwhelming majority of costs, the expensive reagents used in laboratories may constitute a significant share of costs. In this case, the RNA polymerase and dNTPs drive the cost of mRNA isolation up. Also, because of the amount of time it takes to order animals and wait for the proper gestational age, the extra cost to carry these animals ($375) is included. System delays, although very difficult to quantify, are presented in the worksheet as an acknowledgment of their importance. Gathering as many of the relevant costs as possible incurred in redrawing the blood sample is critical.

Internal failure costs are the errors incurred prior to project completion. Simpson and Muthler used the costs of scrap and reworking defects in their analysis. In the research laboratory, similar waste such as the cost of supplies wasted but not consumed would be included. For example, RNA is a very sensitive compound that can denature easily and prove ineffective if warmed or not treated with the proper reagents. The necessity of having to reisolate an RNA sample because it had been reconstituted in tap water rather than DEPC treated water and therefore denatured would be considered an internal failure cost.

In the PCR diagnostic retest example, inconclusive evidence on a gel signifies that an error has occurred. Assuming the proper controls were run and additional experimental samples remain, it would be possible to perform the PCR again without having to redraw a blood sample in the animal facility. These internal failure costs are less expensive than the external failure costs mentioned earlier.

The technician's labor time is cut down, in part because of not having to travel to and engage in the sterile precautions in the animal facility. However, labor, supply, and other costs are incurred in rerunning the PCR, sample preparation, and rerunning the gel (see Exhibit 18–2–2). An additional cost incurred is the amount of time the principal investigator spends interpreting the gel and requesting another test. The disparity in income between the technician and doctor causes this value to be disproportionately high ($2,100) for a low volume of labor hours. System delays are again included in the worksheet. Like internal failure costs in relation to external failure costs, these system delays are smaller as well.

Exhibit 18–2–2 TQM Cost Worksheet: Internal Failure Costs

Subject of TQM Analysis: Recombinant Gene Diagnostic Retests

Part B: Internal Failure Costs
Volume of Failures 650 instances per annum; 125 gels

Type of Cost	Labor × Hours	Average Rate	= Labor Costs	+ Supply Costs	+ Other Costs	= Total Costs
Rerun PCR	113	13	$1,463	$3,250	$1,300	$6,013
Prep samples	14	13	188	325		513
Rerun gel	63	13	813	188		1,035
Order retest	21	100	2,100		35	2,100
System delays						
Total			$4,564	$3,763	$1,335	$9,661

Cost per failure instance: Total failure cost/instances = $9,661/650 = $14.86

Source: Adapted from *Essentials of Cost Accounting for Health Care Organizations,* Aspen Publishers, Inc.

The third type of costs Simpson and Muthler identify is appraisal costs. Appraisal costs are associated with delivering a quality product. As appraisal costs rise, the quality of the product rises as well. The costs of inspecting a product prior to shipping are appraisal costs.

In the PCR example, the principal investigator uses the product produced by the technician. The internal failure costs in the example just mentioned could be avoided if the technician were able to read the gel prior to the principal investigator. The costs incurred to train the technologist in this skill would be considered appraisal costs. The technician may not be able to fully interpret the gel, but may be able to determine whether or not the appropriate information is available. If an error is found, an internal failure has already occurred, but the magnitude of it could be lessened. The downtime between running the gel and conferring with the principal investigator, and the principal investigator's time and effort spent interpreting a faulty gel, could be avoided.

Exhibit 18–2–3 details the labor costs required to train the technician to screen the gel. Also included in the appraisal costs are the time and supplies used to map, prepare, and run controls throughout the experiment. Interpreting the gel for the desired result is only part of the diagnosis. It is also necessary to know whether or not contamination or artifact have tainted the test and if the test is working properly. The PCR is an extremely powerful tool that "grows" DNA and RNA in million-fold quantities. Just a picogram of contaminating DNA can appear on the final gel after a PCR. Including the appropriate controls in an experiment, a positive control (known sample) and a negative control (blank sample), can clarify results and avoid unnecessary reruns.

Like appraisal costs, the fourth type of cost identified by Simpson and Muthler, prevention costs, rises in a direct relationship with quality by reducing the incidence of internal and/or external failure costs. Establishment of an operating procedure is a common prevention cost.

In the PCR example, the costs of technician training, supply checking, and a maintenance plan for the PCR machine are prevention costs. Seminars attended and hands-on training in the laboratory, usually with more experienced lab personnel, constitute $850 of prevention costs associated with technologist training (see Exhibit 18–2–4).

Exhibit 18–2–3 TQM Cost Worksheet: Appraisal Costs

Subject of TQM Analysis: Recombinant Gene Diagnostic Retests

Part C: Appraisal Costs; Total Volume: 22,000 tests

Type of Cost	Labor Hours	×	Average Rate	=	Labor Costs	+	Supply Costs	+	Other Costs	=	Total Costs
Screen gel	37		13		$ 481						$ 481
Map and prepare controls	183		13		2,379		$6,600		$1,200		10,179
Total					$2,860		$6,600		$1,200		$10,660

Source: Adapted from *Essentials of Cost Accounting for Health Care Organizations,* Aspen Publishers, Inc.

Exhibit 18–2–4 TQM Cost Worksheet: Prevention Costs

Subject of TQM Analysis: Recombinant Gene Diagnostic Retests

Part D: Prevention Costs; Total Volume: 22,000 tests

Type of Cost	Labor Hours	×	Average Rate	=	Labor Costs	+	Supply Costs	+	Other Costs	=	Total Costs
Technologist training	50		13		$ 650		$200				$ 850
Supply checking	50		13		650		350				1,000
PCR machine Maintenance contract									$2,500		2,500
Total					$1,300		$550		$2,500		$4,350

Source: Adapted from *Essentials of Cost Accounting for Health Care Organizations,* Aspen Publishers, Inc.

Checking supplies on a regular basis can avoid the problem mentioned earlier of reconstituting RNA in non-DEPC treated water or using enzymes that have lost their effectiveness in the PCR reaction. Also, due to the importance of the PCR machine and the need for exact temperatures to properly perform the reactions, a maintenance plan for the machine ($2,500) is included in the prevention costs.

The summary presented in Exhibit 18–2–5 details the costs of engaging in TQM practices and not engaging in these practices. The cost of undertaking a TQM program is listed on the appraisal and prevention costs lines; the benefits are found in how much the external and internal

failure costs are reduced. This information can be used to determine if the laboratory should engage in a quality improvement program. Frequently, a small expenditure in appraisal and/or prevention costs can have a significant impact in reducing failure costs.

TQM can be combined with cost accounting to improve the quality of output produced. In the biomedical laboratory examined, external and internal failure costs were quantified, as were appraisal and prevention costs. The decision to implement quality improvement measures can be examined by weighing the difference between the costs of improving quality and the costs of incurring failures.

Exhibit 18–2–5 TQM Cost Worksheet: Summary

Subject of TQM Analysis: Recombinant Gene Diagnostic Retests

Type of Cost	Labor Costs	+	Supply Costs	+	Other Costs	=	Total Costs
External Failure Costs (from Part A)	$ 3,857		$ 5,416		$ 575		$ 9,848
Internal Failure Costs (from Part B)	4,563		3,763		1,335		9,661
Appraisal Costs (from Part C)	2,860		6,600		1,200		10,660
Prevention Costs (from Part D)	1,300		550		2,500		4,350
Total	$12,580		$16,329		$5,610		$34,519

Source: Adapted from *Essentials of Cost Accounting for Health Care Organizations,* Aspen Publishers, Inc.

REFERENCES

1. S.A. Finkler, *Essentials of Cost Accounting for Health Care Organizations,* Aspen Publishers, Inc., Gaithersburg, MD, 1994: 343–345.

2. W.O. Cleverley, *Essentials of Health Care Finance,* 3rd ed., Aspen Publishers, Inc., Gaithersburg. MD, 1992: 260–266.

3. S.A. Finkler, 351.

4. J.B. Simpson and D.L. Muthler, Quality costs: Facilitating the Quality Initiative, *Journal of Cost Management for the Manufacturing Industry 1,* no. 1 (Spring 1987): 25–34.

Index

About the Authors

Steven A. Finkler, PhD, CPA, is Professor of Public and Health Administration, Accounting, and Financial Management at New York University's (NYU) Robert F. Wagner Graduate School of Public Service. At NYU, Dr. Finkler directs the financial management specialization in the Program in Health Policy and Management. He is also a member of a National Advisory Council at the National Institutes of Health (NIH). Dr. Finkler is a member of the editorial board of *Health Care Management Review* and served as Editor of *Hospital Cost Management and Accounting,* a monthly publication, from 1984–1997.

Dr. Finkler received a BS in economics and an MS in accounting from the Wharton School, University of Pennsylvania. His MA in economics and PhD in business administration were awarded by Stanford University. An award-winning teacher and author, Dr. Finkler, who is also a CPA, worked for several years as an auditor with Ernst and Young and was on the faculty of the Wharton School before joining NYU.

Among his publications are three other books: *Finance and Accounting for Nonfinancial Managers* (Revised Edition, Prentice-Hall, Inc. 1996), *Budgeting Concepts for Nurse Managers* (Second Edition, W.B. Saunders, 1992), and *Financial Management for Nurse Managers and Executives*, coauthored with Christine Kovner (W.B. Saunders, Second Edition forthcoming 1999).

Dr. Finkler has published more than 200 articles in many journals, including *Healthcare Financial Management, Health Care Management Review, New England Journal of Medicine, Health Services Research, Inquiry, Medical Care, Nursing Economics,* and *The Journal of Nursing Administration*.

Dr. Finkler has consulted extensively and has worked on a wide variety of costing studies in the field of health services research. He conducts seminars on health services financial management, both around the country and abroad.

David M. Ward, PhD, is Assistant Professor of Health Administration and Policy in the Department of Health Administration and Policy and holds a faculty appointment with the Center for Health Care Research at the Medical University of South Carolina. His teaching activities at the Medical University include Financial Management for Health Care Organizations and Healthcare Accounting to students obtaining a Masters in Health Administration. Dr. Ward is a member of AHCPR's Work Group on Nurse Staffing and Quality of Care in Hospitals and a member of the Cost Accounting and Analysis Advisory Panel for the Finance Project.

Dr. Ward received his BA from Colgate University and an MPA and PhD from the Robert F. Wagner Graduate School of Public Service at New York University. Outside of academics, Dr. Ward spent several years as a Supervising Budget Analyst with the New York City Office of Management and Budget.

Dr. Ward's research activities have focused on the use of cost-effectiveness analysis and linear programming for increasing the efficiency of health care spending. Dr. Ward has published in a number of journals, including *Health Care Financing Review, Public Budgeting and Financial Management,* and the *American Journal of Public Health.*

In addition to Dr. Ward's research and teaching activities, he consults and conducts financial management seminars across the country.